**Lecture Notes: Psychiatry**

# Lecture Notes
# Psychiatry

## Paul Harrison

DM (Oxon), FRCPsych
Professor of Psychiatry
University of Oxford

## John Geddes

MD, FRCPsych
Professor of Epidemiological Psychiatry
University of Oxford

## Michael Sharpe

MD, FRCP, FRCPsych
Professor of Psychological Medicine
University of Edinburgh

## Tenth Edition

A John Wiley & Sons, Ltd., Publication

This edition first published 2010, © 2005, 2010 by P.J. Harrison, J.R. Geddes and M. Sharpe
Previous editions 1964, 1968, 1972, 1974, 1979, 1984, 1989, 1998

Blackwell Publishing was acquired by John Wiley & Sons in February 2007. Blackwell's publishing program has been merged with Wiley's global Scientific, Technical and Medical business to form Wiley-Blackwell.

*Registered office:* John Wiley & Sons Ltd, The Atrium, Southern Gate, Chichester, West Sussex PO19 8SQ, UK

*Editorial offices:* 9600 Garsington Road, Oxford OX4 2DQ, UK
    The Atrium, Southern Gate, Chichester, West Sussex PO19 8SQ, UK
    111 River Street, Hoboken, NJ 07030-5774, USA

For details of our global editorial offices, for customer services and for information about how to apply for permission to reuse the copyright material in this book please see our website at www.wiley.com/wiley-blackwell

The right of the authors to be identified as the authors of this work has been asserted in accordance with the Copyright, Designs and Patents Act 1988.

*Library of Congress Cataloging-in-Publication Data*

Harrison, P.J. (Paul J.), 1960–
    Lecture notes. Psychiatry.—10th ed./ Paul Harrison, John Geddes, Michael Sharpe.
        p. ; cm.
    Other title: Psychiatry
    Includes bibliographical references and index.
    ISBN 978-1-4051-9137-1
    1. Psychiatry—Outlines, syllabi, etc.    2. Psychiatry—Examinations, questions, etc.    I. Geddes, John, MD.    II. Sharpe, Michael.    III. Title.    IV. Title: Psychiatry.
    [DNLM:    1. Psychiatry—Examination Questions.    2. Psychiatry—Handbooks. WM 34 H321L 2010]
    RC457.2.H375 2010
    616.89—dc22

                                    2010008383

A catalogue record for this book is available from the British Library.

Set in 8 on 12 pt Stone Serif by Toppan Best-set Premedia Limited
Printed and bound in Malaysia by Vivar Printing Sdn Bhd

1    2010

# Contents

# Preface

Four percent of medical students end up as psychiatrists. This book is aimed equally at the other 96%, because the skills, attitudes and knowledge you will learn by studying psychiatry are relevant to all doctors—and to all other health professionals.

After providing what we hope and believe are convincing reasons why psychiatry is worth studying and how to start (Chapter 1), we take a practical approach to 'doing' psychiatry. Our guide to assessment comprises a brief Core (Chapter 2), followed by more detailed Modules to be used as required (Chapter 3), and a guide to risk assessment (Chapter 4). Chapter 5 describes how to draw everything together and communicate the information to others.

The middle chapters cover the principles of aetiology (Chapter 6), treatment (Chapter 7) and psychiatry services (Chapter 8). We have tried to be evidence based in our treatment recommendations. The main psychiatric disorders of adults are covered in Chapters 9–15, followed by childhood disorders (Chapter 16) and learning disability (Chapter 17). Last, but not least, Chapter 18 discusses the psychiatric assessment and treatment in non-psychiatric medical settings—the place where most psychiatry actually happens.

In writing the book we have tried to make psychiatry both logical and enjoyable. Naturally, it is also intended to help you to pass the end-of-course exam, so we've highlighted important facts in each chapter and have included some multiple choice questions, and suggestions for other sources of information.

We thank Mark Underwood and Digby Quested for expert advice on aspects of mental health law and community care, and are grateful to the many other colleagues who have generously shared their expertise with us.

The book is dedicated to Sandra, Rosie, Charlotte and Grace; Jane and Caitlin; Liz, Joe and Anna.

**PJH, JRG and MCS**

# Chapter 1

# Getting started

Psychiatry can seem disconcertingly different from other specialties, especially if your first experience is on a psychiatric in-patient unit. How do I approach a patient? What am I trying to achieve? Is he dangerous? How does it relate to the rest of medicine? This chapter is meant to help orientate anyone facing the same situation. Like the rest of the book, it is based on three principles:

- Psychiatry is part of medicine.
- Psychiatric knowledge, skills and attitudes are relevant to all doctors.
- Psychiatry should be as effective, pragmatic and evidence based as every other medical specialty.

## What is psychiatry?

'Psychiatry is ... weird doctors in Victorian asylums using bizarre therapies on people who are either untreatably mad or who are not really ill at all.' Although remnants of such ill-informed stereotypes persist, the reality of modern psychiatry is very different and rather more mundane! Psychiatry is, in fact, fundamentally similar to the rest of medicine: it is based upon making reliable diagnoses and applying evidence-based treatments that have success rates comparable with those used in other specialties. Most patients with psychiatric

*Lecture Notes: Psychiatry*, 10e. By Paul Harrison, John Geddes and Michael Sharpe. Published 2010 by Blackwell Publishing Ltd.

illness are not mad and most are treated in primary care. Nor are psychiatric patients a breed apart—psychiatric diagnoses are common in medical patients. And psychiatrists are no stranger than other doctors, probably.

Psychiatric disorders may be defined as illnesses that are conventionally treated with treatments used by psychiatrists, just as surgical conditions are those thought best treated by surgery. The specialty designation does not indicate a profound difference in the illness or type of patient. In fact it can change as new treatments are developed; peptic ulcer moved from being a predominantly surgical to a medical condition once effective drug treatments were developed. Similarly, conditions such as dementia may move between psychiatry and neurology.

The conditions in which psychiatrists have developed expertise have tended to be those that either manifest with disordered psychological functioning (emotion, perception, thinking and memory) or those which have no clearly established biological basis. However, scientific developments are showing us that these so-called psychological disorders are associated with abnormalities of the brain, just as so-called medical disorders are profoundly affected by psychological factors. Consequently, the delineation between psychiatry and the rest of medicine can increasingly be seen as only a matter of convenience and convention.

However, traditional assumptions continue to influence both service organization (with psychiatric services usually being planned and often situated separate from other medical services) and terminology (see below).

## Where is psychiatry going?

Psychiatry is evolving rapidly and three themes permeate this book:
- *Psychiatry, like the rest of medicine, is becoming less hospital based.* Most psychiatric problems are seen and treated in primary care, with many others handled in the general hospital. Only a minority are managed by specialist psychiatric services. So psychiatry should be learned and practised in these other settings too.
- *Psychiatry is becoming more evidence based.* Diagnostic, prognostic and therapeutic decisions should, of course, be based on the best available evidence. It may come as a surprise to discover that current psychiatric interventions are as evidence based (and sometimes more so) as in other specialties.
- *Psychiatry is becoming more neuroscience based.* Developments in brain imaging and molecular genetics are beginning to make real progress in the neurobiological understanding of psychiatric disorders. These developments are expanding the knowledge base and range of skills which the next generation of doctors will need. These developments do not, however, make the other elements of psychiatry—psychology and sociology, for example—any less important, as we will see later.

## Why study psychiatry?

Studying psychiatry is worthwhile for all trainee doctors, and other health practitioners, because its *knowledge*, *skills* and *attitudes* are applicable to every branch of medicine. Specifically, studying psychiatry will give you:
- A basic knowledge of the common and the 'classic' psychiatric disorders.
- A working knowledge of psychiatric problems encountered in all medical settings.

- The ability to assess effectively someone with a 'psychiatric problem'.
- Skills in the assessment of psychological aspects of medical conditions.
- A holistic or 'biopsychosocial' perspective from which to understand all illness.

## Useful knowledge

Formerly, patients with severe psychiatric disorders were often institutionalized and their management was exclusively the domain of psychiatrists. The advent of community care (Chapter 8) means that other doctors, especially GPs, encounter and participate in their management, so all doctors need basic information about these 'specialist' psychiatric disorders. Equally, all doctors need to recognize and treat the more common psychiatric illnesses, such as anxiety and depressive disorders. These are extremely prevalent in all medical settings, yet they are all too often overlooked and ineffectively treated (Chapter 18).

## Useful skills

Most psychiatric disorders are diagnosed from the history, and many treatments are based on listening and talking. So, psychiatrists have had to acquire particular expertise in interviewing patients, in assessing their state of mind and in establishing a therapeutic doctor–patient relationship—with patients who may pose challenges in this respect because of the nature of their problems. These skills remain important in all medical practice. For example, all doctors should be able to:
- Make the patient feel comfortable enough to express their symptoms and feelings clearly.
- Use basic psychotherapeutic skills. For example, knowing how to help a distressed patient and how best to communicate bad news.
- Discuss and prescribe antidepressants and other common psychotropic drugs with confidence.

Without these 'soft' skills, the 'hard' skills of technological, evidence-based medicine cannot be fully effective. An impatient, non-empathic doctor is less likely to elicit the symptoms needed to make the correct diagnosis, and her patient is less likely to adhere to the treatment plan she prescribes.

## Useful attitudes

Psychiatric diagnoses are still associated with stigma and misunderstanding. These stem largely from the misconception that illnesses that do not have established 'physical' (or 'organic') pathology are 'mental', and that such 'mental' illness is not real, represents inadequacies of character, or are the person's own fault. Studying psychiatry will help you to challenge these attitudes. You will see many patients with severe symptoms in whom no 'organic' pathology has been established, but who have real symptoms and disability. You will be repeatedly reminded of the stigma which patients with psychiatric problems experience from the public, and sometimes from their relatives and even, sadly, from health professionals. Finally, you will be confronted with the reality of human frailty. Recognizing these issues and dealing with them appropriately—by developing positive, educated and effective attitudes—is another important consequence of studying psychiatry. You might conclude, as we have done that:

- Suffering is real even when there is no 'test' to prove it.
- Psychological and social factors are relevant to all illnesses and can be scientifically studied.
- Much harm is done by negative attitudes towards patients with psychiatric diagnoses.
- Your own experience and personality will influence your relationship with patients—your positive attributes as well as your vulnerabilities and prejudices.

## How to start psychiatry

### The psychiatric interview

The first, key skill to learn is how to listen and talk to patients, in that order. The *psychiatric interview* has two functions:
- It forms the main part of the psychiatric assessment by which diagnoses are made.

- It can be used therapeutically—in the psychotherapies the communication between patient and therapist is the currency of treatment (Chapter 7).

## Psychiatric assessment

Because of its central importance, the principles of psychiatric assessment are outlined here. The practicalities are described in the next two chapters. Psychiatric assessment has three goals:
- To elicit the information needed to make a diagnosis, since a diagnosis provides the best available framework for making clinical decisions. This may seem obvious, but it hasn't always been so in psychiatry.
- To understand the causes and context of the disorder.
- To form a therapeutic relationship with the patient.

Though these goals are the same in all of medicine, the balance of psychiatric assessment differs:
- The interview provides a greater proportion of diagnostic information. Physical examination and laboratory investigations usually play a lesser, though occasionally crucial, role.
- The interview includes a detailed examination of the patient's current thoughts, feelings, experiences and behaviour (the *mental state examination*) in addition to the standard questioning about the presenting complaint and past history (the *psychiatric history*).
- A greater wealth of background information about the person is collected (the *context*).

Psychiatric assessments have a reputation for being excessively long. We take a pragmatic approach to the *process* of assessment. A *core assessment* is used to collect the essential diagnostic and contextual information (Chapter 2). Then, more detailed *modules* are used if anything has led you to hypothesize that the patient has a particular disorder (Chapter 3).
- This two-stage *core and module* approach considerably shortens most assessments—to 30–45 minutes or less. It also happens to be what psychiatrists actually do—as opposed to what they tell their students to do.

## Diagnostic categories

Solving a problem is always easier when you know the range of possible answers. Similarly, before embarking on your first assessment, it helps to know the major psychiatric diagnoses and their cardinal features. Table 1.1 is a simplified guide. As you gain experience, aim for more specific diagnoses which correspond to those listed in the International Classification of Diseases, 10th revision (ICD-10) which are used in this book (see Appendix 1).

- There is an American alternative to ICD-10, called the Diagnostic and Statistical Manual of Mental Disorders, 4th edition (DSM-IV), widely used in research. The two systems are broadly similar.
- Whatever the classification, remember the underused category of 'no psychiatric disorder'.
- A term such as 'nervous breakdown' has no useful psychiatric meaning—it may describe almost any of the categories in Table 1.1.

## Psychiatric classification

The classification of psychiatric disorders has several problems that you should be aware of before you start:

- *Most diagnoses are syndromes, defined by combinations of symptoms, but some are based on aetiology or pathology*. For example, depression can be caused by a brain tumour (diagnosis: organic mood disorder), or after bereavement (diagnosis: abnormal grief reaction) or without clear cause (diagnosis: depressive disorder). This combination of different sorts of category leads to some conceptual and practical difficulties, which will become apparent later.
- *Comorbidity: many patients suffer from more than one psychiatric disorder* (or a psychiatric disorder and a medical disorder). The comorbid disorders may or may not be causally related, and may or may not both require treatment. As a rule, comorbidity complicates management and worsens prognosis.
- *Hierarchy: not all diagnoses carry equal weight.* Traditionally, organic disorder trumps everything (i.e. if it is present, coexisting disorders are not diagnosed), and psychosis trumps neurosis. This principle is no longer applied consistently, partly because it is hard to reconcile with the frequency and clinical importance of comorbidity.
- *Categories versus dimensions.* The current system assumes there are distinctions between one disorder and another, and between disorder and health. However, such cut-offs are notoriously difficult to demonstrate, either aetiologically or clinically, whereas there is good evidence that there are continuums—for example, between bipolar disorder and schizophrenia, and for the occurrence of psy-

**Table 1.1** A basic guide to psychiatric classification.

| Category | Examples of disorders | Basic characteristics | Common presentations |
|---|---|---|---|
| Organic disorder | Dementia, delirium | Defined by 'organic' cause | Forgetfulness, confusion |
| Psychosis | Schizophrenia | Delusions, hallucinations | Bizarre ideas, odd behaviour |
| Mood disorders | Depression | Low mood | Tearful, fed up, somatic complaints |
| Neurosis | Anxiety disorders | Emotional disturbance | Worried, tired, stressed |
| Somatoform disorders | Somatization disorder | Unexplained physical symptoms | Chronic pain, fear of disease |
| Substance misuse | Opiate dependence | Effects of the drug | Addiction, withdrawal, depression |
| Personality disorder | Dissocial, histrionic | Dysfunctional personality traits | Exacerbation of traits when stressed |
| Learning disability | Down's syndrome, autism | Congenitally low IQ | Developmental delay, physical appearance |

chotic symptoms in 'normal' people. However, clinical practice requires 'yes/no' decisions to be made (e.g. as to what treatment to recommend) and so a categorical approach persists.

• *Psychiatric classification is not an exact science*. All classifications have drawbacks, and psychiatry has more than its share, as illustrated by the above points. Nevertheless, despite the imperfections, rational clinical practice requires a degree of order to be created, and most of the current diagnostic categories at least have good reliability, and utility in predicting treatment response and prognosis.

## After the assessment: summarizing and communicating the information

Completion of the psychiatric assessment is followed by several steps:

• *Make a (differential) diagnosis*, according to ICD-10 categories (Appendix 1), using your knowledge of the key features of each psychiatric disorder.

• *Attempt to understand how and why the disorder has arisen* (Chapter 6).

• *Develop a management plan*, based on an awareness of the best available treatment (Chapter 7), how psychiatric services are organized (Chapter 8) and the patient's characteristics, including their risk of harm to self or others (Chapter 4).

• *Communicate your understanding of the case* (Chapter 5).

---

**Key points**

• Psychiatry is a medical specialty. It mostly deals with conditions in which the symptoms and signs predominantly concern emotions, perception, thinking or memory. It also encompasses learning disability and the psychological aspects of the rest of medicine.

• Knowledge, skills and attitudes learned in psychiatry are relevant and valuable in all medical specialties.

• Be alert to the possibility of psychiatric disorder in all patients, and be able to recognize and elicit the key features.

• The major diagnostic categories are: neurosis, mood disorder, psychosis, organic disorder, substance misuse and personality disorder.

# Chapter 2

# The core psychiatric assessment

## Approaches to psychiatric assessment

The principles and goals of psychiatric assessment were outlined in Chapter 1. A 'traditional' first assessment interview includes both an extensive search for symptoms and detailed, wide-ranging questions about the patient's life history. Though comprehensive, this approach is inefficient and takes well over an hour, which in many situations is unrealistic. Also, the content and conduct of the assessment are largely pre-specified, and hard to modify or abbreviate—probably a reason why psychiatric problems are neglected in general medical practice.

We suggest a more flexible approach to assessment in which screening questions and other basic information (the Core; this chapter) are used to identify possible diagnoses, which are then confirmed or excluded by more detailed assessment (the Modules; Chapter 3). This lessens the time required for assessments and, we think, makes them more satisfying.

- To use the core and module strategy successfully you need a working knowledge of psychiatric disorders and their symptoms, in order to generate the diagnostic hypotheses that guide your assessment. This basic knowledge can be attained

*Lecture Notes: Psychiatry*, 10e. By Paul Harrison, John Geddes and Michael Sharpe. Published 2010 by Blackwell Publishing Ltd.

rapidly. A useful start is to learn Table 1.1 and to browse the key points at the end of Chapters 9–17.

## The mental state examination

All psychiatric assessments include a mental state examination (MSE) as well as the history. Two aspects of the MSE can cause confusion:
- *What is the time frame?* Classically, the MSE is limited to those features present at the time of examination, with everything else being in the history. In practice, the MSE is often also used to assess the patient's report of recent (past hours or days) symptoms. Be aware that some examiners adhere to the division between history and MSE more rigidly.
- *Is the MSE the psychiatric equivalent of the physical examination?* To a degree it is, since it is where the *signs* of psychiatric disorder (i.e. observations made by the interviewer—'patient keeps looking anxiously around') are elicited. However, the MSE also includes *symptoms* (experiences reported by the patient—'I can hear an alien over there') and in this respect it overlaps with the history (Figure 2.1).

### The 'core and module' psychiatric assessment

The *core* is a 'stripped down' assessment designed to:

**Figure 2.1** A comparison of medical and psychiatric assessments, showing the relationship of history, functional enquiry, mental state examination (MSE) and physical examination. Note the overlap between the components of the psychiatric assessment. For example, recent suicidal thoughts might be detected in the history or MSE; akathisia (Chapter 7) may be elicited as a symptom in the history or MSE or as a sign in the physical examination.

- Obtain a clear account of the patient's main problem(s).
- Screen rapidly but systematically for evidence of psychiatric disorder.
- Provide the background 'contextual' information needed to guide immediate management.

An assessment may then proceed to use one or more *modules* according to:
- The diagnostic suspicion(s) raised by the core assessment or other available information.
- The need to exclude a disorder that, though unlikely, would be clinically significant.

The modules cover cognitive function, psychosis, mood disorder, neurosis, eating disorder, substance misuse, somatic symptoms and the unresponsive patient. Each is designed to confirm whether a disorder in that category is present and, if so, to establish the specific diagnosis. Each module also covers contextual information needed for the overall understanding of the case.
- Assessment of childhood disorders, learning disability and sexual functioning are covered in their respective chapters. Risk assessment is described in Chapter 4.

The way the interviewer moves from core to module, and the number of modules that are needed, will differ from case to case. It may also change as the interviewer becomes more experienced (i.e. becomes better at generating good diagnostic hypotheses). Three examples show how the assessment may develop:

*A woman complains of tiredness and feeling fed up. The core assessment reveals evidence of depression and a recent increase in alcohol intake, but not of suicidal intent, psychosis or cognitive impairment. You proceed to the mood and substance misuse modules which confirm the presence of a depressive disorder, but no significant alcohol problem.*

*A wife reports her 70-year-old husband is getting confused. Your initial suspicions are of dementia, so you administer the cognitive module. However, though his concentration is poor, he does not appear demented. Returning to the core, you find evidence of depression, so you move to the mood module which shows that he is suffering from a severe depressive episode.*

*A man is brought in having been found standing in the road naked, screaming at passers-by to stop irradiating him. On this basis, you proceed to the psychosis and risk assessment modules regardless of what he may report during the core assessment (since he may initially deny symptoms in case you are part of a conspiracy). Given that illicit drugs can produce this kind of behaviour, you also use the substance misuse module.*

If no modules have been triggered by the core assessment and review of the case, it may be concluded that there is no evidence that the person has a psychiatric disorder.

## Interviewing skills

Effective psychiatric assessment comes from knowing what questions to ask when, and how to ask them—as well of course from knowing how to interpret the answers. So, before proceeding to the content of the assessment we outline the skills needed to obtain the necessary diagnostic information rapidly and accurately—and which will help you develop a therapeutic relationship with the patient.

## Before the interview

• Find a suitable location. You will be discussing intimate, and sometimes distressing, topics. The room should be comfortable, and as sound-proof as possible. This can be challenging, especially on medical wards.
• Always consider safety, since occasionally patients may become disturbed or violent (Chapter 4). Discuss with a senior member of staff (e.g. should you have a chaperone?). Check local procedures (e.g. are there panic buttons?). Arrange seating so you are closer than the patient to the door. Safety is a particular issue when carrying out domiciliary assessments.
• Arrange the setting. Chairs are best arranged at ninety degrees to each other. If a desk is required for making notes, this should not be directly between the patient and the interviewer.
• Arrange not to be interrupted—turn off mobile phones and pagers whenever possible.
• Read any referral letter and previous notes. These may provide a preliminary diagnostic hypothesis, clarify the reason for the referral and suggest lines of questioning.

## Beginning the interview

• Introduce yourself, check the identity of the patient and make him comfortable.

• Sit in a relaxed and slightly forward posture.
• Describe the reason for the interview, the time available and the procedure to be followed.
• Emphasize confidentiality. If notes are to be taken, explain why.

## Progress of the interview

• Begin by asking an open question such as: 'How have you been feeling?' or 'Could you start by telling me a bit about what you think is the problem?' Closed (but not leading) questions are used to clarify the responses (e.g. 'You say you're not sleeping well: is it that you can't get to sleep, or that you wake too early?').
• Encourage the patient to list their main problems and describe each in his own words. Ensure you understand the nature of the current problem, before asking when it started.
• Keep control of the interview, yet allow the patient sufficient time to answer questions fully and in his own way. This balance can be the hardest skill to learn.
• Get answers that are as precise as possible—for example, estimates of symptom duration.
• As well as responding to what the patient says, be sensitive to non-verbal clues—for example, the patient's facial expression, demeanour, posture and tone of voice.

## Ending the interview

• Summarize what you've been told back to the patient. This helps ensure you've gained an accurate picture, and reinforces to the patient that you have been listening carefully.
• Ask if anything major has been overlooked.
• Give the patient an opportunity to ask questions.
• Explain what you plan to do next.

## The core psychiatric assessment

The core psychiatric assessment covers the essence of the topics in Table 2.1 and is outlined below. It consists of a core history, a core mental state examination, and some core contextual questions.

**Table 2.1** The core psychiatric assessment.

> *Core history*
>    Reason for referral
>    Presenting complaint(s), and their history
>    Psychiatric and medical history
>    Alcohol and drug use
>
> *Core mental state examination*
>    Appearance and behaviour
>    Mood
>    Speech
>    Thoughts
>    Perceptions
>    Cognition
>    Insight
>
> *Core contextual information*
>    Family history
>    Personal history
>    Current circumstances
>
> *(Risk assessment)*
>
> *(Core physical examination)*

- The accompanying notes provide background and rationale to the questions, plus a glossary of important terms.

## The core history

### Reason for referral

Who made the referral? Why?

**Notes**

- Clarify what questions the referrer wants addressed. This may give clues about the best way of approaching the interview and suggest initial diagnostic possibilities.
- Identify the best *informant* available—someone to supplement and corroborate the history.

### Presenting complaint(s) and their history

What does the patient think is the main problem or problems?

Does the patient have any other problems? List them.

Assess the nature, duration and progression of the symptom(s).

Are there any precipitating and relieving factors? Has any treatment already been tried?

Assess the degree of functional impairment: effect on relationships, work, sleep, etc.

**Notes**

- Getting a list of the patient's problems allows you to start generating diagnostic hypotheses. Some problems will be symptoms (e.g. agitation); others will represent the patient's predicament or provide the context of the disorder (e.g. homelessness).
- The diagnostic importance of a particular psychiatric symptom is affected by its characteristics (intensity, fluctuation, duration, etc.) and associated features (e.g. concurrent symptoms). Knowing the relevant information to elicit comes rapidly with increasing knowledge and experience.
- Don't ignore 'medical' symptoms. A brief functional enquiry to elicit these should be included.

### Psychiatric and medical history

Nature of any previous psychiatric contact. Diagnosis? Treatments tried, and their effect.

Current medication and allergies.

Any serious medical illnesses or operations?

**Notes**

- About 50% of psychiatry referrals have had prior psychiatric contact. A previous diagnosis is best seen as a strong hypothesis (i.e. it has a high pre-test probability) to be tested. Equally, keep an open mind since the new problem may be different, or the previous diagnosis might be wrong. Past history may also provide useful information about prognosis and the patient's attitude to his disorder and its management.
- Psychiatric and medical disorders have many overlaps, hence the need to elicit any significant past or current medical history. A medical history is also essential because physical illness is common in people with psychiatric disorders, and often undiagnosed. For example, patients with schizophrenia have high rates of diabetes mellitus and hyperlipidaemia.

### Alcohol and drug use

How much does the patient drink in an average week? Record in units of alcohol.

If the patient drinks alcohol regularly, ask the four FAST questions (Box 2.1). They take about 20 seconds.

> **Box 2.1  The FAST questionnaire for alcohol problems**
>
> The four FAST questions:
> 1. *How often do you have eight or more drinks on one occasion?*
> 2. *How often during the past year have you failed to do what was normally expected of you because of drinking?*
> 3. *How often during the past year have you been unable to remember what happened the night before because you had been drinking?*
> [For these questions, score 0 for never, 1 for less than monthly, 2 for monthly, 3 for weekly and 4 for daily or almost daily].
> 4. *Has a relative, friend, doctor or other health worker been concerned about your drinking or suggested you cut down?*
> [For this question, score 0 for never, 2 for yes but not in past year, 4 for yes, in the past year].
>
> Notes:
> - Maximum score =16. A score of 3 or more indicates hazardous drinking.
> - The answer to Q1 may make the other questions unnecessary: if the answer is 'never', (s)he is not a hazardous drinker and they can be omitted; conversely, a score of 3 or 4 means (s)he is considered a hazardous drinker—so move straight to the substance misuse module and the AUDIT (Chapter 3).

### Notes

- Alcohol and other drugs may be a cause, a component or a consequence of many psychiatric disorders. All are common, so substance (mis)use should always be briefly ascertained.
- The recommended limits for alcohol intake are 21 units per week for men and 14 for women. (1 unit is half a pint of beer, a single measure of spirits, or a small glass of wine.)
- The CAGE is an alternative and widely used alcohol screening tool. Its four questions are: Have you ever felt you ought to **C**ut down on your drinking? Have people **A**nnoyed you by criticizing your drinking? Have you ever felt **G**uilty about your drinking? Have you ever had a drink first thing in the morning (an '**E**ye-opener')? If three or more yes answers are given, the likelihood ratio for problem drinking is 250. Repeat questions for any illicit drugs used.

### The core mental state examination

The core MSE concentrates on aspects of the recent mental state which are commonly affected by psychiatric disorder and which have diagnostic weight.
- Much of the core MSE will have been covered in the history, from observations made in passing, or as part of a module already administered. However, the MSE is still useful to ensure that the presence or absence of all important recent phenomena are established and documented.

The headings of the core MSE are:
- *Appearance and behaviour*—much can be gleaned from careful observation of the patient's manner, movements and dress. An underestimated source of diagnostic information.
- *Mood*—depressive symptoms are very common. This section covers them, and the associated issue of suicidal risk.
- *Speech*—abnormal speech may be present in neurological, psychotic and mood disorders.
- *Thoughts*—thought content, and the way thoughts flow, are affected in many psychiatric disorders. The nature of the abnormalities gives important diagnostic clues.
- *Perceptions*—mainly affected in psychotic and organic disorders. Lesser alterations in sensory experiences also occur in neurosis.
- *Cognition*—cognitive impairment is characteristic of dementia and delirium, but can also occur in some other disorders. If severe, it may prevent a useful history from being taken (see the cognitive function module in Chapter 3).
- *Insight*—lack of awareness of illness is classically a sign of psychosis or organic disorder. In all disorders, the patient's views as to the nature and significance of their problems are important, not least since it may affect their views about the need for (and choice of) treatment.

## Appearance and behaviour

Note the attitude of the patient to the interview and the rapport made.

Is the patient tearful, anxious, overactive or underactive?

Are there any unusual movements or eccentric behaviour?

Note the patient's physical appearance and dress.

**Notes**

- Many psychiatric disorders are accompanied by characteristic changes in manner, emotional expression or physical appearance. These often provide the first diagnostic clue. So, from the moment you meet, observe closely. For example:
  - In the waiting room, you see the patient is garishly dressed, pacing around and trying enthusiastically to engage other patients in conversation. Is he manic? Intoxicated? Disinhibited due to a frontal lobe tumour?
  - The patient is avoiding eye contact and with little facial expression—is he depressed? Is he parkinsonian?
  - A woman has a tremor. Could it be Parkinson's disease? Is she taking antipsychotic drugs or lithium?
  - A young woman looks gaunt and is wearing a baggy sweater on a warm day. Could it be anorexia nervosa?
  - A man keeps breaking off in mid-sentence and looking over his shoulder. Is he hearing voices? Does he think the room is bugged? Both could indicate paranoid schizophrenia.
  - A woman keeps grimacing and making a strange movement of her arms. Are these movements suggestive of catatonic schizophrenia? Or Huntington's chorea?
  - A young man is trying to hide plasters on both his wrists. Has he been self-harming?

## Mood

Disturbances of mood usually are in the depressive direction (low mood), but can also be manic (elevated mood). Usually the likely direction of any alteration will be apparent before you reach this stage of the interview, and questions can be focused accordingly.

- How have you been feeling in yourself recently?
- How would you describe your mood? On a scale of 1–10?
- Have you been low in spirits or depressed?
- Can you still enjoy the things that you normally enjoy?
- Or is life particularly good/more enjoyable?

Ask about suicidal ideation (see Chapter 4). Use cues from the patient to broach the subject. For example:

- It sounds as if life's a bit of a struggle at the moment. Have you felt life isn't worth living?
- Have you actually thought of harming yourself in anyway?
- Have you made any plans to end your life?

**Notes**

- Record both how the patient reports their mood (*subjective* mood) and also how it appears to you (*objective* mood). The two can be discrepant (see Chapter 9).
- Always screen for mood disorders. They are common and some patients may not be aware of, or do not complain of, mood symptoms.
- The best screening questions for depression concern the presence of persistent low mood, and the loss of pleasure (*anhedonia*).
- Always assess suicidal intent (Chapter 4). There is no evidence that asking about suicide increases the risk of it—probably the opposite.
- The mood section of the MSE can also reveal anxiety symptoms. Usually, however, these are detected more from appearance and thoughts sections.

## Speech

Does the patient speak spontaneously or only in response to questioning?

Is the patient's speech hard to understand? If so, is it because of articulation (dysarthria) or content (dysphasia)?

What is the rate and volume of speech?

**Notes**

- Quiet speech which tails off or is monosyllabic is typical of depression; the opposite occurs in mania.
- Dysarthria suggests a neurological disorder or side-effect of antipsychotic drugs.
- Dysphasia suggests a focal neurological disorder or thought disorder.
- Abnormalities in the content or flow of what is said are recorded in the next section.

## Thoughts

Ask the patient to describe their current preoccupations and worries.

● Do you have particular things on your mind at the moment? If so, what?

Is the patient's train of thought difficult to follow? Try and describe how?

● Do you feel that people are against you or trying to harm you in some way?

● Do you feel that something strange is going on?

● Do you keep having the same thought or worry going round and round in your mind?

● Are you having any problems thinking clearly?

### Notes

Abnormalities of thoughts and thought processes occur in many psychiatric disorders, and the precise form of the abnormality can be diagnostically important. Distinguish between the *content*, *nature* and *flow* of thoughts:

● **Thought content.** Record the presence and topic of predominant thoughts. For example:

  o recurrent worries about physical health in hypochondriasis.

  o a general theme of persecution in a delusional disorder.

  o a preoccupation with weight in an eating disorder.

● **The nature of the thoughts.** Three types of abnormal thought are recognized. Each has a very different diagnostic significance:

  o A *delusion is a false belief. It is firmly held despite contrary evidence and is out of keeping with the patient's cultural or religious background.* For example, a patient is absolutely convinced that he is an assassin's target and so has locked himself in his flat and adopted a disguise. There may be one delusion or many, and they may be persistent or fleeting. Delusions carry special weight in the diagnosis of psychosis, so their recognition is an important skill (see the psychosis module, Chapter 3). During the development and treatment of psychosis, delusions may be *partial*, in that the patient realizes they might be false.

  o An **obsession** *is a recurrent thought, impulse or image that enters the subject's mind despite resistance.* The patient realizes that it originates from their own mind and may not be true, but they cannot resist thinking it and often have to act upon it (a *compulsion*). For example, obsessional thoughts about having dirty hands, the compulsion being to wash repeatedly. These symptoms characterize obsessive–compulsive disorder (OCD) and also occur in depression.

  o An **overvalued idea** is a belief not held quite as strongly as a delusion, and is typically more 'understandable'. It is typified by the belief of a malnourished girl with anorexia nervosa that she is fat.

● **The flow of thinking.** Even if the content and nature of thoughts are normal, the flow (form) of thinking may not be. This is called *thought disorder* or *formal thought disorder*. It is often first detected if the patient is given time to reply at length to an open question, whereupon the interviewer realizes he is having problems following the train of thought. Write down a sample of what is said. Different sorts of thought disorder characterize schizophrenia and bipolar disorder.

## Perceptions

Do you see or hear things that other people can't?

Have you ever heard voices speaking when there was nobody there?

Do things or people seem different from normal?

### Notes

● A **hallucination** *is a perception experienced as real in the absence of a stimulus.* For example, hearing a voice in the corner of the room when no-one is there. Like a delusion, the person is absolutely convinced (at the time) that the experience is real. True hallucinations are pathognomonic of psychosis. They can occur in any modality; auditory hallucinations are the most common; visual hallucinations suggest an organic psychosis. Like partial delusions, there are also partial hallucinations—usually called *pseudohallucinations*—which are perceived inside the head; they have little diagnostic significance. Similarly, hallucinations are common whilst falling asleep (*hypnogogic*) or waking up (*hypnopompic*), and are not abnormal.

● An **illusion** *is a misperception*—for example, seeing someone in the shadows when there's no-one there. They have an 'as if' quality and in isolation have no diagnostic significance (and so an illusion must be distinguished clearly from hallucination).

● **Depersonalization** *is a feeling of detachment from the normal sense of self*—'as if I am acting'. *Derealization* is similar, a feeling of detachment from the external world. Both are a feature of neurosis but can be mistaken for the perplexity of psychosis.

## Cognition

Is the patient orientated in time, person and place?

Is there 'clouding of consciousness'?

Show the patient three items (e.g. watch, pen, shoe) and ensure they have registered them; test for recall 2 minutes later. If the patient can recall the three items, the likelihood ratio for cognitive impairment is 0.06.

### Notes

● Cognitive impairment is the hallmark of organic disorders—especially dementia and delirium. It can also occur as a feature of depression, especially in the elderly (sometimes called *pseudodementia*) and in schizophrenia (hence its previous name of *dementia praecox*).
● In delirium there is *clouding of consciousness* (usually manifested as decreased responsiveness to, or awareness of, surroundings); in dementia there isn't (Chapter 13). See cognitive function and unresponsive patient modules.
● If significant cognitive abnormalities are detected, physical examination and the cognitive function module are essential.

## Insight

Do you think anything is wrong with you? If so, what?

Do you need any treatment? If so, what sort?

### Notes

● Insight is not all or nothing, but a matter of degree, and it fluctuates according to the mental state.
● Insight has several components. It includes the person's ability to recognize:
   ○ abnormal mental experiences as abnormal.
   ○ that the person is suffering from a psychiatric disorder.
   ○ the need for, and benefits of, treatment. This aspect has particular implications when considering compulsory treatment under the Mental Health Act (Chapter 8).

## Core contextual information

Recording key details of the person's background and current circumstances is part of the core assessment because they provide a *context* for the patient's problems. This helps in several ways:
● It enhances the therapeutic relationship by demonstrating an interest in the patient as a person.
● It helps identify causal factors (e.g. a bereavement, childhood abuse).

● It identifies potentially modifiable contributory problems (e.g. financial worries).
● It reveals personal factors which affect management (e.g. the presence of a supportive partner to supervise medication).
● It sometimes helps diagnostically. For example, asking about employment reveals that a depressed man lost his job for being repeatedly late; further questioning showed this to have resulted from an unrecognized alcohol problem.

How much contextual enquiry is needed depends on the nature of the patient's problems, and what is already known. For example, in general practice the patient's circumstances will usually be well known; for a woman newly referred to your out-patient clinic, extensive questioning might be needed to clarify the relationship of her failing marriage and business to her depressive disorder.

Core contextual information falls into three broad categories: *family history*, *personal history* and *current circumstances*.

## Family history

Family tree—at least parents, siblings, children. Their ages, occupations, health.
   Nature of the family relationships.
   Family psychiatric and medical history.

### Notes

● Problems in family relationships are commonly associated with psychiatric disorder.
● A positive family history is a risk factor for most psychiatric disorders, for genetic and environmental reasons.

## Personal history

Childhood—health problems, maltreatment, school record.
   Personality—the patient's usual attitudes, mood, beliefs, and interests.
   Relationship(s)—number, duration, type, gender.
   Employment history (nature of work, problems).
   Criminal offences?

**Notes**

- Aspects of childhood can be associated with subsequent psychiatric disorder (e.g. conduct disorder with dissocial personality disorder; childhood abuse with later depression and neurotic disorders).
- The premorbid personality shapes the risk, type and prognosis of psychiatric disorder. Ask simple questions about relationships, interests and prevailing mood. Offering alternatives may be helpful—for example, 'Would you describe yourself as a loner or very sociable?'
- A patient's view of their personality and life may be distorted during psychiatric illness. For example, a depressed person will report themselves in an unduly negative light. Always corroborate personality details from a close informant.
- The pattern of past relationships can give diagnostic clues—for example, an absence of close relationships in schizoid personality disorder or many turbulent ones in borderline personality disorder.
- The nature of employment gives clues to the patient's level of functioning. A deteriorating or disrupted work record may reflect a psychiatric disorder or a personality trait, respectively.
- Having a 'forensic history' (i.e. a criminal record) may be directly related to a psychiatric disorder or a coincidence. A history of violence will affect management regardless—see risk assessment (Chapter 4).
- Questions on sexual history and functioning may be necessary at this stage, but detailed or especially sensitive discussion on this topic may better be deferred until a later stage (see Chapter 11).

## Current circumstances

Current relationships. Who is there to support the patient, and who is dependent on the patient?

Current employment.

Current worries—finances, housing, relationship, etc.

**Notes**

- The current relationship is an important factor: it may have contributed to the disorder or have been damaged by it. Having a supportive partner improves outcome and assists management. Check the partner's gender.
- All patients with severe psychiatric disorder should have an assessment of needs (Chapter 8). Detailed information about the current circumstances is an essential component of this.

- Ongoing worries and stresses can perpetuate psychiatric disorder; their resolution is often part of management (e.g. helping the patient sort out a housing problem).

## The core physical examination

The physical health of a psychiatric patient is important because:

- Medical conditions can present with psychological symptoms. For example, lethargy and low mood may signify anaemia or carcinoma.
- Patients with psychiatric disorders have increased rates of medical illness, either because of a common aetiology or because the psychiatric disorder leads them to neglect their health.

So, in every assessment take account of the patient's physical appearance, as well as their age, symptoms, medical history, etc., and always consider what examination is required. This may include a brief examination of all systems. However, there is no pre-specified physical examination in the psychiatric assessment since it depends upon the setting, the patient, the disorder and the treatment.

*The setting.* For example:

- A full examination is performed on every psychiatric admission because the psychiatrist takes medical responsibility whilst the patient is in hospital.
- In an emergency assessment, have a low threshold for examination since the possibility may not have been considered in the rush to refer the patient.
- In primary care, the GP may have examined the patient thoroughly before referral.

*The patient.* For example:

- Full examination if the patient has not been seen by a doctor recently.
- Full examination if homeless, since at risk of tuberculosis, malnutrition, etc.
- Examine relevant systems if there is a known history of a medical disorder, or if functional enquiry revealed significant symptoms.

*The disorder and its treatment.* For example:

- If alcohol misuse is suspected, examine for the physical signs which accompany it.

- Patients on antipsychotic drugs long term should be examined for tardive dyskinesia.
- Patients with somatic symptoms.

For patients receiving psychiatric care in the community, the responsibility for the patient's medical health should be agreed between psychiatrist and GP; usually it resides with the latter.

## Core investigations

Core medical investigations do not exist in psychiatry, other than the convention that routine blood tests are performed on admission to an inpatient ward. Elsewhere, investigations should be used to test a specific diagnostic hypothesis arising from the history, MSE or physical examination. For example:

- A urine drug screen in suspected drug-induced psychosis.
- Extensive biochemical, imaging and genetic investigations in a 30-year-old with dementia.
- A brain scan in someone with delirium and a history of a fall.
- Thyroid function tests in a patient with anxiety, palpitations and weight loss.

## Shrinking the core: a 'one minute screen' for psychiatric disorder

The core assessment is portable for use in all settings, not just in specialist psychiatry. However, there are occasions when only a moment can be spent on psychiatric assessment. Even this is worthwhile. The seven questions in Table 2.2 screen rapidly for psychiatric disorders common in general practice or the general hospital.

- A positive response to any question should lead to a core and module assessment.

**Table 2.2** A 'one minute screen' for common psychiatric disorders.

| During the past month: | Screening for: |
|---|---|
| 1. Have you felt low in spirits? | *depression* |
| 2. Do you enjoy things less than you usually do? | *depression* |
| 3. Have you been feeling generally anxious? | *neurosis (anxiety)* |
| 4. Are you worried about your health or other specific things? | *neurosis (health anxiety)* |
| 5. Has your eating felt out of control? | *eating disorder* |
| 6. Do you drink alcohol? If so, ask FAST or CAGE questions (p. 10) | *alcohol problem* |
| 7. Present 3 items and ask patient to recall them after 2 minutes. | *dementia/delirium* |

### Key points

- The aim of psychiatric assessment is to gather sufficient information to make a diagnosis and set it in context.
- Most information comes from the history and mental state examination, though physical examination and investigations are sometimes important too.
- Diagnostic hypotheses should be made early in the assessment and then tested using more specific questioning.
- A flexible approach can be achieved by combining a core assessment with specific modules (Chapter 3) which are only used when the likelihood of a specific diagnosis is raised.
- Psychiatric disorder can and should be rapidly screened for in all medical settings.
- Interviewing skills allow you to gather information efficiently and form an effective alliance with the patient.

# Chapter 3

# Psychiatric assessment modules

## Using assessment modules

The purpose of the core assessment (Chapter 2) was to screen efficiently for features associated with a high probability of psychiatric disorder. The modules are used to confirm, refine or refute these diagnostic hypotheses. The modules focus on: cognitive function, psychosis, mood, neurosis and related disorders, eating disorders, substance misuse and the unresponsive patient.

- Each module contains general advice about the areas to cover, suggestions for specific questions, and explanatory notes and definitions of key terms. There is no distinction between the history and MSE in the modules; different headings are used as required to suit the module.
- The clinical features of psychiatric disorders are covered in Chapters 9–15. Refer to the relevant chapter in conjunction with the module.
- An adequate assessment often requires more than one module.
- Other aspects of assessment are covered elsewhere: risk (Chapter 4), sexual functioning (Chapter 11), children (Chapter 16) and learning disability (Chapter 17).

*We do not suggest reading this chapter in one go. Instead, read through a module as you come across a clinical problem requiring its use.*

*Lecture Notes: Psychiatry*, 10e. By Paul Harrison, John Geddes and Michael Sharpe. Published 2010 by Blackwell Publishing Ltd.

## Assessment of cognitive function

*Cognitive function* comprises attention, memory and language. It is the first module, since impairment in these areas interferes with the psychiatric assessment, occasionally to the point that no useful history can be obtained from the patient.

---

**Key questions addressed by the cognitive function module**

- *Is clinically significant cognitive impairment present?*
- *If so, what is its cause?* The major causes are *dementia* (chronic; normal level of consciousness) or *delirium* (acute; consciousness impaired). Both have a range of specific causes, which are then investigated (Chapter 13).
- *The disorders causing cognitive impairment include a range of neurological and general medical disorders (e.g. intracranial tumours and other space-occupying lesions, infections), and so the module also includes a detailed medical history, neurological examination and relevant investigations.*

**Triggering the module**

The suspicion of cognitive impairment may have arisen for many reasons. For example:
- The patient has scored poorly on the core cognitive screen.
- The patient is muddled, as judged by their manner or response to initial questions.
- A history of forgetfulness.
- The patient is old (e.g. >20% of 80 year olds have dementia).

---

**Related modules**

If the person can't or won't answer questions or engage in the assessment, use the *unresponsive patient* module. The *mood* module is often needed because depression can cause mild cognitive impairment. The ability to self-care may be impaired, so *risk* assessment is necessary.
- If poor cognitive functioning is life long, consider *learning disability* (Chapter 17).
- Deafness is a classic, but hopefully rare, cause of a misdiagnosis of dementia.

## The cognitive function module

Before proceeding, revise the cognition section of the core assessment (Chapter 2). First, ask whether the patient (or their informant) has noticed a problem with memory, and characterize this. While doing so, note the patient's understanding and use of language, and their ability to attend to the questions.
- Do you find yourself forgetting things? Can you give me some examples?
- When did it begin? Any idea what might have happened?
- What aspects of life are affected? (e.g. work, cooking, shopping).
- Do you have any problems finding words, or understanding what people say to you?

Sometimes it is useful to ask the patient to describe the main events and chronology of their day (especially if you can corroborate the history).
- If they give an implausible story, consider *confabulation* (the fabrication of recent events to cover gaps in memory) that occurs in *amnesic syndrome* (Chapter 13).

Then, tell the patient you want to ask some questions to assess their memory. This makes people anxious, so emphasize it's not a pass or fail kind of test. Questions should test a range of memory domains:
- Orientation questions (e.g. What day of the week is it? Which town are we in? What kind of place is this?).
- Questions of general knowledge (e.g. Who is the Prime Minister?).

- Semantic knowledge (e.g. point to objects and ask the patient to name them).
- Ask the patient to spell a five-letter word backwards, or 'serial sevens'—take 7 from 100 and keep taking 7 away).
- Can the patient respond to practical instructions. (e.g. Pick up the pencil from the table and put it on the floor).
- Recall can be tested by asking the patient to recall the objects named, or the word spelt backwards, a few minutes later.
- Draw a circle and ask the patient to imagine it's a clock, and to put the numbers in and draw the hands pointing to a particular time (e.g. 9.30).
- Ask the patient to write a simple sentence of their own choice.
- Test abstract reasoning. For example, What's similar between a dog and a cat?

Ensure the patient has registered each question—don't be misled by sensory problems, and try to note any lack of attention or motivation.

There are also formal tests of memory function, comprised of questions such as those listed here, which are used in the routine assessment of dementia. The choice of scales and screens varies between clinicians and settings.
- The scale which is most widely used, including by non-specialists, is the *Mini-Mental State Examination (MMSE)*, not to be confused with the mental state examination. It is also used to determine which patients are eligible for cholinesterase inhibitor drugs for Alzheimer's disease. It consists of 12 questions. The maximum score is 30; normal score is 26–30; 21–25 suggests dementia (likelihood ratio = 5), and 20 or less is highly suggestive (likelihood ratio = 8).

## Assessing the cause of cognitive impairment

Assess for features of delirium.
- Is the person drowsy? Are they fully aware of their surroundings?
- Are they distractable? Irritable?
- Do they seem to be hallucinating?
- When did the problems start?
- Any obvious cause (e.g. post-ictal, septic).

Administer the depression module.

Check (again) for any symptoms or signs suggesting a neurological or general medical disorder or focal lesion.

### Notes

- The hallmark of delirium is '*clouding of consciousness*'—drowsiness, distractibility, fleeting delusions, and visual hallucinations. There is usually an acute onset and fluctuating course.
- Depression can also cause cognitive impairment and may present because of it.
- If neither delirium nor depression is present, the diagnosis is almost certainly dementia.
- Unawareness of self-identity is rare, even in severe dementia, and raises the possibility of a dissociative disorder (Chapter 10).

## Other components of the module

Do a careful physical examination. Look for evidence of vascular disease, thyroid status, alcohol abuse or infection. The neurological examination should include testing of cranial nerves and evaluation of cortical functions (e.g. apraxias, hemineglect, primitive reflexes).

### Notes

- If dementia is diagnosed, proceed to assess: (a) its likely cause, (b) its effect on daily living and (c) any associated problems. These issues are covered in Chapter 13.
- Delirium is due to a variety of medical conditions, many of which need urgent treatment (Chapter 13).
- Talk to the informant first if the impairment is severe.

## Assessment of psychosis

The cardinal features of psychosis (delusions, hallucinations and lack of insight) were defined in the core assessment (Chapter 2) and relate mostly to the disorders covered in Chapter 12.

---

**Key questions addressed by the psychosis module**

- *Is the person suffering from a psychosis?* Some people with strange ideas or strange behaviour may turn out to have a neurosis, a personality disorder or no diagnosis at all. Similarly, some people can appear and behave entirely normally despite having a psychosis. Detection of a psychosis is therefore sometimes difficult, not least because people may be frightened of their experiences, or what will happen to them if they tell you.
- *If so, which psychosis is it?* The main disorders in which psychotic symptoms occur are: schizophrenia, severe depression, mania, drug-induced psychoses, delusional disorders and organic psychoses (e.g. in dementia or delirium).

**Triggering the module**

Psychosis may be suspected for diverse reasons, such as:
- Possible delusions elicited in the core assessment.
- Bizarre or inexplicable behaviour.
- History of amphetamine use.
- A young adult found in a neglected state.
- A man heard talking to himself in a police cell.

**Related modules**

The module is usually accompanied by the *mood* and *substance misuse* modules because of the overlap of these conditions. *Risk assessment* is needed as psychoses commonly lead to a risk of harm to self and, much less often, to others.

## The psychosis module

The diagnosis of schizophrenia and other psychoses relies on detailed evaluation of a number of symptoms and signs, especially concerning abnormalities of thought content and form, so the module is quite long.

## Appearance and behaviour

Note manner, dress, posture and movements.
- Are there mannerisms or stereotypies?
- Is the patient dressed unusually? Is there evidence of self-neglect?
- Is the patient restless?

### Notes

- Manner—patient may be suspicious (you may be part of his conspiracy theory), distracted (by hallucinations) or distant and uninterested (?negative symptoms of schizophrenia).
- Dress—some people with schizophrenia may dress idiosyncratically. For example, a man wore a silver foil hat to prevent his thoughts being extracted.
- Motor abnormalities occur in psychosis and as common side-effects of antipsychotic drugs, especially the older 'typical' ones. The side-effects include *dystonia, parkinsonism, akathisia* and *tardive dyskinesia* (Chapter 7).
- A *mannerism* is a repetitive movement or gesture which is complex and seemingly purposeful. A repeated simple and purposeless one is a *stereotypy*. Both occur in schizophrenia.
- *Catatonia* describes a group of motor signs which are rare but characteristic of the subtype of catatonic schizophrenia, although they can also occur in organic disorders or as an isolated 'catatonia syndrome':
  - *Echopraxia/echolalia* (the patient imitates the interviewer's every action or word).
  - *Automatic obedience* (compliance with all instructions regardless of consequence).
  - *Ambitendency* (tentative movements back and forth—as if unsure what to do).
  - *Posturing* (*catalepsy*) (the maintenance of inappropriate or bizarre postures).
  - *Waxy flexibility* (limbs held in externally imposed positions—muscle tone is increased).
  - *Negativism* (seemingly motiveless resistance to all instructions or attempts to be moved).

## Mood

Does the overall mood seem normal? Is it responsive?

Is the emotional expression appropriate with the topic being discussed?

### Notes

- Psychosis can occur with severe depression and in mania. In this instance, the mood abnormality is usually readily apparent. Here, only the abnormalities of mood occurring in schizophrenia are mentioned.
  - *Flattened affect* is a decrease in emotional responsivity and expression, even when emotionally charged topics are discussed. It is a negative symptom of schizophrenia. Needs to be distinguished from depression and parkinsonism.
  - *Incongruous affect:* emotion not in keeping with the topic being talked about.

## Speech

Are made-up words (*neologisms*) used, or words and language used idiosyncratically?

### Notes

- A *neologism* is a made-up word, usually invested with a personal meaning. Be sure the patient doesn't just have a larger vocabulary than you …
- If the patient's sentences, or overall answers, don't quite make sense or seem puzzling or unexpected, it may signify thought disorder, as outlined below.

## Thoughts—content

Is there any evidence of delusions?
- Is anything bothering you at the moment?
- Do you believe or understand things differently from other people?
- Do people have a special interest in you? Are people against you? How do you know?
- Is anything on the TV referring to you particularly?
- When did you first realize this (i.e. the delusional belief) was true? How?

## Notes

- Because, by definition, a delusion is believed to be true, its detection requires you to be receptive to clues and sometimes to 'go along' with implausible statements in order to elicit more details. For example, a man matter-of-factly asked one of us how we were affected by the Bulgarian mafia—the first hint of his psychosis. A non-committal reply led him to elaborate and reveal his persecutory delusional system.
- Different sorts of delusions are recognized:
  - A *delusional perception* is a delusional interpretation of a normal perception. For example, a man saw a woman sneeze and knew this meant he must leave town. It is sometimes preceded by a sense of unease or perplexity that something strange is going on (*delusional mood*).
  - In a *delusion of reference*, an event or message (often on TV) has a unique meaning for the person. An *idea of reference* is similar, but not delusional in intensity (and thus not a true psychotic symptom); it may occur in paranoid personality disorder.
  - A *secondary delusion* is one that arises understandably from another mental state abnormality (e.g. delusions of guilt in depression); a *primary* delusion doesn't.
  - Delusions may be classified by content. The most common are *persecutory* delusions (sometimes incorrectly called *paranoid delusions*), in which the person believes they are the victim of perceived injustice or conspiracy. *Grandiose* delusions are seen in mania, *nihilistic* ones in depression.

## Thoughts—flow and possession

Is it difficult to follow the meaning of what the patient is saying? Write down a representative sample.

Do the person's thoughts seem to flow normally?

- Do your thoughts sometimes stop suddenly? (*thought block*).
- Are your thoughts sometimes removed from your head? (*thought withdrawal*).

Does the person feel in control of their thoughts and actions?

- Do your thoughts get put into your head from outside? (*thought insertion*).
- Can other people directly influence your thoughts or actions? (*passivity; thought control*).

Are the thoughts experienced unusually?

- Are other people aware of your thoughts? (*thought broadcasting*).

- Do any of your thoughts get repeated in your mind like an echo? (*thought echo*).

## Notes

- *Thought disorder* (also called *formal thought disorder*) occurs in schizophrenia. The connections between thoughts and ideas are obscure and there is a rambling quality. Descriptive terms include *knight's move thinking* and *loosening of associations* and, in rare severe cases, *word salad*. For example, in response to a question about what the person had been up to before the appointment: 'I got on the bus when I saw the man from the hostel, in the next street where I was. Like it was that dog again, you know? Still, doctor, what do you think? …'. A different type of thought disorder occurs in mania.
- In schizophrenia, abnormalities also occur in the perceived source, ownership and fate of thoughts:
  - *Thought insertion:* thoughts originate elsewhere and are put into the patient's head.
  - *Thought withdrawal:* the experience of thoughts being removed from one's mind.
  - *Thought broadcast:* the subject experiences his thoughts being available to and heard by others.
  - *Thought block:* the flow of thoughts abruptly ends. Distinguish from thought withdrawal and from simple loss of concentration.
  - *Passivity:* thoughts, feelings or actions are experienced as being under external control. For example, a schizophrenic who killed her son described being unable to resist carrying out this act because of the 'force' controlling her. Passivity phenomena are important in risk assessment (and in how resulting crimes are dealt with).

## Perceptions

Does the person seem to be hearing things that are not there?

- Do you hear voices when there doesn't seem to be anyone present? (*auditory hallucinations*).
- Are the voices inside (*pseudohallucinations*) or outside (*hallucinations*) your head?
- What are they talking about?
- Do they talk directly to you or about you? (*second* and *third person hallucinations*, respectively).
- Do they comment on what you're doing? (*running commentary*).
- Do they want you to harm yourself or other people?

Repeat similar questions for hallucinations in other modalities.

**Notes**

● The characteristic hallucinations of schizophrenia are *third person auditory hallucinations* (i.e. hearing the voice talking *about* you). Sometimes these take the form of a *running commentary* by two or more voices.

● *Somatic hallucinations* (e.g. buzzing sensations due to a beehive in the chest) and hallucinations in other modalities also occur. *Visual hallucinations* suggest an organic psychosis. *Olfactory hallucinations* occur in temporal lobe epilepsy.

● Auditory hallucinations in psychotic mood disorders are *mood congruent*—that is, critical and derogatory in severe depression; grandiose in mania—whereas those in other psychoses are not.

## Cognition

Is the patient disorientated?

**Notes**

● An acutely psychotic patient may be distracted by his experiences, or be worried that your questions are trying to trick or harm her, and therefore she may perform poorly on cognitive testing. Try and distinguish this from the perplexity of delirium.

● Patients with chronic schizophrenia may have genuine cognitive impairment as part of their illness; they characteristically underestimate their age by several years, and perform worse than expected on most psychometric tests. This can be exacerbated by lack of motivation, and by some forms of medication.

## Other components of the module

Check insight.

● Do you think you are ill in any way? Do others? Do you need help? What sort?

Ask about complications of pregnancy or delivery, place of upbringing, academic achievements and social interests.

Ask about family history of psychosis.

Ask about past or current substance abuse.

Ask about premorbid personality and level of functioning.

Corroborate the history from an informant.

Carry out a physical examination, concentrating on the neurological system.

Consider laboratory investigations and magnetic resonance imaging (MRI) scan (see Chapter 12).

**Notes**

● Insight is characteristically lost in psychosis, but in practice it is affected to varying degrees (see Chapter 2). *Distorted awareness of reality* is a related term which conveys what is often apparent to the interviewer.

● Family history, obstetric complications, an urban upbringing and problems at school are all associated with schizophrenia.

● Alcohol and illicit drugs can induce psychosis. Consider the substance abuse module.

● A decline in level of functioning (intellectually and socially) is common before and during the onset of schizophrenia.

● Organic disorders of many kinds can produce psychosis (see Chapter 12), hence the relevance of medical history and physical examination.

## First-rank symptoms of schizophrenia

A number of symptoms in this module are called *first-rank symptoms*, and are accorded great significance in the diagnosis of schizophrenia. They are summarized in Table 3.1.

**Notes**

● For definitions of first-rank symptoms, see above (p. 20).

● The likelihood ratio for schizophrenia is >4 if a first-rank symptom is present. However, they are not pathognomonic—first-rank symptoms occur in other psychoses, and not all schizophrenics have had one.

● They are sometimes called *Schneiderian* symptoms after Kurt Schneider, the psychiatrist who described them.

**Table 3.1** First-rank symptoms of schizophrenia.

*Delusions*
    Delusional perception

*Hallucinations*
    Thought echo (audible thoughts)
    Third person auditory hallucinations
    Running commentary

*Thought flow and possession*
    Thought withdrawal
    Thought insertion
    Thought broadcasting

*Passivity*
    Passivity of thought, feelings or actions

• Listing and defining first-rank symptoms is a favourite exam question.

## Assessment of mood

There are separate modules for lowered mood (*depression*) and for elevated mood (*mania*), described here in turn.
• First, review the relevant sections of the core assessment.

## Assessment of depression

---

**Key questions addressed by the depression module**

• *Is the person depressed?* Depression must be distinguished from normal sadness.
• *If so, is the diagnosis a depressive disorder, or are the depressive symptoms part of another disorder?* They can occur secondarily in, for example, schizophrenia and neuroses.
• *If the diagnosis is a depressive disorder, what type is it?* Depression can be a single episode, recurrent or part of bipolar disorder. It may include psychotic symptoms. It can be caused by many organic disorders and by drugs, both prescribed and illicit.

**Triggering the module**

Examples of the triggers for this module include:
• Detection of a depressive symptom or suicidal thought in the core assessment.
• Unexplained fatigue.
• Any of the presentations in Table 9.2.

**Related modules**

Depression overlaps and coexists with so many diagnoses that any of the other modules may be necessary. The presence of mood disturbance requires risk assessment (mainly for suicide) as well.

---

## The depression module

### Appearance and behaviour

Does the patient look depressed? Is he crying? Is he agitated?
    Does he exude a sense of gloom?
    Is there good eye contact?

Is there a normal range of emotional expression?

**Notes**

• In depression there is often decreased eye contact and a lack of expression and movement—called *psychomotor retardation*. Other depressed people are *agitated*, pacing to and fro or wringing their hands.

### Speech

Is the speech normal in speed, loudness and amount?

**Notes**

• In severe depression, speech is slow, quiet and sparse. Sentences tail off, as though the patient cannot summon the energy or concentration to continue.

### Mood

Has the patient noticed a change in mood, enjoyment or in energy?
• How have you been feeling in your spirits?
• Do you still enjoy the things that you usually do? If not, can you give some examples?
• How is your energy level? Do you feel more tired or fatigued than usual?
    Then:
• How long have you felt this way?
• Did anything seem to trigger it off?
• Is your mood lower at a particular time of day? How do you feel first thing?
• Do you often feel like crying?
• Do you easily get irritable?
• In the past, have you had periods of better than usual mood, or boundless energy, or have behaved out of character?

**Notes**

• The duration, pervasiveness and severity of these symptoms affect the diagnosis and management.
• *Anhedonia*, the lack of pleasure from normally enjoyed activities, is a key symptom of moderate and severe depression.
• *Reactivity of mood*: in severe depression, the normal reactivity of mood to circumstances is lost.

- *Diurnal variation of mood*: mood is typically worst early in the morning, improving as the day goes on.
- The predominant subjective feeling in depression may be sadness, irritability, fatigue, lethargy or lack of energy (*anergia*).
- The last question above may give a clue to mania in the past, and thus to a possible bipolar mood disorder. If there is any hint of a positive response, use the mania module.
- Depressive symptoms are common in the bereaved and can be hard to distinguish from normal grief (Chapter 9).

## Sleep, appetite and other bodily functions

- How are you sleeping at the moment? Do you have problems getting to sleep, interrupted sleep or of waking early? Or are you sleeping more than usual?
- What is your appetite like? Do you enjoy your food? Have you lost weight?
- Are you constipated? (Are your periods regular?)
- Has your interest in sex changed recently?

### Notes

- Biological rhythms and drives are frequently impaired in depression. The presence of 'biological' or 'somatic' symptoms is one way to define the boundary between mild depression and more severe cases—the latter sometimes called *melancholia*.
- Sleep is affected in several ways. *Initial insomnia* is common when there is accompanying anxiety. Sleep is shallow and unrefreshing. *Early morning waking* is the most characteristic change, often occurring with diurnal variation of mood, so the patient is awake and at his most desperate when the rest of the world is asleep. Increased sleep and sluggishness can also occur.
- Appetite is reduced with resulting weight loss and contributing to constipation.
- Irregular periods or amenorrhoea occur in women.
- There is a general loss of energy and libido.

## Thoughts—content

- What things are on your mind at the moment? Anything particular bothering you?
- Do you see things getting better? What might improve things?
- Do you feel guilty about anything you have done?
- Do you feel that you are of value?

- Do you have worries about your physical health?
- Do you feel that people are getting at you? If so, is it justified?

   Make sure to ask in detail about suicidal thoughts and intent (Chapter 4).

### Notes

- Prevailing thoughts (or 'cognitions') have a negative colouring, centring upon perceived failures, worthlessness, low self-esteem, and so on.
- Hopelessness and guilt feelings are important, not only because they are distressing but also because they may lead to suicidal thoughts and intentions.
- The content of thoughts (and the person's appearance) may suggest accompanying anxiety—covered in the neurosis module.
- Worries about health and complaints of physical symptoms are common in depression, as well as in neurotic syndromes.

## Thoughts—nature

Are any of the thoughts obsessional in nature?
- Do you find yourself checking things repeatedly?
- Do you like things especially clean and tidy?

   Are any of the thoughts delusional?
- Use the criteria and approach described in the psychosis module.

### Notes

- Obsessional thoughts and ruminations are common in depression; if prominent, consider OCD and use the neurosis module.
- Delusions are rare in depression as a whole, but characterize psychotic depression. They tend to be *mood congruent* and *nihilistic*.

## Perceptions

Are there hallucinations? What are they like?

### Notes

- Hallucinations sometimes occur in psychotic depression—usually second person voices saying derogatory things.
- Depressed people may describe that sensations are less intense than usual and they feel isolated from the normal emotions and activities of the outside world.

## Cognition

Is concentration impaired?
- What is your concentration like?
- Can you read a paper or follow a TV programme?

Is there objective evidence of cognitive impairment? (See cognition module).

### Notes

- Depression, especially in the elderly, can produce apparent cognitive impairment, sometimes called *pseudodementia*. This is a mixture of lack of motivation and poor concentration. It must be distinguished from dementia, as it responds to treatment of the depression.

## Other components of the module

Does the patient think they are depressed?

Identify past and current stressors—marital strife, unemployment, etc.

How has the patient tried to cope with the problems?

Is there a past history of mood disorder? What has its course been? What treatment worked?

Does the person have depressive or neurotic traits in their personality?

Is there a family history of psychiatric disorder or suicide?

### Notes

- Severely depressed patients may deny that their mood is abnormal and decline treatment.
- At its most severe, patients may stop eating, drinking and even moving. *Depressive stupor* is life threatening and an indication for emergency electroconvulsive therapy (ECT).
- Stressors (*life events*) can precipitate depression; identifying them helps make sense of the depression—and can be therapeutic.
- Coping strategies adopted by patients may lead to additional problems. For example, use of alcohol.
- Many patients have had previous episode(s) of mood disorder. Ask about their nature, treatment and outcome.
- Depressive personality traits may affect the risk and outcome of depressive disorders. An informant should provide the personality information.
- A positive family history is a risk factor for depressive disorder and suicide.

## Assessment of mania

> ### Key questions addressed by the mania module
>
> - *Is the person manic?* Mania is a pathological elevation of mood that causes substantial impairment in occupational and/or social functioning. Mania is the key syndrome in bipolar disorder. Milder manic symptoms do not necessarily cause impairment and are called *hypomania*. In hypomania, functioning may be improved but it can also precede a manic relapse.
> - *Has the person been manic in the past?* Even if she is currently depressed or euthymic (normal mood), a history of mania is important because of its diagnostic and therapeutic implications (Chapter 9).
>
> ### Triggering the mania module
>
> The mania module may be triggered by:
> - A hint of manic symptoms in the core assessment or depression module.
> - Recent grandiose, disinhibited or disorganized behaviour.
> - A past history of bipolar disorder.
> - A family history of bipolar disorder.
>
> ### Related modules
>
> Most patients with an episode of mania will have had a history of depression, and some have current depressive symptoms (a '*mixed affective state*'), so always use the *depression* module. Mania can be associated with *substance misuse*.

## The mania module

### Appearance and behaviour

Note manner and dress.

Is the patient elated, distractable, or irritable?

Is the patient overactive?

### Notes

- Clothes and make up may be bright and garish or dishevelled.
- Look out for flamboyant or disinhibited gestures. The patient may try and hug you, snatch your notes or challenge your qualifications.
- A manic person may be unable to concentrate enough to give useful or consistent answers. If so, focus on observing and eliciting current symptoms and signs. Take the rest of the history later or from an informant.

- The predominant emotion can be euphoria and infectious gaiety, or sudden and extreme irritability.
- Determine if the patient's behaviour is causing them any problems in areas such as work, relationships, etc.

## Speech

Is the speech fast? Excessive in amount? Loud? Hard to interrupt?

**Notes**

- Speech in mania is fast, loud, expansive and hard to interrupt (*pressure of speech*). It reflects the underlying pressure of thoughts and the person's attempts to share their many wonderful ideas.

## Mood

Has the patient noticed a change in mood or energy level recently? Can they describe it?
- Do you feel happier than usual? More confident?
- Are you feeling full of energy?
- Have you been very irritable or impatient?
- How long has this been the case?

**Notes**

- Some people with mania deny their mood is elevated, or are too busy to think about it.
- Mood can be labile or *mixed*—simultaneous depressive and manic features.
- An increase in energy level and drive to do things almost always occurs.
- In some people, the elevated mood can be experienced as irritability.
- The duration of symptoms of elevated mood is important in making the diagnosis, and in the distinction of mania from hypomania (see Chapter 9).

## Sleep, appetite and other bodily functions

- How are you sleeping? More or less than usual?
- How's your appetite?
- Has your interest in sex, or other activities, changed?

**Notes**

- Tiredness and sleep drive are decreased. A manic patient may stay up all night working or playing.

- Appetite may be increased, or the patient may be too busy to eat.
- Libido tends to be enhanced and sexual activity uninhibited.

## Thoughts—content

- What's on your mind at the moment?
- Do you have special powers or abilities?

**Notes**

- Thoughts are expansive and grandiose. There may be a single, preoccupying scheme (e.g. to build a football stadium in their garden), but usually there is a kaleidoscope of incomplete, jumbled ideas.

## Thoughts—nature

Are the thoughts delusional?

Is there any evidence of reckless or dangerous ideas?
- Have you got plans to buy anything?
- Can you do things which most people might find difficult or even impossible?

Does the train of thought jump from one topic to another?

**Notes**

- In mania, the grandiose ideas may become delusional. Religious themes are common—for example, the patient knows he is the Messiah. Sometimes delusions are dangerous—the belief that one can drive excessively fast, fly or borrow unrealistic amounts of money. Take these risks seriously—the unpredictability of mania means they may suddenly be acted upon.
- *Flight of ideas* is a type of thought disorder characteristic of mania. Thoughts jump rapidly from one thing to another, with understandable, if unusual, connections between them. The links are often based on puns, rhymes and other associations—for example, 'I'm fine, a fine wine, whining and moaning like Jonah … Jonah the whale … in Wales …'. Write down a snippet.

## Perceptions

Is there any evidence of hallucinations?

**Notes**

● Mood-congruent auditory and occasionally visual hallucinations occur. For example, voices telling the person what special powers they have and how they can save humanity.

## Other components of the module

Does the patient think they are unwell or need treatment?

Corroborate recent history, especially with regard to unusual and inappropriate beliefs and actions.

Assess the degree of dysfunction being caused by the symptoms.

Check recent use of illicit drugs or alcohol.

Ask about past history of mania or depression.

Has the patient ever been prescribed lithium or other mood stabilizer? Is he supposed to be taking it now? Has he been compliant?

Ask about family history of mood disorders.

Do a physical examination.

**Notes**

● Insight fluctuates in mania. A person may seem aware of their condition and agree the need for treatment one moment but not the next.
● An informant usually paints a more dramatic picture of recent behaviour than does the patient. Gather evidence of specific dangerous or out-of-keeping behaviours, since they affect management—for example, whether the patient should be detained, or needs a pregnancy test.
● Manic episodes can be caused by drugs, such as amphetamines and steroids, and sometimes by alcohol.
● Bipolar disorder is often treated long term with lithium to prevent relapse, and sudden discontinuation can precipitate mania. Ask the patient if they take lithium, and check the plasma level.
● Bipolar disorder is strongly familial.
● Physical examination is indicated since mania can be due to an organic disorder (e.g. frontal lobe tumour), especially if the first episode occurs in middle age or beyond.

## Assessment of neurosis (including stress-related and somatoform disorders)

Neuroses are emotional disorders, usually involving anxiety in some form as their central feature, and manifesting as psychological, cognitive and physical (somatic) complaints. As discussed in Chapter 10, for various reasons the neuroses are classified together with *stress-related disorders* (where neurotic symptoms are attributed to a particular stressor) and *somatoform disorders* (where medically unexplained physical symptoms predominate). However, it is easier to divide them up here in terms of modules: the first concerns neurotic and stress-related disorders; the following one covers somatoform disorders.

● This is a notoriously confusing area, diagnostically speaking, and we suggest you read Chapter 10 in conjunction with these modules.

## Assessment of neurosis and stress-related disorders

**Key questions addressed by the neurosis and stress-related module**

● *Does the person have a neurosis?* A distinction must be made from (a) worries and emotional distress which are within normal limits or are part of the person's personality, and (b) from neurotic symptoms occurring in depression or other diagnostic categories.
● *If a neurosis is present, which one?* There are many types of neurosis, including panic disorder, phobias, OCD and hypochondriasis (Table 10.1). Occasionally, but importantly, anxiety disorders can be organic in origin (e.g. phaeocromocytoma).

**Triggering the module**

Neurotic symptoms are extremely common. The module might be triggered, for example, by:
● A woman who is preoccupied or clearly worried about something.
● A person distressed by a recent trauma.

**Related modules**

Neurotic symptoms often coexist with depression, so the *depression module* will nearly always be necessary. Use the *substance misuse* module if there is evidence of alcohol or drug use as a cause of, or response to, the symptoms. Worries about food or body image will trigger the *eating disorders* module. If the presentation is predominantly with somatic concerns (e.g. pain, fatigue) use the *somatoform disorders* module.

## The neurosis module

### Appearance

Does the patient look tense, anxious or worried?

**Notes**

- Anxiety is a state of arousal and may be apparent from the person's appearance and behaviour. With practice, it is usually possible to distinguish this from the agitation of depression.

### Anxiety

Start with open questions:

- Have you been worrying a lot about things recently? What about?
- Do you feel wound up or tense?
- Do you suffer from aches and pains?
  Characterizing the anxiety:
- Are the feelings there most of the time, or only in specific situations? If so, what things or situations make you anxious?
- Do you get sudden 'attacks' of anxiety? How does your body feel then?
- Can you put your worries out of your mind?
- Do you avoid doing things because of your worries?

**Notes**

- Anxiety consists of *psychological* symptoms (e.g. tension, fear) and *bodily* symptoms (e.g. palpitations, sweating), described in detail in Chapter 10. Either can predominate.
- Anxiety is usually *situational* (*phobic*), occurring in response to a specific stimulus. Less commonly it is *generalized* or *free floating*.
- Anxiety can also be paroxysmal—a *panic attack*: a discrete episode of severe anxiety which builds rapidly then gradually subsides over about an hour.
- People rapidly learn to *avoid* situations in which they feel anxious or uncomfortable. They may first present for help because of the practical problems which avoidance produces.

### Obsessions and compulsions

- Do you get repeated unpleasant images or thoughts coming into your mind?

- Do you have to keep checking things, or keep things very clean and tidy? What do you do? How often?
- Do you try to resist the thoughts or the urge to respond to them? If so, what happens?

**Notes**

- *Obsessions* and *compulsions* are characteristic of OCD and also occur in depression and anankastic personality disorder.
- Severe obsessions can, in practice, be difficult to distinguish from delusions. Stick to their strict definitions (Chapter 2).

### Other symptoms of neurosis

Enquire about somatic symptoms:

- How is your health generally?
- Do you suffer from severe tiredness or exhaustion?
- Have you ever lost your memory, sight or the use of part of your body?
- Have you felt detached or distant from yourself or your surroundings?

**Notes**

- Unexplained physical symptoms (e.g. palpitations) are common in anxiety disorders, and in depression. If they are prominent, and not explained by depression, then consider a *somatoform disorder* (see below).
- Medically unexplained fatigue is the main feature of *neurasthenia* (*chronic fatigue syndrome*). Fatigue and lethargy also occur in depression.
- *Dissociative disorders* are rare neuroses in which there is loss of function (e.g. amnesia, paralysis). They are usually encountered in medical settings (e.g. after admission for neurological investigation).
- Feelings of detachment from self or surroundings (*depersonalization–derealization*) are a common symptom of neurosis, may occur in healthy people when tired and are occasionally a diagnosis in its own right. Such feelings are hard to describe (e.g. 'It's as if there is glass between me and the world') and must be distinguished from psychotic symptoms.

### Other components of the module

When did the symptoms start? Did they seem related to recent events?

How has the person coped? Have they had any treatment?

How do the symptoms interfere with daily life?

Is there a family history of neurosis?

• Have there been major events or difficulties in your life recently?

• Have you ever been in a major accident or trauma? If so, how has it affected you?

### Notes

• Many people have had neurotic symptoms for years before seeking help. If similar symptoms have been present since adolescence, consider personality disorder.

• Whilst all neuroses are made worse by stress, sometimes the symptoms are best understood as a response to a major stress or life change—a *stress-related disorder*. If the stress was within the past few days, then consider an *acute stress reaction*. If the stressor was weeks or months ago, the category is *adjustment reaction*. *Post-traumatic stress disorder* (*PTSD*) is a form of stress-related disorder in which a *significant* event (e.g. rape, serious accident) is followed by reliving of the trauma in flashbacks or nightmares, and avoidance of similar situations.

• People turn to alcohol and other maladaptive strategies (e.g. avoidance) to cope with anxiety and other neurotic symptoms—these responses may exacerbate the situation and should be dealt with as part of the treatment.

• The presence of dysfunction is one criterion used in diagnosing neurosis, so assess the symptoms' effects—for example, on relationships and work performance.

• There is a modest genetic contribution to neurosis, and there may also be relevant learned behaviours from neurotic relatives.

## Assessment of somatic symptoms and somatoform disorders

Somatic symptoms and concerns about health can of course be a presentation of a medical condition and should be assessed accordingly. They may also occur in any psychiatric disorder, particularly neuroses. *Somatoform disorders* really apply to patients where the somatic symptoms are most prominent, and none of these other categories seems applicable (Chapters 10 and 18).

---

### Key questions addressed by the somatic symptoms and somatoform disorders module

• *Are the patient's somatic symptoms medically unexplained?*

• *If so, is the diagnosis somatoform disorder, or are the symptoms part of another neurosis or depressive disorder?*

• *If the diagnosis is somatoform disorder, what type is it?* Somatoform disorders can manifest predominantly with somatic symptoms, or predominantly with concerns about health or appearance.

### Triggering the module

Examples of triggers include:

• Detection of somatic symptoms that appear unexplained by a medical condition in the core assessment.

• Preoccupation with health or disease.

• Repeated and excessive seeking of medical assessment or treatment.

### Related modules

Because somatic symptoms can occur in many disorders, any other module may be needed, especially those covering *neurosis*, *depression* and *eating disorder*s.

---

## The somatoform disorders module

### Appearance and behaviour

Does the patient emphasize somatic complaints?

Are they bothered by chronic unexplained pain? Do they take regular painkillers?

Are they unduly preoccupied with their health?

Do they have evidence of many previous operations?

Do they hide aspects of their body or appearance?

Are they repeatedly seeking reassurance from you that they do not have disease?

Is there evidence that they have deliberately made themselves ill (e.g. by picking open a wound or omitting their insulin)?

## Notes

● In somatoform disorders the patient emphasizes somatic symptoms and downplays psychological ones, and often seeks tests and treatments that are not medically indicated.

● Chronic pain is a common form of somatoform disorder. It can be difficult to manage and may lead to harm from long-term analgesic use.

● Patients with chronic *somatization disorder* may have had many unnecessary operations.

● Repeated reassurance seeking about disease suggests *hypochondriasis*.

● Patients with *body dysmorphic disorder* (*dysmorphophobia*) may seek to hide aspects of their appearance because they perceive themselves as ugly.

● Rarely, patients deliberately make themselves ill (or apparently so) to justify medical care—called *factitious disorder*, or in order to gain some advantage (e.g. money)—*malingering*.

## Mood

Is there evidence of depressed or anxious mood?

## Notes

● Depressed mood or anxiety are often apparent or suspected, but may be denied by the patient. If you conclude either is present and significant, then the somatic symptoms will usually be viewed as symptoms of a depressive or anxiety disorder, and treated as such.

## Sleep, appetite and other bodily function

● How is your health?

● Do you have many aches and pains, or other bodily symptoms?

● Do you have medical problems your doctor(s) can't explain?

## Notes

● Patients with somatoform disorder typically perceive their health as poor even when it is objectively good.

● Many bodily concerns and symptoms may be reported. The more somatic symptoms they have the less likely they are to have a medical condition. Many chronic symptoms suggest somatization disorder.

## Thoughts—content

● What do you think causes your symptoms?

● Are your fearful that you have a particular medical condition?

● What do you think about your appearance?

● What do you think should be done about your symptoms?

## Notes

● Patients may have unlikely theories about what causes their symptoms, but these should not be delusional—if so, the patient has a psychosis of some kind.

● A strong fear of a medical condition is typical of *hypochondriasis*.

● Preoccupation with appearance suggests *body dysmorphic disorder*.

● The patient with a somatoform disorder will often want extensive investigation, and may not be reassured by negative results.

## Other components of the module

What is the nature and quantity of the medical history?

Will the patient cooperate with a psychiatric assessment?

What does the patient want done?

## Notes

● A frequent medical attender and 'thick notes' suggest a chronic somatization disorder.

● Many patients want medical not psychiatric treatment. They may minimize distress to lessen the probability of a psychiatric diagnosis. The assessment usually proceeds more smoothly if you pay due attention to and make it clear that you accept their somatic symptoms before asking about psychological ones.

● Patients do not necessarily want treatment. Some want validation that they are ill; others want you to complete insurance claims. Others may want treatment that you consider inappropriate (e.g. a further surgical referral) and decline treatment you do recommend (e.g. psychological therapy). The potential for conflict can be reduced if you ask what they want, without necessarily acquiescing to it.

## Assessment of eating disorders

### Key questions addressed by the eating disorders module

- *Does the patient have an eating disorder?* The core feature is an overevaluation of shape and weight. The disorders must be distinguished from problems of weight, shape or diet occurring in other psychiatric disorders or secondary to a medical disorder.
- *If so, is the diagnosis anorexia nervosa or bulimia nervosa?* The former is characterized by low body weight, the latter by repeated binges which punctuate the dietary restriction. However, many patients with an eating disorder do not fit into either of these classic categories, or shift between them.

When using the module, note that:

- People with eating disorders can be difficult to engage and tend to minimize their problems, so take the opportunity (and the time) to form a good relationship, and plan to corroborate the history.
- Physical complications of anorexia nervosa are serious and can be life threatening.
- The disorders do occur in men.

### Triggering the module

The eating disorder module may be triggered by:

- A patient saying she has problems controlling her eating.
- Medically unexplained weight loss.
- A teenage girl with fatigue or amenorrhoea.
- A patient who looks thin or is wearing several layers of clothes on a hot day.

### Related modules

The *depression* and *neurosis* modules will invariably be necessary given the overlap between these conditions. Risk assessment is important since deliberate and accidental self-harm can occur.

## The eating disorder module

### Eating, bingeing and weight

Ask about diet:

- Describe a typical day's food intake.
- Are you on a diet? If so, what sort? How strict?

Ask about binges:

- Do you ever feel out of control and eat a large amount of food rapidly ('binge')?

- If so, what do you eat in a binge? Afterwards, how do you feel? What do you do?

Ask about weight:

- What is your current weight? How often do you weigh yourself?
- Have you ever been very overweight or underweight?

### Notes

- A description of a typical day's intake is an informative way of discovering the patient's eating patterns and the quantity and type of food being consumed. But, as with alcohol histories, interpret with caution.
- Dieting in someone who is not overweight raises suspicion of an eating disorder.
- A person's response to being asked about their diet or current weight can itself give clues.
- A past history of obesity and dieting is common.
- Bingeing followed by induced vomiting is the main feature of bulimia nervosa.

### Attitude to weight and shape

- Do you think you are fat? How much would you like to weigh?
- How do you feel about your body? How would you like it to be?
- Do other people say you're too thin? Do you believe them?

### Notes

- *Preoccupation with weight and diet* and *distortion of body image* are key diagnostic features, so explore fully her views on the subject. The woman may be convinced that she is overweight despite being demonstrably underweight. These beliefs are overvalued ideas (p. 12).
- A low body weight is seen as an accomplishment not a problem to a person with anorexia nervosa. Asking how the person would feel if she weighed a normal amount [a body mass index (BMI) of 18 or more; see below] can be useful.

### Physical symptoms of weight loss

Ask about menstrual history (check if taking oral contraceptive pill):

- Are your periods regular?
- When was your last period?
- When did your periods begin?
- Have you been more tired or weaker than usual?

## Notes

● Amenorrhoea (or scanty, irregular periods) is a feature of anorexia nervosa. If the disorder began in her early teens, menarche may never have occurred.

● Fatigue, lethargy and weakness are consequences of starvation and should alert the doctor to the need for physical examination and investigation.

## Additional methods of weight control

Has the patient tried other ways of losing (or maintaining) weight?

● What exercise do you do? How often?

● Do you use laxatives, diuretics or slimming pills, or drink large amounts of coffee?

## Notes

● Misuse of diuretics increases the risk of hypokalaemia, which is one of the causes of death in eating disorders.

## Physical examination

Weigh the patient and measure them. Calculate the BMI.

Examine the mouth and hands. Are there calluses? Poor state of teeth?

Check the cardiovascular system.

Note secondary sexual characteristics.

Is there lanugo hair?

Are there scars suggestive of self-cutting?

## Notes

● Patients may wear very baggy clothes, or ensure they have a full bladder, to give a misleading impression of their weight. Weigh them in their underwear (in the presence of a chaperone if necessary).

● The *BMI* is weight (kg)/[height (m)]$^2$. BMI should be 18–25. In anorexia nervosa, the BMI is below 17.5—sometimes well below.

● Always examine the *cardiovascular* system. Arrhythmias occur due to hypokalaemia. *Bradycardia* and *peripheral oedema* are common in anorexia.

● There are various signs in the skin, mouth and teeth of people with an eating disorder (Chapter 11). Lanugo is fine downy hair on the arms, back and face in anorexia nervosa.

● Self-cutting occurs in a some people with an eating disorder, especially those with bulimia nervosa.

## Other components of the module

Obtain a history of the development of the eating disorder.

Ask about past medical and psychiatric history.

Ask about personality.

Ask about academic and other achievements and intentions.

Corroborate history from an informant.

Perform relevant investigations.

## Notes

● People with eating disorder often minimize their problems. Always try and confirm the history about dieting, bingeing, etc.

● The medical differential diagnosis of eating disorder includes inflammatory bowel disease, hypopituitarism and neoplasms. Each is rare, but important.

● The psychiatric differential diagnosis includes depression and body dysmorphic disorder.

● Eating disorders are more common than expected in people with diabetes mellitus.

● Investigations may be needed to rule out other causes of anorexia and weight loss and to check for *complications* of weight loss (Chapter 11).

● Perfectionism is a common personality trait in eating disorder, especially anorexia nervosa.

● Personal risk factors include ballet dancing, modelling and participation in other activities where thinness and fitness are valued.

## Assessment of substance misuse

Use of alcohol and illicit drugs is common. Substance misuse can be a diagnosis and a problem in its own right, as well as contributing to the cause and persistence of many other psychiatric disorders.

● Note that you cannot psychiatrically assess (nor detain) someone who is intoxicated by alcohol or other drugs. Though you may be pressured to do so (e.g. by nursing staff in the emergency department), it must be deferred till the person is sober.

---

**Key questions addressed by the substance misuse module**

• *Which substance(s) are misused and in what way?* This includes establishing the duration, quantity and pattern of use.
• *Is the person dependent on the drug?* Physical dependence on alcohol, opioids and some other drugs is the most serious form of misuse.
• *What are the complications of the misuse?* Substance misuse produces diverse medical, psychiatric and social harms.

**Triggering the module**

Examples of triggers for this module include:
• Identification of significant alcohol intake in the core assessment.
• Insomnia in a stressed and depressed executive.
• Acute psychotic symptoms in a young person.
• Unexplained recurrent episodes of irritability or low mood.
• Perinasal inflammation or needle marks.

**Related modules**

The module will be used particularly in association with the *psychosis*, *mood* and *cognitive function* modules, given the diagnoses that arise from or coexist with substance misuse. *Risk assessment* is also necessary as substance users have high rates of deliberate and accidental self-harm.

---

## The substance misuse module

*The questions below refer to alcohol; modify for other substances as required.*

## The quantity and the pattern of consumption

• How much do you drink in the average week? What do you drink?
• Do you sometimes drink much more than that?
• Do you drink every day?
  Ask the patient to describe a typical day.
  Ask about how long the current pattern has been present.

### Notes

• Self-reports of consumption are underestimates (by half, as an unproven rule of thumb). The description of a typical day can be more revealing and accurate. Also ask about the associated behaviours and feelings.
• Check the type of beer drunk—the alcohol content varies considerably.
• Some people misuse alcohol in a steady fashion, others do so intermittently.
• Regular drinking that began in early adolescence is common amongst alcohol misusers.
• Use the AUDIT screening questionnaire (Box 3.1). It takes about 2 minutes. Note that the FAST questions asked in the core assessment (Chapter 2) are modified and extracted from the AUDIT.

## Dependence and withdrawal

• Do you have to drink more than you used to in order to get the same effect?
• Have you ever got into trouble due to your drinking?
• Have you tried to cut down the amount you drink? What happened?
• Do feel that you have lost control over your drinking?
• Do you drink more than you intend to?
• Do you ever have a drink in the morning to get you going?
  Ask the patient to rate the importance of drinking compared with other activities.
  Identify if the patient continues to drink despite awareness that it is harmful.

### Notes

• *Dependence* describes a cluster of physiological, behavioural and cognitive features arising from sustained use of alcohol, opioids, amphetamines and some other drugs (Chapter 14). Its features include: a *compulsion* to take the substance, *tolerance* (the need for increasing doses of the substance to achieve the same subjective effect) and *withdrawal*. Dependence is associated with serious medical and psychiatric complications.
• Withdrawal symptoms are a physiological reaction to lack of the dependent substance. They can arise from some prescribed drugs, including benzodiazepines and some antidepressants.
• The features of alcohol withdrawal include tremor, retching, sweating and muscle cramps. If severe, it is called *delirium tremens*.

---

**Box 3.1 Alcohol Use Disorders Identification Test (AUDIT)**

1. *How often do you have a drink containing alcohol?*
   (0) never. (1) monthly or less. (2) 2–4 times a month. (3) 2–3 times a week. (4) 4 or more times a week.

2. *How many drinks containing alcohol do you have on a typical day when you are drinking?*
   (0) 1 or 2. (1) 3 or 4. (2) 5 or 6. (3) 7–9. (4) 10 or more.

3. *How often do you have six or more drinks on one occasion?*
   (0) never. (1) less than monthly. (2) monthly. (3) weekly. (4) daily or almost daily.

4. *How often during the past year have you found that you were not able to stop drinking once you had started?*
   (0) never. (1) less than monthly. (2) monthly. (3) weekly. (4) daily or almost daily.

5. *How often during the past year have you failed to do what was normally expected of you because of drinking?*
   (0) never. (1) less than monthly. (2) monthly. (3) weekly. (4) daily or almost daily.

6. *How often during the past year have you needed a first drink in the morning to get yourself going after a heavy drinking session?*
   (0) never. (1) less than monthly. (2) monthly. (3) weekly. (4) daily or almost daily.

7. *How often during the past year have you had a feeling of guilt or remorse after drinking?*
   (0) never. (1) less than monthly. (2) monthly. (3) weekly. (4) daily or almost daily.

8. *How often during the past year have you been unable to remember what happened the night before because you had been drinking?*
   (0) never. (1) less than monthly. (2) monthly. (3) weekly. (4) daily or almost daily.

9. *Have you or has someone else been injured as a result of your drinking?*
   (0) no. (2) yes, but not in the past year. (4) yes, during the last year.

10. *Has a relative, friend, doctor or other health worker been concerned about your drinking or suggested that you cut down?*
    (0) no. (2) yes, but not in the past year. (4) yes, during the last year.

AUDIT scoring and interpretation: numbers in parentheses are scores for each question, so maximum score is 40.
- 8 or more indicates a strong likelihood of hazardous or harmful alcohol consumption.
- 20 or more suggests dependence.

---

## Associated psychosocial problems

Ask whether drinking has caused any psychological or social problems.
- Have you got into financial problems due to your drinking?
- Have you ever missed work or lost a job due to your drinking?
- Has drinking interfered with your relationships?
- Have you ever been in trouble with the police (e.g. drink driving) due to your drinking?

### Notes

● This section is a really an example of an extended *contextual history* (Chapter 2). It is necessary because substance misuse leads to many psychosocial problems.

## Psychiatric and medical complications

- Has drinking affected your physical health? For example, jaundice, shakes, hepatitis?
- Have you ever had blackouts while drinking?
  Ask about the patient's medical and psychiatric history.

### Notes

● Misuse of alcohol and other substances leads to a range of psychiatric and medical disorders, the characteristics of which depend on the substance being misused.
● Psychiatric disorders associated with alcohol misuse include depression, psychosis, delirium and dementia, as well as suicide and sexual dysfunction. Use screening questions from core assessment and then other relevant modules to investigate these areas.

## Physical examination

Examine the patient for the stigmata of alcohol dependence (Chapter 14).

### Notes

- A physical examination, focusing on liver disease and neurological signs, is essential with alcohol misuse because of its many effects on the body.
- Many medical disorders result from unsuspected alcohol misuse.
- Opioid use produces its own physical signs.

## Investigations

Many may be indicated—for example, breath or blood alcohol, full blood count (FBC), liver function tests (LFTs), urine or hair analyses.

### Notes

- Medical problems of alcohol misuse, suspected from the history or physical examination, may need investigation and liaison with the GP or a physician.
- The mean corpuscular volume (MCV) and hepatic $\gamma$-glutamyl transpeptidase (GGT) are raised in 60–70% patients with alcohol misuse. If other causes of their elevation are excluded, they are useful markers of alcohol misuse and for monitoring progress.
- Testing for hepatitis B and C, and human immunodeficiency virus (HIV), should be considered in intravenous users.
- Urine screens pick up some drugs or their metabolites, for varying lengths of time after use. Hair analyses are more sensitive (and cover a longer time frame) but are not widely available.

## Use of other substances

The same kinds of question should be repeated for each class of misused drug.

### Notes

- Many people who misuse one drug misuse at least one other.
- Use similar questions to those used for alcohol to establish the drugs used, the pattern of use and the associated problems.
- Ask about the route of administration.
- Patients may need reassurance about confidentiality when discussing drug use.

- Not all misused drugs are illegal—for example, analgesics.

## Assessment of the unresponsive patient

By unresponsive, we mean a person who does not participate in the assessment, not one who is unconscious. Such people may be seen in a psychiatric clinic or ward, or a psychiatric consult is requested in a general hospital or other medical setting.

---

**Key questions addressed by the unresponsive patient module**

- *Why is the person unresponsive?* Lack of cooperation with the assessment, due to inability or unwillingness, is uncommon but causes obvious problems. The main diagnostic questions are:
  - *Is there clouding of consciousness?* If so, consider delirium, stupor and their various causes.
  - *If not, is there evidence of psychosis, severe mood disorder or dissociative disorder?* These disorders can all present with unresponsiveness.
  - *Is the person intentionally uncooperative?* This may be a sign of malingering or simply a belief that they are better off keeping quiet.

Note that:
- Because the module is for use when communication is limited, it focuses on appearance, behaviour and physical examination.
- Unresponsive patients can be aggressive, and any physical examination will be without their consent. So, ensure the environment is safe and be accompanied—you may need a witness to confirm what took place.

**Triggering the module**

By definition, the module will be triggered when a patient does not cooperate (fully) with the assessment. For example:
- A patient found standing rigidly in the street staring at the sky.
- A patient who sits there but does not speak.
- An aggressive patient who does not reply to any questions and demands to leave.

**Related modules**

Complete the assessment when the patient becomes responsive. The *cognitive function* and *psychosis* modules will almost certainly be needed.

---

## The unresponsive patient module

### Background information

Is there an informant? Get as many details as possible, covering:

- Onset, course and duration of current episode.
- Past medical and psychiatric history.
- Medication, drug and alcohol history.

Check person's pockets and possessions for other clues.

Check hospital and GP records in case there is a past history.

### Notes

- Your problems are largely solved by a good informant or past records. For example, the patient may be known to have catatonic schizophrenia, a recent head injury, or be wanted by the police.

### Level of consciousness

Is the patient responsive to her surroundings?

Ask her to nod or open her eyes.

Does she move? Do her eyes follow a moving object? Is she paying attention to what's going on?

### Notes

- Establishing if there is clouding of consciousness is crucial since it indicates delirium and the need for urgent medical treatment.
- *Stupor* describes a condition in which the patient does not speak, move or respond, but appears fully conscious. Amongst psychiatric in-patients, stupor is caused mainly by catatonic schizophrenia, severe depression, organic disorders such as drug-induced states, akinetic mutism, and by dissociative disorder. In other populations (e.g. neurology wards) the proportions—and even the meaning of the word stupor—are different.

### Facial expression and communication

Does her expression change?

Does she seem fearful, depressed, preoccupied or hostile?

Does she speak spontaneously or in response to questions?

Can she communicate in other ways—for example, by writing or hand signals?

### Notes

- Facial expression and behavioural responses give diagnostic clues. For example, the characteristic appearance of a severely depressed patient; perplexity and fear in someone with psychosis or delirium; the focused hostility of someone with a personality disorder who does not want to be interviewed.
- In *elective mutism*, usually seen in children, the unresponsiveness is limited to speaking—other forms of communication are intact.

### Motor system

Is posture abnormal? Is it awkward or bizarre?

Is muscle tone normal? Is there resistance when you try and make a movement?

Is there spontaneous movement?

Are there stereotyped movements or mannerisms?

### Notes

- These questions are aimed mainly at detecting *catatonia* (see psychosis module), which usually occurs in catatonic schizophrenia but is also caused by some rare neurological syndromes.
- Increased muscle tone, decreased consciousness and hyperthermia suggest neuroleptic malignant syndrome (Chapter 7).
- Surreptitious observation may reveal that the patient behaves differently when unaware she is being observed—indicating feigned unresponsiveness.

### Other components of the module

What is the patient's attitude to being examined?

Do a neurological examination in addition to aspects mentioned above—include cranial nerves, reflexes.

Do a general physical examination—for signs of recent hygiene, trauma, intoxication, etc.

### Notes

- Examine the neurological system in as much detail as possible. Consider asking for an urgent neurological or general medical consultation if no clear psychiatric cause for the unresponsiveness is found.

**Key points**

- Each module allows the suspicion of a psychiatric disorder, raised by the core assessment (Chapter 2), to be confirmed, or dispelled. It also fleshes out the relevant contextual information to help explain the causes and correlates of the disorder.
- There are modules for cognitive impairment, psychosis, depression, mania, neurosis, somatoform disorders, eating disorder, substance misuse and the unresponsive patient.
- A given patient may need one or several modules in the assessment.
- As you become more competent at interviewing, and more knowledgeable about the disorders, the core and module approach will become more intuitive, more effective and quicker to complete.

# Chapter 4

# Risk: harm, self-harm and suicide

## Risk in psychiatry

In psychiatry, *risk* refers to the probability that an adverse event such as self-harm, suicide or harm to others will occur. Public and professional concern about such events makes *risk assessment* and *risk management* an important part of psychiatric practice. A brief evaluation of risk, especially of suicide, is always part of the core assessment, but often a more detailed risk assessment is required. For example, in someone with:

- Current suicidal intent.
- A history of mood disorder, psychosis or substance abuse.
- A history of self-harm or violence to others.

This chapter covers the assessment and management of risk in general, and self-harm and danger to others in particular.

- Harmful outcomes can never be eliminated. However, competent risk assessment and management can decrease their likelihood.

## Risk assessment

When assessing the risk of harm to self or others, look for features associated with an increased risk. Try and gather the information from different sources—patient, informants, medical records, social services, police, etc.

In the *history*:
- Previous harm to self or others—the past is the best predictor of the future.
- Recent actions suggestive of impending harm (e.g. buying a hosepipe, making a will).
- Recent major stresses or losses.
- Depressive disorder, psychosis, substance abuse or personality disorder.

In the *mental state*:
- Suicidal or violent thoughts.
- Significant mood disturbance.
- Psychotic symptoms, especially passivity.

In the *context*:
- Demographic factors (Table 4.1).
- Abuse of drugs or alcohol.
- Social restlessness or *anomie*—for example, few relationships, frequent changes of address.
- Easy access to potential weapons or victims.

## Formulation of risk

After completing the risk assessment, document the findings:
- What potential harmful outcome, if any, has been identified?
- What is your estimate of its probability?
- How immediate and long lasting is the risk?
- What factors may increase or decrease the risk?
- What can be done to reduce the risk?

*Lecture Notes: Psychiatry*, 10e. By Paul Harrison, John Geddes and Michael Sharpe. Published 2010 by Blackwell Publishing Ltd.

**Table 4.1** Risk factors for suicide.

| Factor | Comment |
|---|---|
| *Demographic factors* | |
| Male | |
| Increasing age | Though the rate in young males has increased |
| Living alone | |
| Unemployed | |
| Recent life crisis | |
| Previous deliberate SH | Increases suicide rates 100-fold |
| Occupation | High rate in vets, doctors, nurses, pharmacists, farmers |
| *Illness-related factors* | |
| Chronic medical problems | |
| Psychiatric disorder | Present in 70% of suicide victims, usually depression |
| Depressive disorder | 15% suicide rate in severe depression |
| Schizophrenia | >10% commit suicide |
| Substance misuse | Especially alcohol and opioid dependence |
| Personality disorder | Higher suicide rate, especially borderline type |
| Being in psychiatric care | 75% of suicides have been in psychiatric treatment |
| In-patient | 5% of suicides |
| Recently discharged | |
| *Mental state factors* | |
| Depressed mood | |
| Expressed wish to be dead | |
| Detailed suicide plans | |
| Hopelessness | |
| Lack of reason to go on living | e.g. Bereavement |

*Mr J is referred for a psychiatric opinion because he has threatened to kill his wife and himself. He has convictions for bodily harm and theft. You find no evidence of depressive disorder, psychosis or violent thoughts. However, he admits to drinking heavily at weekends, whereupon he becomes threatening and low in mood. His wife and the police (with his permission) corroborate the history. Your preliminary conclusion is of an alcohol-related problem and possibly personality disorder. His risk of harm or self-harm is low when sober but quite high when intoxicated or stressed. This fluctuating pattern of risk will continue as long as his drinking problem does. Marital strife is the other factor increasing risk.*

## Risk management

Risk management aims to:
- Reduce the level of immediate risk.
- Maintain it at an acceptable level.

- Set up a process for reviewing the risk.

Risk management strategies can be divided into immediate and longer term interventions.

*Immediate interventions* may include:
- Psychiatric admission, if necessary under the Mental Health Act.
- Acute sedation.
- Ensuring adequate community support.
- Lowering of tension and the provision of reassurance as a result of the assessment.
- Making the family and significant others aware of the risk.
- Removing access to weapons.
- Notifying the police.

*Longer term interventions* include:
- Effectively treating associated psychiatric disorder.
- Implementing the care programme approach (Chapter 8).

- Alleviating social stresses.
- Enhancing positive coping strategies.

In all cases, ensure that:

- The management plan is documented and communicated to all others involved in managing the case (Chapter 5).
- A date is set for reviewing the case and the plan—this may be within hours for an acutely suicidal in-patient, or every year in a stable patient in the community.

> You discuss Mr J with your colleagues and draw up a risk management plan. A copy is also given to Mr J, his wife and GP. Mr J is given advice to help him cut down his drinking. The couple refer themselves to Relate to try and reduce conflicts between them. It is made clear to Mr J that he will be held responsible should he harm his wife. He agrees to record his alcohol intake and to return in 6 weeks.

## Suicide and self-harm

### Definitions

- *Self-harm (SH)* or *deliberate self-harm* is the umbrella term for self-inflicted non-fatal harm. Self-cutting is the most common form, though self-poisoning accounts for 90% of medical presentations of SH.
- *Attempted suicide* is a term that may be used where there was a definite attempt to take one's life, and *parasuicide* when the degree of suicidal intent associated with the act is not clear.
- *Suicide* is the taking of one's own life. Although suicide is clearly defined by death, establishing intent retrospectively is often difficult—some suicides were acts of SH in association with distress that went tragically wrong.

### Self-harm

SH is important because:

- *It is common.* There are about 150 000 presentations to general hospitals in the UK with SH each year. SH accounts for 10% of all acute medical admissions. It is the most common reason for acute admission of women and the second most common for men. A GP may expect five of his/her patients to commit acts of SH each year.
- *It is a risk factor for further acts of SH and for suicide.* About 20% present with further acts of SH, and 1–2% will commit suicide in the following year.
- *It can be the presenting feature of serious psychiatric disorder.* However, most patients seen because of SH have a mild depressive disorder, adjustment reaction, personality disorder or no psychiatric diagnosis. Substance misuse is common.

Motivations for SH are various and mixed. Only a minority have clear and sustained suicidal intent. Many acts are an impulsive response to what is perceived as an intolerable situation, or an attempt to influence the behaviour of others. SH often occurs under the influence of alcohol.

- SH can also represent a failed outcome of a determined attempt at suicide. Though rare, recognition of this small group is important.

### Suicide

Though not a common cause of death, suicide is the third biggest cause of lost years of life because it often affects young adults. People who commit suicide are often depressed, and perceive the future as both intolerable and hopeless. Occasionally, this perception may be shared by others (e.g. in cases of terminal cancer), but usually it is strongly biased by depressed mood. Suicides are usually planned. The risk factors for suicide are shown in Table 4.1.

- There is an increased risk of suicide in the weeks after discharge from a psychiatric hospital. This should be taken into account when planning management over this period.
- Suicide rates in young men increased in the UK in the 1980s and 1990s, before plateauing. The reason is unknown.
- In depressed patients, suicide may occur during the initial recovery phase—some people are so depressed that, until then, they lack the motivation to kill themselves despite a wish to be dead. Suicide risk assessments and interventions should not stop when improvement has begun.

## Assessment of suicide risk

Assessing suicide risk is part of the core psychiatric assessment. If present, a full assessment is then essential. This follows the general principles of risk assessment, taking into account the risk factors for suicide (Table 4.1). Particular attention is paid to:

- The person's expressed intent.
- Their mental state.
- Recent acts of SH.

*Never* omit to assess suicide risk because you think (a) it might precipitate suicide or (b) someone really planning to kill himself will deny it. Neither is true—the evidence is that recognition and active management may prevent suicide. Many people who kill themselves have been in contact with a doctor in the days before the fatal act.

## Assessment following SH

All patients who have self-harmed should be psychiatrically assessed, even if only briefly, to determine their risk of a repeat attempt and to identify the presence of a significant psychiatric disorder. Certain characteristics of the act of SH predict a higher suicidal intent, and a higher risk of subsequent suicide:

- The attempt was planned.
- Affairs were put in order beforehand.
- The person took precautions to avoid discovery.
- They did not seek help afterwards.
- They used a method that they believed to be dangerous.
- They left a suicide note.

## Management after SH

### General management

The number of patients seen because of an act of SH is large, and their management presents a challenge to medical and psychiatric services, especially if these are not well integrated (Chapter 18).

- For most cases, no specialist care is indicated, and the patient is discharged to their GP. It is therefore important to ensure the GP receives clear and prompt communication about the outcome of the assessment (Chapter 5).

> *Ms S was seen in A&E having taken 20 paracetamol tablets earlier that night. She had been drinking and had taken them after a row with her boyfriend. She had not planned to kill herself and now felt foolish about her behaviour. She was unaware that paracetamol could be lethal. She was offered an appointment for out-patient counselling but declined, preferring to see her GP.*

- A minority of patients are found to be at acute risk of suicide and require immediate and intensive management. The priority is to keep the person safe. This may be achieved by psychiatric admission, sometimes under the Mental Health Act. Serious suicidal intent is sufficient grounds for admission under the Act, even if the presence of a psychiatric disorder has yet to be established. If admission is not used, it is important to ensure that relatives are aware of the severity of the situation and know how to contact services urgently if necessary.

> *Mr P was found in his fume-filled car in an isolated field. After being resuscitated he expressed anger at being saved and said that he still wanted to die. He was found to be suffering from psychotic depression and had previously taken a serious overdose. He was admitted to hospital under the Mental Health Act and treated with ECT.*

- Recognizing and treating depression effectively is a priority, given the importance of depression as a factor in suicide—though there is little evidence that doing so does decrease suicide rates.
- Many SH patients have personal, relationship or social problems for which they may be offered help—for example, by counselling or problem-solving therapy, or by referral to community mental health psychology services.

## Management of patients who repeatedly self-harm

A small number of people, mostly young women, present repeatedly with SH by overdosing or wrist

**Table 4.2** Prevention of suicide.

*Individual interventions*
Better detection and management of:
    suicidal intent in patients attending medical services
    depressive disorder
    substance misuse

*Population interventions*
Public education and discussion
Education of doctors and others (e.g. teachers)
Easy, rapid access to psychiatric care or support
    groups (e.g. Samaritans)
Make it harder to commit suicide, e.g. by:
    limiting access to paracetamol—smaller bottles,
      blister packs
    withdrawal of the analgesic coproxamol—especially
      dangerous in overdose
    make it harder to fix a hose over exhaust pipes
    safety nets around high buildings and bridges
Decreasing societal stressors—unemployment,
    domestic violence, etc.
Decreasing substance misuse

cutting. A diagnosis of personality disorder (dramatic cluster; Table 15.1) is often made, and a history of childhood sexual abuse or other trauma may emerge. Management includes:

• Providing psychological support which is not contingent on acts of SH.

• Checking for emergent depressive disorder.

## Suicide as a public health problem

Prevention of suicide in the population has been a priority for health policy, but it is difficult to achieve, in part because social and political factors, and not just medical ones, are important (Table 4.2).

## Risks to others

Despite the public perception, psychiatric patients are more likely to be recipients than perpetrators of violence, and the vast majority of aggressive acts are committed by people in the absence of a psychiatric disorder. Nevertheless, knowing when and how to assess and manage potential harm to others is an important aspect of psychiatric practice.

• In response to public concerns, the UK government proposed the category of *dangerous and severe personality disorder* (Chapter 15).

## Assessment of risk to others

The psychiatric disorders most associated with increased risk of violence are substance abuse, schizophrenia and mania, as well as some personality disorders. These disorders act cumulatively—so the risk is greater in a person with more than one of these diagnoses.

• Harmful acts are occasionally *directly* due to the disorder. For example, passivity experiences in schizophrenia, or nihilistic delusions in psychotic depression, may lead to harm to others. More commonly, violence results *indirectly* from the same combination of frustrations and personality that determine such acts in anybody. The disorder merely decreases the threshold (and perhaps increases the chances that the aggressor is caught.)

• As with most behaviour, the strongest predictor of future violent behaviour is previous violent behaviour.

## Management of risk to others

After identifying a risk to others, the clinician should do all they reasonably can to prevent the harmful outcome.

• Check access to weapons and whether there are specific plans or identified victims.

• Warn a potential target—the risk to others can over-ride patient confidentiality—for example, in cases of *morbid jealousy* (pp. 140–1).

• Discuss the risk with a forensic psychiatrist.

• If there is known or suspected psychiatric disorder, consider admission, if necessary to a secure unit.

• Conversely, if psychiatric assessment reveals no evidence of psychiatric disorder, this conclusion should be clearly recorded.

## Key points

- Risk in psychiatry refers to the risk of self-harm, and the risk of harm by the patient to others.
- Assessment of suicide risk should be included in every psychiatric assessment.
- Detection of risk should lead to active management of the risk.
- Deliberate SH is very common. All patients who have recently self-harmed should be screened for suicidal risk and for psychiatric disorder.
- The majority of people committing suicide have depressive disorder or other chronic psychiatric disorder. However suicide also occurs in people with no known psychiatric history, especially in young men.
- Most psychiatric patients are not violent. Most violence is not committed by psychiatric patients.
- Substance misuse, personality disorder, schizophrenia and mania are all associated with increased risk of harm to others, especially if they coexist.

# Chapter 5

# Completing and communicating the assessment

## Completing the assessment

The process of psychiatric assessment described in Chapters 2–4 provides diagnostic information and an understanding of the patient in context. These facts are now combined to allow you to:

- Make a (differential) diagnosis [using ICD-10 terms (Appendix 1)].
- Identify factors which have contributed to the disorder.
- Plan your initial management, and think about the longer term management.
- Think about the prognosis.
- Summarize and present the case, in a variety of formats.

This chapter covers these areas in turn. An overview of the process is given in Figure 5.1.

- Remember that making a psychiatric diagnosis is not a neutral act—it has drawbacks (e.g. stigmatization) as well as benefits (e.g. effective treatment).

## The diagnostic process

Assuming the core and module approach has worked, you will have eliminated most possible diagnoses for your patient. Sometimes, one overwhelmingly likely diagnosis will remain, but usually there is a differential diagnosis that requires further investigation. Either way, draw up a list of the key features in favour of, and against, each plausible diagnostic possibility.

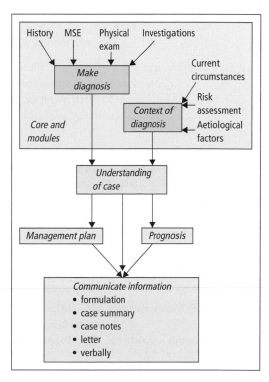

**Figure 5.1** Psychiatric assessment and communication of information.

*Lecture Notes: Psychiatry*, 10e. By Paul Harrison, John Geddes and Michael Sharpe. Published 2010 by Blackwell Publishing Ltd.

- Weighing the diagnostic evidence helps clarify your own thoughts about the case. It is also useful to others who may refer back to your assessment—for example, if there is a subsequent review of the diagnosis.
- Throughout the chapter, a single vignette will be used, to show how different aspects of a case are highlighted depending on the stage in the diagnostic process and the clinical situation.

*Mr K, 55, was referred after a suicide attempt. You have elicited many depressive symptoms, some anxiety symptoms and an alcohol intake of 40 units/week. There are no features suggestive of psychosis or personality disorder, nor of imminent suicide risk. Your provisional diagnosis is a depressive disorder (moderate severity), plus alcohol misuse.*

It is now time to add in the contextual information collected during the core and modules, particularly those factors that appear to help explain the origins and evolution of the disorder.

## The context and cause of the case

When considering causative factors in psychiatry, the two key variables are:
- The *type* of factor—usually divided into biological, psychological and social.
- The *time* at which the factor operates. A useful mnemonic for this is 'the three Ps': predisposing, precipitating and perpetuating.
- Usually all three types of factor, and all three time points, are relevant.

## Types of causes: biological, psychological and social

The development of psychiatric disorders is influenced by biological (genetic and environmental), psychological and social factors (Chapter 6). Sometimes one predominates, sometimes another, but all three always contribute something. Hence the *biopsychosocial model* of psychiatry, which requires that due attention is paid to all three areas and which encourages an equally eclectic approach to treatment.

**Table 5.1** Biological, psychological and social factors for Mr K.

*Biological*
Genetic predisposition
Cerebrovascular disease
Alcohol misuse

*Psychological*
Stress of being gay (a secret?)
Recent breakdown in a serious relationship
Guilt about recent sexual liaisons

*Social*
Social isolation (has his stroke stopped him driving?)
Unemployment affecting his self-esteem or causing financial worries

- The biopsychosocial model should seem obvious and essential. However, psychiatry has at times been guilty of focusing too closely on one or other of its components. This has led to mindless psychiatrists (who see only the molecules) and brainless psychiatrists (who see only minds and the social issues). We hope we are neither, but we could be both.

*Mr K was made redundant 6 months ago. He is gay and his long-term partner left him around the same time, after which he had several casual sexual encounters. He has no close friends or relatives. Mr K had a stroke 2 years ago which left him with a mild hemiparesis. He has had two past depressive episodes. His father committed suicide when Mr K was 5.*

Applying the biopsychosocial approach to Mr K, several causative factors can be proposed, based on evidence from what is known about the origins of mood disorder (Chapters 6 and 9). Not all factors may be relevant, and some may be not be 'provable' facts, but all merit consideration (Table 5.1).

## Timing of causes: predisposing, precipitating and perpetuating

In terms of timing, causal factors can be:
- *Predisposing:* factors which exert a long-term or distant causal effect, such as family history and early childhood experiences.

- *Precipitating:* factors which explain why the disorder has occurred now. They include recent life events, injuries and new medical conditions, and discontinuation of medication.
- *Perpetuating (or maintaining):* factors affecting the course of a disorder. Ongoing marital and social problems and non-adherence with treatment are two common ones. The nature of the disorder itself is also relevant—for example, Alzheimer's disease requires no external perpetuating factors.

Table 5.2 summarizes the causative factors for Mr K according to the three Ps.

- Note that the same factor (in this case alcohol) can be involved in all three aspects of aetiology.
- In practice, a useful tip is to combine the 'type' and 'timing' approaches to causative factors in a $3 \times 3$ box. This provides a template that can be filled in as details of the case emerge.

Having hypothesized the causal factors, try and substantiate them. For example, in this case:

- Examine for neurological deficits.
- Find out more about his alcohol misuse.
- Discover his views on his sexuality.
- Consider an HIV test.
- Investigate how he feels about the redundancy, and its financial consequences.

**Table 5.2** Predisposing, precipitating and perpetuating factors for Mr K.

*Predisposing*
    Genetic predisposition
    Psychological effects of father's suicide
    Guilt about his sexuality
    Alcohol misuse
    Stroke
    Past history of depression

*Precipitating*
    Ending of long-term relationship
    Increased alcohol intake
    Being made redundant

*Perpetuating*
    Social isolation
    Stressors continue
    Excess alcohol intake

- Get hold of his case notes and review his past history.

*You find that Mr K has only minimal physical impairment, but does have mild hypertension and a carotid bruit. He has misused alcohol intermittently for many years; the recent increase in consumption seems to have been a response to his low mood. His sexuality conflicts with his religious beliefs. He feels he was made redundant unfairly because he had taken sick leave, and has been left with serious financial problems. He is HIV negative. His notes reveal a similar clinical picture during previous depressive episodes, with a good response to antidepressants. In one episode, he also developed psychotic symptoms (delusions of guilt) and had a course of ECT. You conclude that he has a recurrent moderate to severe depressive disorder.*

Another way to clarify the role of causal factors and the interplay between them is to create a *life chart*. This is most useful when the history is long and complex, to show whether illness episodes, or recovery from them, are related to specific factors, and whether there is any pattern of treatment response. Table 5.3 shows a life chart for Mr K.

- A life chart can be time consuming to compile, but is usually worthwhile.

## The future context

Having: (a) made a diagnosis and (b) investigated the causative factors, it is time to consider the management and the prognosis—the *future context*. This will follow directly from your current understanding of the case, and both will need to be mentioned in the summary, letter or phone call which will follow the assessment.

## Management

Management in psychiatry involves making a number of decisions, several of which need to be made soon after the initial assessment. For example:

- *Is treatment indicated?* Some assessments produce no evidence of psychiatric disorder, and/or no indication for treatment—other than reassurance and a clear statement of your conclusions.

**Table 5.3** A life chart for Mr K.

| Age | Events | Psychiatric disorder | Treatments |
|---|---|---|---|
| 0 | Complicated delivery | | |
| 5 | Father commits suicide | | |
| 10 | Mother remarries | | |
| 17 | Turbulent home life | Depression, moderate | Amitriptyline 150 mg, 6 months |
| 20 | Joined navy; binge drinking | | |
| 25 | 'Came out'; left navy | | |
| 30 | Met current partner | | |
| 35 | Became storeman | Depression, severe | ECT × 6; fluoxetine 20 mg, 12 months |
| 40 | Mother dies | | |
| 45 | | Intermittent heavy drinking | Counselling |
| 50 | Hypertension | | β-Blocker started, use continues |
| 53 | Mild stroke | | Physiotherapy |
| 54 | Made redundant | | |
| 55 | Relationship ends | Current depressive episode | |

- *How urgent is the problem?* Acute psychosis and severe mood disorders generally need immediate treatment. Serious risk of self-harm or harm to others is a major determinant of urgency. Is the patient sufficiently ill or at risk to need compulsory treatment?
- *Where should treatment take place, and from whom?* Most psychiatric disorders are treated by GPs; some will be referred to psychiatrists; a very few need admission.
- *What management is indicated?* Treatment decisions depend primarily on the diagnosis. However, they are also affected by the context—another reason why contextual information was collected in the assessment. For example, is the patient motivated enough for a psychological treatment? Does his job mean that sedative antidepressants should be avoided? What drug did she respond to last time?

## Prognosis

Once you have a diagnosis and a reasonable understanding of the context, a provisional judgement about prognosis should be possible. Together with the diagnosis, it's the prognosis that is of most concern to the patient, their relatives and the referrer.

- *Short-term* prognosis depends mainly on the natural history of the disorder and, particularly, the treatment response. It is usually possible to give a rough estimate of the likelihood of improvement and its timing.
- *Long-term* prognosis is much more difficult to predict, and opinion on this issue may be deferred. It may be easier to estimate after an initial response to treatment has been observed. There are several non-specific factors which identify people at higher risk of a poor outcome:
  - Insidious onset.
  - Longer duration of disorder prior to treatment.
  - Comorbid personality disorder.
  - Comorbid substance misuse.
  - Lack of close relationships.
  - History of poor adherence to treatment.

## Summarizing and communicating cases

In the assessment process, you have generated and tested diagnostic hypotheses, collected contextual information and have considered the management and prognosis. If it is to be useful, the understanding of the case that you have obtained must be communicated effectively to others. These are the GP and other agencies, those who may use the information in the future and, last but not least, the patient. When planning this communication, ask yourself:

● *What does the recipient want and need to know?* This can vary from a detailed discharge summary for the psychiatric case notes, to a brief letter informing a GP that the dose of a drug has been changed. Avoid unnecessary information—it obscures the important bits. On the other hand, always include important negatives (e.g. 'He is not suicidal', 'She is not psychotic', 'Medication is not indicated'), and it is usually helpful to state the diagnosis and the current treatment in any letter. Similar rules apply to oral presentations.

● *What does the recipient know already?* If you are summarizing a person's tenth admission, information about the previous nine is likely to be available to and known by everyone, and may not need to be repeated. Conversely, a psychiatric court report should be written assuming that the recipient knows nothing about the person and nothing about psychiatry (or psychiatric terminology).

● *What does the patient need to know?* Informing the patient (and family) of the outcome of the assessment is the beginning of effective management. Patients are entitled to know what is written about them; indeed, as a rule, all correspondence will be copied to the patient. This has many potential benefits, but may be particularly challenging in psychiatry because of the nature of the patient's illness or the content of the letter (e.g. in an acute psychosis, or if there is a potential risk to others). In these (rare) circumstances, you may prefer to convey the information to others by phone.

Here we outline different types of communication—a formulation, a case summary, a problem list and a GP letter.

## Formulations

A formulation is a concise, informative way of summarizing a psychiatric assessment. It is also educational for the reader since it involves weighing up the evidence and showing how you came to your conclusions. The formulation consists of:

● *An opening statement*—patient's name, age, occupation, presenting complaint and *brief* summary of main findings.

● *The differential diagnosis*. Put the most likely diagnosis first. Include the factors for and against each diagnosis. Remember that more than one diagnosis may be justified (comorbidity).

● *The context and cause of the problem*. Summarize the causative factors and relevant context. This can be done in different ways, as outlined above.

● *The management plan*. This should be clear and indicate the role of each party in implementing it. Include investigations and immediate interventions.

● *Prognosis*. Short and longer term.

An example of a formulation, for Mr K after his admission, is shown in Box 5.1.

## Case summaries

A psychiatric case summary is equivalent in most respects to a medical one. It is useful:

● At the end of a psychiatric admission.
● On discharge from psychiatric care.
● When the patient is being transferred to other psychiatric services.

Suggested headings are shown in Table 5.4—they overlap with those of the core assessment.

## Problem lists

Once the background to a case is familiar, the emphasis usually switches to current problems and their solution. *Problem lists* ensure that the key issues are identified and dealt with. A problem list for Mr K is shown in Table 5.5.

## Letters between psychiatrists and GPs

Letters from psychiatrists to GPs should be as concise as possible. Remember you are usually offering the GP advice, not giving instructions. Also bear in mind that the GP will often know more than you about the person's history and circumstances. Take into account the purpose of the referral: was it for an opinion or for continuing care? Has the GP asked a specific question or

**Box 5.1 A psychiatric formulation for Mr K**

**Opening statement**

Mr K is a 55-year-old unemployed storeman, seen in clinic last week following an overdose and admitted voluntarily because of suicidal intent and many depressive symptoms. Relevant factors included recent redundancy, relationship break up and alcohol abuse.

**Differential diagnosis:**

1. *Depressive disorder.*
   - For: subjectively and objectively low mood, suicidal ideation, recent self-harm, poor sleep, loss of appetite, feelings of guilt and worthlessness; two prior depressive episodes.
   - Against: his depressive symptoms could be secondary to diagnoses 2–4.
2. *Anxiety disorder.*
   - For: worrying about his health, feeling tense, socially phobic and lies awake worrying.
   - Against: the depressive symptoms began first, and are clearly more prominent.
3. *Alcohol misuse.*
   - For: drinking 40 plus units/week; long history of harmful intake; describes withdrawal symptoms when in the navy (30 years ago).
   - Against: intake over past few years has averaged 25 units/week; recent increase post-dated onset of symptoms; normal LFTs and MCV.
4. *Organic mood disorder.*
   - For: stroke 2 years ago.
   - Against: first episode preceded the stroke; severity of stroke seems insufficient to explain his symptoms.

**Diagnosis:**

Recurrent depressive disorder, current episode severe.

**Context and cause:**

- *Predisposing:* father committed suicide when Mr K aged 5. Alcohol misuse. Guilt about his sexuality. Stroke 2 years ago. Two other depressive episodes (age 17, 35), one requiring ECT.
- *Precipitating:* partner left him 3 months ago after 25 years. Increased alcohol intake. Made redundant 6 months ago.
- *Perpetuating:* social isolation—no close friends or family. Feeling guilty about recent casual homosexual affairs. Continuing high alcohol intake. Financial worries.

**Management plan:**

1. Further investigations: repeat LFTs and HIV test (last done 10 years ago); get old notes; phone GP for background. Needs a medical opinion regarding hypertension and its treatment.
2. Monitor mental state daily. Continue nursing observations whilst actively suicidal.
3. Observe for signs of alcohol withdrawal.
4. Start antidepressant (specify drug and dose). Benzodiazepine if required for sleep or sedation.
5. As mental state settles, assess further the current stressors—employment, finance, sexuality.
6. Longer term will need continuing support—begin care programme approach assessment.

**Prognosis:**

His history predicts a good response to antidepressants. However, if stressors continue, recovery will be compromised and he will be vulnerable to relapse.

requested a particular intervention? Generally the GP is most interested in:

- The diagnosis.
- A specific management plan, including the date of review and what he or she is expected to do.
- What the patient/relative has been told, and whether they have been copied into the correspondence, as mentioned above.
- What the patient and GP should do if matters unexpectedly deteriorate (or improve).

**Table 5.4** Headings for a psychiatric case summary.

Demographic details
  Name, age, sex, occupation
  Dates: of referral, assessment, admission, discharge,
    Mental Health Act status
Presenting complaint(s)
  Nature, onset, progression, treatments to date
Mental state at presentation
Past psychiatric history
  Diagnoses, admissions, treatments
Personal history
  Childhood, academic and job record, relationships,
    children
  Premorbid personality
  Use of alcohol and drugs
Mental state examination
Risk assessment
Physical examination
Investigations
Differential diagnosis
Management and progress
  Current symptoms and problems
Prognosis

### Box 5.2 Psychiatric discharge letter to GP

*Dear Dr,*
*Re: Mr J.K., d.o.b 1.1.54, 24 Easy Street, Anytown*

***Diagnosis: recurrent depressive disorder, current episode severe***

#### Course and current situation

*Mr K has made a good recovery from his illness as detailed in the summary sent to you on his discharge from the ward 6 months ago, although as you know, he required augmentation with lithium for full recovery. At review in clinic today he was entirely free of symptoms.*

#### Management and prognosis

*Thank you for prescribing his medication (amitriptyline 150 mg nocte; lithium carbonate 800 mg nocte), which he has taken as prescribed. His lithium level should continue to be checked every 6 weeks and maintained at 0.5–0.8 mmol/l—it was stable at 0.72 mmol/l last week. He should continue on the medication for at least another 6 months. At that time he intends to stop it, but he is aware that his risk of relapse will be lower if he remains on amitriptyline. When he does decide to stop, it should be tailed off gradually, over several weeks.*

*Mr K is fully aware of the diagnosis and our formulation of its causes (especially the relationship break-up, and his alcohol intake). We have addressed these issues, and they appear largely resolved. His drinking is now within normal limits, and he has begun a new relationship, which is going well. His financial worries have evaporated having been left money in an aunt's will.*

*We have not arranged to see him again. Please get in touch if you wish to discuss his case further, or if problems recur.*

*Yours etc.*
*cc Mr J.K.*

**Table 5.5** A problem list for Mr K.

| Problem | Action | Agent | Review |
|---|---|---|---|
| Suicide risk | Close observation | Nursing staff | Daily |
| Depression | Start amitriptyline 50 mg | Psychiatrist | One week—plan to increase dose |
| Insomnia | Sleep hygiene; hypnotics | Psychiatrist | One week |
| Social isolation | Investigate supports | Social worker | One week |
| Sexual guilt | Get contact number of local gay groups | Social worker | One week |
| HIV status | Consider HIV test | GUM clinic for advice | Two weeks |
| Alcohol misuse | Counselling | Specialist nurse | Unspecified |

As a final visit to Mr K's case, Box 5.2 is a letter to his GP, a year later.

Letters from GPs to psychiatrists should follow the same principles. The psychiatrist wants to know:

- The presenting complaint(s), the chronology and the GP's provisional diagnosis.
- What is the reason for the referral—for a diagnostic opinion, treatment advice, ongoing care, etc?
- Is there an acute crisis? If not, why refer now?
- Past psychiatric and medical history.
- Key personal and social details (e.g. recent stressors, drug misuse).
- Any specific issues to be aware of (e.g. language difficulties, history of violence, vulnerable dependants).

---

**Key points**

- Completing the psychiatric assessment involves using the information you have collected to make a diagnosis, understand its likely causes, plan management and estimate prognosis.
- When thinking about why the disorder has arisen, divide the factors according to type (biological, psychological and social) and timing (predisposing, precipitating and perpetuating).
- A formulation is a useful way of summarizing a case. It comprises: an introductory statement, the diagnoses and evidence for and against each differential diagnosis, the causative factors, the management plan and the prognosis. It is also a good intellectual exercise when developing skills or practising for an examination.
- Tailor the content and format of any communication to the needs of the recipient. Be concise, structured and emphasize the points relevant to diagnostic and management decisions.

# Chapter 6

# Aetiology

## Thinking about aetiology in psychiatry

In this chapter we examine the general principles and approaches relevant to understanding the aetiology of psychiatric disorders. A key point is that psychiatric disorders, like all illnesses, are caused by multiple and diverse influences—some known, many unknown. A corollary of this is that very few 'causes' are either necessary or sufficient; rather, each factor acts to alter the risk of disorder. The contribution of specific 'causes' of course differs from patient to patient, but as a rule each of the major psychiatric disorders is characterized by a well-established set of risk factors.

For example, we might hypothesize that a teenager's eating disorder arises from:

- Inheritance of a genetic predisposition.
- Childhood obesity.
- Wanting to be a ballerina.
- Peer and media pressure to be thin.
- Disturbed 5-HT (5-hydroxytryptamine) neurotransmission.
- A hypothalamic tumour.

The study of aetiology in psychiatry has to be equally diverse (Table 6.1).

*Lecture Notes: Psychiatry*, 10e. By Paul Harrison, John Geddes and Michael Sharpe. Published 2010 by Blackwell Publishing Ltd.

- The only exceptions to the 'multifactorial' rule are a few, very rare, familial dementias which are caused by single gene mutations.
- A given causal factor often contributes to several different disorders.
- Longitudinal, prospective studies, starting with healthy but 'at-risk' individuals and following them up until illness develops in some, are a powerful design. They help distinguish 'state' from

**Table 6.1** Approaches to studying the aetiology of psychiatric disorders.

| Field | Approaches |
|---|---|
| Epidemiology | Prevalence and incidence studies |
| | Risk factor studies |
| Sociology | Life events |
| | Family influences |
| | Cultural factors |
| | Illness behaviour |
| Psychology | Behavioural theories |
| | Cognitive theories |
| | Psychodynamic theories |
| | Personality theories |
| | Neuropsychology |
| Biology | Genetics |
| | Biochemistry and pharmacology |
| | Brain imaging |
| | Neuropathology |
| | Animal models |

'trait' changes, and other problems of retrospective or cross-sectional studies of illness. Obviously they are more feasible in some situations than others.

• Aetiological conclusions should be just as evidence based as therapeutic and diagnostic ones.

## Epidemiology

Epidemiological methods can be applied to social, psychological or biological studies. They have contributed in two main ways to psychiatry:

• Population surveys have provided good information about the *prevalence* and *incidence* of the major psychiatric disorders, their sex and age distribution, and so on. This basic demographic information underpins most other kinds of aetiological research.

• Cohort and case–control studies have identified *risk factors* for psychiatric disorders—ranging from urban birth to autoimmune diseases to viral infection and drug side-effects. An example is the finding that head injury increases the risk of dementia. Sometimes, as in this example, the causality of an epidemiological finding is fairly clear, but often it is not (e.g. the association of unemployment with depression), and further studies must be carried out to see which way the causal arrows point.

## Social factors

Social factors are important in both the cause and shaping of psychiatric disorder. They can operate at different levels:

• *The immediate environment.* One's surroundings act as non-specific risk factors for illness. For example, psychiatric disorders are twice as common in those living in deprived conditions as in those living in affluent conditions. Many mechanisms are probably involved, including social conflict, substance misuse, noise and overcrowding; there may also be underlying factors that contribute independently to poverty and psychiatric disorder. In addition, having a psychiatric disorder may make it harder for the person to improve their circumstances and make continuing poverty more likely.

• *Life events.* Things happening to us and our environment can serve as stressors and precipitants.

• *The social and family group.* Parents, siblings and others close to us are important influences on our development and functioning—for better and worse. For example, childhood emotional deprivation predisposes to later depression, whereas being in a close relationship protects against the effect of stressors.

• *The wider environment.* Environment in a broader sense is also relevant. For example, societal attitudes contribute to the prevalence of eating disorders, whilst political decisions affect the types and quantities of substances misused. Sociologists have also investigated transcultural differences in the occurrence of psychiatric disorders—many are universal, but some are much more common in particular populations.

• Some of these apparently 'social' influences actually involve genes too—because genes and environment interact. In other words its 'nature plus nurture', not 'nature versus nurture'.

## Life events

Life events are specific external stressors. They include marriage, bereavement, unemployment and moving house. Life events, especially negative ones, lead to an increased risk of psychiatric disorder, notably depression, in succeeding months.

• The impact of the life event on the hypothalamo-pituitary–adrenal (HPA) axis is often implicated to explain this relationship, since the HPA axis, including cortisol production, is integral to the stress response, both normal and abnormal.

• If a recent life event is the predominant, understandable trigger for a psychiatric disorder, the diagnostic category of *stress reaction* or *adjustment reaction* may be appropriate (Chapter 10).

## The social origins of depression

A classic example of the role of social factors in psychiatry concerns depressive disorder. Researchers wondered why depression was particularly common in women of low socio-economic status, and why some women did not get depressed despite similar circumstances. They identified several factors (examples of the 'three Ps' approach to causation introduced in Chapter 5):

• Women who as children had suffered emotional deprivation or death of a parent were at greater risk of depression. Other *vulnerability (predisposing) factors* included not having a supportive partner or close friend, and being stuck at home with several young children.

• In the women who had one or more of the vulnerability factors, depressive disorder was *precipitated* by a single major life event or by an accumulation of minor stressors.

• Continuing stress and lack of support acted as *perpetuating* factors.

• The key researchers were Brown and Harris, sociologists working in London in the 1970s. The basic findings have been replicated by others, in other environments and populations.

## Family theories

Family theories view psychiatric disorder in one member as reflecting an abnormality in the whole family. They are applied particularly to childhood psychiatric disorders, where the theories have inspired a treatment approach—*family therapy*. However, it has been hard to confirm the aetiological role of the family, for two main reasons:

• Recent research shows that resemblances between family members are influenced by genes at least as much as by the family environment. An example where family factors (in a sociological sense) were wrongly invoked is autism, which was attributed to parents being aloof or obsessional, whereas in fact it is highly genetic.

• How do you show that family abnormalities are causal? In the 1950s, schizophrenia was explained in terms of parenting styles (the 'schizophreno-genic mother') and patterns of family communication ('double bind', 'schism and skew'). Such abnormalities, if they occur, seem more likely to be the result, not the cause, of having a son or daughter with schizophrenia in the house.

## The sick role and illness behaviour

The *sick role* describes four processes that occur when someone is ill:

• Exemption from normal obligations (such as earning a living).

• A right to receive care.

• An obligation to cooperate with care.

• A desire to recover.

*Illness behaviour* refers to the behaviour of the person in the sick role.

Both the sick role and illness behaviour are sociological concepts that describe normal processes. They can also be excessive or maladaptive, and then are relevant to understanding the presentation and persistence of psychiatric (and medical) disorders.

• People differ markedly in their response to symptoms—that is, they vary in their illness behaviour and readiness to adopt the sick role. Some are stoical and are reluctant to complain, while others dramatize symptoms and have a low threshold for medical consultation. These individual differences are compounded by society's views about psychiatric disorder—including stigma and ignorance about their nature and treatability. As a result, psychiatric patients may have more difficulty than medical patients in negotiating a sick role.

• Patients with medical complaints who appear to adopt the sick role unnecessarily or excessively (i.e. have *abnormal illness behaviour*) may have depression or a somatoform disorder.

• The benefits of the sick role (sometimes called *secondary gain*) play an especially important role in dissociative and somatoform disorders (Chapter 10).

## Antipsychiatry

Some sociologists, and some psychiatrists, have argued that psychiatric disorders are not medical illnesses, but merely social constructs to label and deal with deviant behaviour. This thesis—*antipsychiatry*—was influential in the 1960s, with Thomas Szasz, an American psychotherapist, being a leading figure. Whilst anti-psychiatry was important in drawing attention to the limitations of psychiatric knowledge and the dangers of stigmatization and institutionalization, there is little evidence to support its tenets, and it is not helpful to ill patients.

• A related stance ('*critical psychiatry*') is currently advocated in some quarters. It sees psychiatric disorders as predominantly social in origin and requiring psychosocial interventions. It is influenced by particular philosophical beliefs, and marked by scepticism as to the importance of medical and neuroscientific aspects of causation and management.

## Psychological factors

There are various psychological models of psychiatric disorder, differing in their theoretical background and experimental support, but sharing two features:

• They are extensions of theories of normal psychological processes.

• The theory is complemented by a psychological treatment that arises from it.

### Behavioural theories

Many of our actions are explicable in terms of learned behaviours or *conditioning*. There are two types of conditioning, *classical* and *operant*. These underlie contemporary *behavioural theories* of normal and abnormal behaviours.

• Behavioural theories gave rise to *behavioural therapy*, which is an effective intervention in its own right for several childhood disorders and anxiety disorders (see Chapter 7).

### Classical conditioning

In classical conditioning, we unconsciously associate two stimuli that regularly occur together. In Pavlov's classic experiments, dogs were given food when a bell was rung. After a while the dogs began to salivate when the bell rang, even if no food was there. This conditioning gradually wears off (*extinction*). People are classically conditioned in many ways—for example, a person may become aroused at the sight of lingerie if they have come to associate it with impending sexual gratification.

• Conditioning is important in the development of some psychiatric disorders. For example, agoraphobia developing in a woman who was twice assaulted in the street; she associates leaving the house with the fear of attack, which she avoids by staying at home.

### Operant conditioning

A behaviour will occur more frequently if it is rewarded (*positive reinforcement*), and decreases if it is not (*negative reinforcement*) or if it has unpleasant consequences (*punishment*). This is called *operant conditioning*. Rats learn to press a lever if it gives them food but not to press it if it doesn't, or if they receive a painful shock. Children will shout and scream if they learn that this behaviour gets them an ice cream; on the other hand they learn to be polite if that is effective in obtaining one. Adults are equally conditionable, though might not like to think so.

• *Learned helplessness* is an example of operant conditioning. Animals subjected to inescapable stresses (electric shocks) eventually give up trying to avoid them. A similar mechanism is proposed to explain why childhood adversity predisposes to depression in adulthood.

### Cognitive theories

The core assumption of cognitive theories is that cognitions (thoughts, patterns of thinking and ways of processing information) influence our mood, behaviour and physiology, and that inaccurate or distorted cognitions can lead to inappropriate or abnormal mood and behaviour.

• Cognitive theories of depression and anxiety disorders are especially well developed. The cognitive model explaining how panic disorder develops is summarized in Figure 6.1.

*A woman gets a twinge of chest pain whilst reaching for a tin of beans in the supermarket. She has the thought that it might be a heart attack, even though in fact it's a*

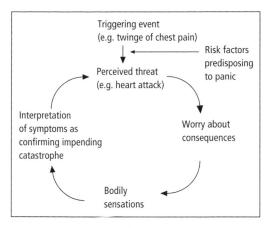

**Figure 6.1** Cognitive model of a panic attack.

*muscle strain from overdoing it at the gym that morning. Having had the thought, she becomes more anxious about the possibility of a heart attack, and all that entails, and beings to experience the physiological changes associated with anxiety—such as palpitations, sweating … and chest tightness. She interprets these sensations as confirming that she is having a heart attack, the anxiety increases and she has a panic attack. Although it passes, the next time she is in the supermarket she recalls the episode, becomes hypervigilant for bodily sensations and a second panic attack occurs more readily than before. As the cycle continues, her cognitions and the associated symptoms are repeated until she has established panic disorder.*

- In the equivalent cognitive model of depression, the central abnormality is the presence of dysfunctional assumptions and negative thoughts that lead to a vicious cycle of lowered mood and more negative thoughts.
- Cognitive distortions can arise for different reasons. For example, the lady above may be concerned about a heart attack because of an episode of childhood myocarditis, the recent death of a relative from a heart attack or from watching an item on the news on heart disease in women.
- Cognitive theories are well validated and are clinically important because they have led to an effective and widely used form of psychotherapy— *cognitive therapy* (Chapter 7).

## Psychodynamic theories

*Psychoanalysis,* associated with Sigmund Freud and his followers, is a complex theory of psychological processes and the origins of psychiatric disorders, especially neurosis. It also refers to the therapy inextricably linked to the theory. Psychoanalysis has changed a lot since the time of Freud, and the generic term *psychodynamic* is usually used to describe theories that combine Freudian elements with later ideas. Key features include:

- Feelings and memories of which we are unaware, especially those arising from very early in life, shape our current thoughts, feelings and actions.
- The mind is partitioned; some is conscious but much is unconscious. In Freud's final model, the components of the mind were the *ego, superego* and *id*: the ego is the part of us in contact with reality; the superego is like our conscience; and the id is our instinctive drives and desires. The energy of the id is called *libido,* which is primarily sexual in nature.
- Neuroses result from a failure to progress through normal stages of mental development.
- We use unconscious *defence mechanisms* to reduce tensions which exist between our conflicting desires (Table 6.2). These mechanisms may be healthy or dysfunctional.

Psychodynamic theories have been influential but are much less prominent or important in psychiatry than previously, for several reasons:

- They are not true scientific theories, in the sense of being empirically testable or refutable.
- When elements of the theories have been tested, they have not been well supported by evidence.
- Psychodynamic psychotherapies are still of unproven efficacy—and are now of very limited availability in most health care systems, including the NHS.

Nevertheless, psychodynamic insights are still clinically useful in:

- Emphasizing that early experiences, and unconscious processes, can affect our feelings and actions—whatever the mechanisms involved.
- Outlining psychological defence mechanisms— strategies we automatically use to cope with real or perceived stresses (Table 6.2).

**Table 6.2.** Defence mechanisms.

| Defence mechanism | Definition |
| --- | --- |
| Repression | Suppressing desires and memories from consciousness |
| Denial | Behaving as though genuinely unaware of external reality |
| Projection | Attributing your own feelings to someone else |
| Displacement | Shifting emotions from the appropriate object or person to a more acceptable target, e.g. kicking the dog rather than your father |
| Reaction formation | Behaving in a way opposite to your (unacceptable) instincts |
| Regression | Returning to an earlier pattern of behaviour, e.g. to become more dependent on others |
| Sublimation | Finding a socially acceptable alternative outlet for emotions |
| Intellectualization | Thinking about your emotions rather than feeling them |

- Identifying *transference* and *counter-transference*, relevant to all doctor–patient relationships (Chapter 7).

## The role of personality

Personality describes our persistent pattern of thoughts, attitudes and behaviours. As such, it is critical to psychiatric disorder (as introduced in Chapter 5), but the very fact that the two are so intertwined makes it hard to identify the specific aetiological relationships between them. It is clear, though, that:

- Different personality types predispose to different psychiatric disorders.
- Personality affects the clinical picture of psychiatric disorder (i.e. acts as a *pathoplastic* factor).
- Personality affects the prognosis of psychiatric disorders.

Personality can itself be abnormal (*personality disorder*), and interact with and coexist with psychiatric disorders. These issues are discussed in Chapter 15.

## Biological models

### Genetics

A genetic contribution to a psychiatric disorder may be suspected, as with any medical disorder, for one of four reasons:

- If the disorder clusters in families. Familial aggregation can be shown to reflect shared genes not shared environment if twin studies show a higher concordance rate in monozygotic (MZ; identical) than dizygotic (DZ; non-identical) twin pairs, because MZ twins have essentially identical genomes, but DZ twins share 50% of genes. These studies establish the *heritability* of a disorder (or trait)—see below.
- If the incidence of the disorder remains increased in adopted-away children (though this doesn't control for prenatal environment—which may be relevant for some disorders, such as schizophrenia).
- If there is a known chromosomal (*cytogenetic*) aberration—for example, Down syndrome or fragile X syndrome.
- If there is a known pathological or biochemical abnormality, then the underlying gene is a *candidate gene* for the disorder. For example, in Alzheimer's disease, the β-amyloid protein in senile plaques led to the discovery of amyloid gene mutations. The lack of definitive lesions in most psychiatric disorders means there are few convincing candidate genes.

Apart from a few dementias (e.g. Huntington's disease) and developmental disorders (e.g. tuberous sclerosis), psychiatric disorders are not caused (determined) by gene mutations following Mendelian inheritance patterns. Instead, there are genetic variants (*polymorphisms*) that act as risk factors, significantly but slightly increasing susceptibility to the disorder.

**Table 6.3** Approximate heritability of psychiatric disorders.

| Disorder | Heritability (%) |
| --- | --- |
| Addiction | 40 |
| Alzheimer's disease | 50 |
| Anxiety disorders | 30 |
| Autism | 80 |
| Bipolar disorder | 80 |
| Depressive disorder | 40 |
| Schizophrenia | 80 |

*Heritability* refers to the size of the genetic predisposition; it describes the proportion of the disorder in the population that is attributable to genes. It is best measured in large-scale twin studies. Heritability estimates for psychiatric disorders (for which good data are available) are shown in Table 6.3.

• Heritability is a population average figure. Any given individual's disorder may be much more or less 'genetic'.

• The rest of the 100% not explained by heritability denotes the environmental contribution, usually divided into individual-specific and shared environmental factors.

Although there is a substantial heritability for many psychiatric disorders, it is proving difficult to complete the next step (Figure 6.2)—to locate the chromosomal loci and susceptibility genes themselves. There are several possible reasons for this:

• There are many genes, each conferring on their own only a small amount of the risk for a psychiatric disorder.

• The genes interact with each other (*epistasis*), and with environmental factors (gene × environment or GE), in ways which are very hard to detect and measure.

• The disorder may be caused in different people by different genes (*genetic heterogeneity*) or different variants of the same gene (*allelic heterogeneity*).

• The causative genes may not map onto the currently defined clinical syndromes—that is, the wrong patients, genetically speaking, are being grouped together.

Nevertheless, the search is worth pursuing since identification of genes gives clues as to the core

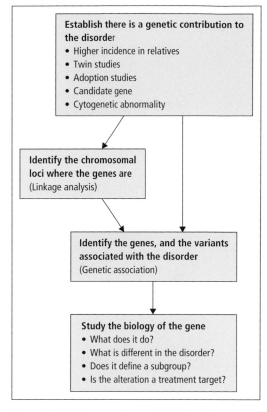

**Figure 6.2** Finding genes for psychiatric disorders.

biological basis for an illness, and potentially for its effective treatment (e.g. several current treatment trials to correct the β-amyloid abnormality of Alzheimer's disease).

## Biochemistry and pharmacology

Biochemical theories propose that psychiatric disorders are caused by a biochemical abnormality, usually affecting the level or activity of a neurotransmitter, or the enzymes which metabolize it, or the receptors which it binds to, or the transporters which regulate its levels in the synapse. For example, the 5-HT (serotonin) theory of depression includes variants implicating $5\text{-HT}_{1A}$ receptors, 5-HT transporters and tryptophan hydroxylase.

• Many of these theories were based originally on the mechanisms by which psychotropic drugs work. For example, antipsychotics treat schizophrenia and were found to block dopamine receptors; this observation led to the dopamine hypothesis of schizophrenia (Chapter 12). Forty years later, there is now evidence it is true, to some degree, but the line of reasoning is flawed: diuretics treat heart failure, but heart failure is not usually due to renal disease.

## Measurements in the brain

Biochemical studies of the brain after death were crucial in the understanding of Alzheimer's disease; in particular, the discovery of cholinergic deficits and the β-amyloid protein. Similar approaches have revealed abnormalities in other psychiatric disorders, including schizophrenia, mood disorders and autism, though no comparably clear picture has emerged. Part of the problem is that studies of post-mortem brains have many limitations, such as the effects of dying, death and a bias towards old, medicated and chronically ill cases. This makes it difficult to establish whether alterations occurred early or late in the disease, and to exclude ageing or treatment effects.

Now, a range of *functional imaging* techniques are available which overcome these problems and allow the living brain to be studied (and by using first-episode and unmedicated subjects, the confounds mentioned above can be avoided).

- Positron emission tomography (PET) and single photon emission computed tomography (SPECT) use radioactive ligands to measure brain receptors or metabolites. They have shown, for example, that people with schizophrenia do not have elevated dopamine $D_2$ receptors (as one version of the dopamine hypothesis had proposed). The methods are limited by the radioactivity involved, and a lack of suitable ligands for many molecules of interest (e.g. glutamate receptors).
- PET and SPECT, together with functional magnetic resonance imaging (fMRI) and magnetoencephalography (MEG), can also be used to measure regional brain metabolism and activity. Such information points to the specific brain regions that may be involved in the pathophysiology of a disorder.

## Peripheral markers

The brain is relatively inaccessible, so many biochemical measurements have been made in cerebrospinal fluid (CSF), blood or urine. A robust finding is that people who are impulsive and aggressive have low CSF levels of the metabolite of 5-HT, suggesting impaired functioning of the central 5-HT system. However, it is often unclear whether peripheral markers reflect the situation in the brain.

- In a *neuroendocrine challenge test*, a substance known to produce a change in the plasma level of a hormone is administered. The size of the change is used as a marker of the sensitivity of the system which mediates the response in the brain. For example, in the *dexamethasone suppression test* (DST), plasma cortisol is measured after a dose of dexamethasone, to assess HPA axis function. Many people with severe depression fail to suppress cortisol—leading to a 'steroid hypothesis' of depression
- The study of body fluids in psychiatry is of renewed interest in the current search for *biomarkers* —that is, biological indices (such as levels of gene expression, or of metabolites) that can help predict onset, progression or treatment response of a disorder, or help in its differential diagnosis.

## Brain structure

### Structural brain imaging

Computed tomography (CT) and MRI allow brain structure to be investigated *in vivo*. For example, they show that patients with schizophrenia have enlarged lateral ventricles, and that the hippocampus is smaller in those with recurrent depressive disorder.

- Longitudinal MRI studies are increasingly used. For example, they show that some differences in brain structure long precede the onset of symptoms in schizophrenia, whilst others develop as the illness does.
- MRI methods can now also identify the white matter pathways that connect one part of the brain with another—many people think the anatomical basis of psychiatric disorders is not to be found in

any one place, but in how the brain is wired up, in both a structural and a functional sense.

## Neuropathology

Many dementias have a known neuropathological basis—indeed, neuropathology provides the diagnostic criteria. Most other psychiatric disorders do not. Nevertheless, recent studies using sensitive and molecular techniques suggest that there are histological changes in schizophrenia, mood disorder and autism.

## Animal models

No one would suggest that a rat can get schizophrenia—and how would we know if it did? However, animal studies have contributed to psychiatric research in various ways—Pavlov and learned helplessness have already been mentioned—and they continue to be of use:

• To assess the effects of an experimental intervention (e.g. maternal separation, neonatal hippocampal damage) upon relevant behaviours (e.g. cognitive performance, social interactions) and biology (e.g. receptor sensitivity).

• *Transgenic* animals allow the role of specific genes in brain function and dysfunction to be investigated. For example, mice containing a mutated human amyloid precursor protein gene develop cognitive impairment and histological features of Alzheimer's disease; mice without a prion protein gene are resistant to prion disease (Chapter 13).

• Animals, usually rats, are still widely used to test potential psychotropic drugs.

---

**Key points**

• The cause of most psychiatric disorders is multifactorial. It involves biological, psychological and social factors.

• There is a genetic predisposition to most disorders, and sometimes a large genetic contribution. However, the number and identity of the genes involved in most disorders remain unknown.

• Other biological aetiological factors are diverse and include head injury, infections and drug side-effects.

• Important psychological factors are early experience, cognitive style and conditioning.

• Social influences include childhood deprivation, relationship problems, family structure and unemployment.

## Chapter 7

# Treatment

Psychiatric treatments may be categorized as *biological*—drugs and ECT; *psychological*—the psychotherapies; and *social*. A combination of approaches is usually used. Sometimes *compulsory* treatment is given.

- This is the longest and most 'fact-packed' chapter. We suggest you read about a particular treatment as you encounter it in your clinical work.
- Table 7.1 gives a chronology of the major treatments currently in use.
- Chapter 8 considers how treatments are delivered and services organized.

## Evidence-based treatment

As in the rest of medicine, there is excellent evidence for some psychiatric treatments and rather less for others. We have tried to use an evidence-based approach to our recommendations—highlighting NICE (National Institute for Health and Clinical Excellence) recommendations where appropriate—and to point out areas where the evidence is lacking and there is clinical uncertainty.

- Appendix 2 summarizes useful sources of evidence regarding psychiatric treatments.

---

*Lecture Notes: Psychiatry*, 10e. By Paul Harrison, John Geddes and Michael Sharpe. Published 2010 by Blackwell Publishing Ltd.

## Drug treatments

The study of psychiatric drugs—their mechanisms, uses, effects and side-effects—constitutes *psychopharmacology*.

## Principles and practice of prescribing

Drugs used in psychiatry can be grouped into eight main categories (Table 7.2).

- Consult a more detailed text for complete information about individual drugs, doses, side-effects, drug interactions and contraindications.
- Always check the *British National Formulary* or similar before prescribing any drug with which you are not wholly familiar.
- Box 7.1 summarizes the important principles that govern the prescription of all psychiatric drugs. Bear these in mind as you read on, and try to put them into practice.
- Many patients—maybe even the majority—do not take their drugs regularly. This key issue is variously called *compliance*, *adherence* or *concordance*, and the lack of it is a major reason for apparent non-response to medication. Box 7.2 lists the main reasons for the problem and how to minimize it.

## Antidepressants

Antidepressants are effective, readily available and a first-line treatment for depressive disorders. Some

**Table 7.1** When current psychiatric treatments entered regular use.

| | Physical therapies | Psychotherapies |
|---|---|---|
| 1900s | | Psychoanalysis |
| 1930s | Psychosurgery<br>Electroconvulsive therapy | Group therapy |
| 1950s | Antipsychotics<br>Monoamine oxidase inhibitors<br>Tricyclic antidepressants | Brief psychodynamic therapy |
| 1960s | Benzodiazepines | Family therapy<br>Behavioural therapy |
| 1970s | Lithium | Cognitive therapy |
| 1980s | Selective serotonin reuptake inhibitors | Cognitive behavioural therapy (CBT) |
| 1990s | Atypical antipsychotics<br>Acetylcholinesterase inhibitors | |
| 2000s | | Psychoeducation |

**Table 7.2** Drug treatments in psychiatry.

| Type | Example | Main indications |
|---|---|---|
| *Antidepressants* | | Depression, neuroses |
| SSRIs | Fluoxetine, sertraline | |
| TCAs | Amitriptyline | |
| MAOIs | Phenelzine | |
| SNRIs | Venlafaxine | |
| Other | Mirtazapine | |
| *Mood stabilizers* | | Bipolar disorder |
| Lithium | | |
| Valproate | | |
| Lamotrigine | | |
| Carbamazepine | | |
| *Hypnotics and anxiolytics* | | Anxiety, insomnia |
| Benzodiazepines | Diazepam | |
| *Antipsychotics* | | Schizophrenia, other psychoses |
| Typical antipsychotics | Haloperidol | |
| Atypical antipsychotics | Clozapine, olanzapine | |
| *Anticholinergics* | Procyclidine | Extrapyramidal side-effects of antipsychotics |
| *Stimulants* | Methylphenidate | Attention deficit disorder |
| *Drugs for dementia* | | Alzheimer's disease (moderate to severe) |
| Cholinesterase inhibitors | Donepezil | |
| NMDA receptor antagonist | Memantine | |
| *Drugs used in substance dependence* | | Detoxification, abstinence |
| Alcohol | Disulfiram, acamprosate | |
| Smoking | Bupropion | |
| Opiates | Methadone | |

SSRIs: selective serotonin reuptake inhibitors; TCAs: tricyclic antidepressants; MAOIs: monoamine oxidase inhibitors, SNRIs: selective serotonin and noradrenaline reuptake inhibitors; NMDA: *N*-methyl-D-aspartate.

## Box 7.1 Principles of psychiatric prescribing

- *Choose the right drug.* This requires an adequate assessment, diagnosis and consideration of other factors such as comorbid medical conditions.
- *Give the right dose.* Antidepressant doses are often inadequate, antipsychotic doses excessive. Each poses risks: lack of efficacy and unnecessary side-effects, respectively.
- *Give the drug for the right duration.* Antidepressants tend to be given for too short a period and anxiolytics for too long. Again, the trade-off is between incomplete response and adverse effects, including the potential for dependence.
- *The efficacy and side-effects of drugs within a class may differ.* The choice of drug is determined largely by previous experience in any specific patient, side-effects (e.g. sedative profile), strength of evidence and your own experience. Other things being equal, use well-tried drugs with solid evidence of efficacy and known safety rather than the latest fashion.
- *Avoid combinations of drugs from the same class.* There is no evidence for greater efficacy, and often more side-effects.
- *Psychiatric drugs are better than placebo … but not always by much.* Due humility is essential, along with a clear grasp of how and when to prescribe appropriately—and an awareness of, and willingness to use, alternative strategies.

## Box 7.2 Non-compliance in psychiatry

**Major causes are:**

- Reluctance to accept the need for treatment.
- Lack of belief in drug efficacy.
- Concern about drug side-effects, including worry about becoming 'addicted'.
- Stigma.
- Forgetfulness.
- Expense.
- As an effect of the disorder being treated—for example, a psychotic patient may be convinced you want to poison him; a severely depressed person may feel they do not deserve to recover.

**Improve compliance with medication by:**

- Establishing a good therapeutic relationship.
- Discovering the patient's own views about their illness and its treatment. Correct any misapprehensions, but respect their views if they disagree with yours.
- Sharing of information about the evidence for (and against) the drug. Give simple, clear advice and figures—for example, 'You have a 60% chance of being a lot better after a month'; 'There is a small chance you'll feel nauseous at first'. Give the patient a chance to ask questions or dispute the evidence. And make sure that you include discussion about the risks and benefits of *not* taking the treatment.

are also used to treat other disorders. The major classes are shown in Table 7.2. The efficacy of antidepressants is well established. Selective serotonin reuptake inhibitors (SSRIs) and tricyclic antidepressants (TCAs) have similar efficacy, with about 60% of patients responding after 6 weeks. Over the same period, 30–40% respond to placebo.

- Patients often want to stop antidepressants too soon. Antidepressants usually produce some reduction in symptoms by 4–6 weeks, but it may take many months for the patient to recover fully. Continued treatment maintains the improvement in the medium term (6 months after getting better). Prolonged use halves the chances of relapse in those at risk.
- All antidepressants are thought to work by enhancing activity of the monoamine neurotransmitters noradrenaline (NA) and/or serotonin

(5-HT; Figure 7.1). The various classes achieve this in different ways.

- The focus here is on the drugs; see other chapters for discussion about their use in management. Chapter 9 discusses the treatment of depression, including combination therapies and treatment resistance.

## Selective serotonin reuptake inhibitors (SSRIs)

SSRIs are the usual first-line antidepressant.
- *Mode of action.* Selectively inhibit synaptic 5-HT reuptake transporters, thereby increasing synaptic 5-HT concentration (Figure 7.1).
- *Practical usage.* Usual to start at full dosage, once daily with breakfast. Like all antidepressants, they take 7–14 days for onset of antidepressant efficacy.

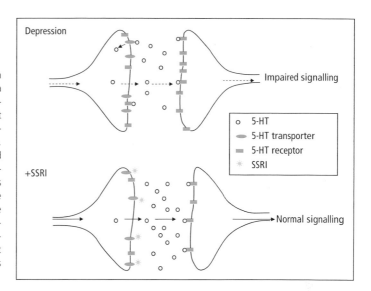

**Figures 7.1** How SSRIs work. In depression, there is thought to be a relative 5-HT deficiency, and upregulation of 5-HT receptors. The net effect is abnormal signalling and functioning of the postsynaptic neuron. SSRIs block the 5-HT transporter, and increase 5-HT in the synapse. The antidepressant effect takes several days to occur, because other adaptive changes also have to occur (to restore normal firing of the neuron, downregulate receptors, and other secondary effects). TCAs work similarly, but act upon the presynaptic receptors and noradrenergic synapses too.

However, side-effects (see below) occur in the first few days—remember to warn the patient of this. Consider giving a hypnotic for the first few weeks to aid sleep. Always withdraw an SSRI slowly at the end of treatment.

- *Individual SSRIs.* There are some modest differences in properties between SSRIs. A good first choice is *sertraline* (50–100 mg/day) which is effective, well tolerated and has a 'clean' profile, few interactions with other drugs, and maybe a lower incidence of sexual dysfunction. *Escitalopram* (10 mg/day) is also well tolerated although still not available generically and therefore more expensive. *Fluoxetine* (20–40 mg/day) has a long half-life, so is useful if compliance is poor, and withdrawal reactions are rare (but drug interactions persist longer).

- *Side-effects.* Usually well tolerated, though 15% have nausea, abdominal discomfort, diarrhoea, insomnia and agitation, mainly in the early stages. Sexual dysfunction (lack of libido, anorgasmia) is common in women and also occurs in men. SSRIs may increase the risk of upper gastrointestinal bleeding and hyponatraemia. Some people experience discontinuation symptoms (insomnia, nausea, dizziness, agitation) when stopping the drug; hence withdraw over a few weeks.

- *SSRIs and suicide.* There can be an increase in suicidal thoughts and behaviour with SSRIs in the early stages of treating depression, particularly in younger adults and children. Patients should always be monitored for suicide risk carefully at this time. However, any such risk must be set against the benefits of effective treatment in reducing the unequivocal suicide risk associated with depression.

- *Overdose.* Few effects; rarely if ever fatal.

- *Cautions and contraindications.* Few. May increase seizures in epilepsy. Coadministration with serotonergic drugs (including monoamine oxidase inhibitors (MAOIs), L-tryptophan, lithium and St. John's Wort) may lead to *serotonin syndrome*, a potentially life-threatening condition that includes tachycardia, shivering, sweating, hyperthermia and hyper-reflexia, progressing to shock and renal failure.

## Tricyclic antidepressants (TCAs)

Despite the overall advantages of SSRIs, TCAs retain an important role, especially for people intolerant of, or unresponsive to, SSRIs. They may also have slightly greater efficacy in severe depression and in chronic pain.

- Not all drugs in this class are actually tricyclic in structure. Semantically strict people call them *heterocyclic antidepressants*.

• *Mode of action.* Inhibit presynaptic NA and 5-HT transporters. Some TCAs are more selective for one monoamine than another—for example, clomipramine mainly acts on 5-HT; desipramine on NA. Unlike SSRIs, TCAs also block various receptors, contributing to their side-effect profile (Table 7.3).

• *Practical usage.* Usually given at night (due to their sedative action) or in divided doses. Delayed onset of action as for SSRIs, though reduction in anxiety (anxiolysis) and sedation occur rapidly. To minimize initial side-effects, start at a low dose and increase over 10 days.

• *Side-effects.* See Tables 7.4 and 7.5. The ability to drive and use machinery may be impaired due to drowsiness.

**Table 7.3** Receptor blockade by TCAs and their associated side effects.

| Receptor blocked | Side-effect produced |
| --- | --- |
| Muscarinic cholinergic | Dry mouth, urinary retention, constipation, blurred vision, glaucoma, tachycardia, delirium, sexual dysfunction |
| Alpha-1 adrenergic | Postural hypotension, drowsiness, sexual dysfunction |
| Histamine $H_1$ | Drowsiness, weight gain |
| Other or unknown | Arrhythmias, seizures |

**Table 7.4** Chemical structures of antipsychotics.

| Chemical class | Example |
| --- | --- |
| Phenothiazines | |
|   Aliphatic side chain | Chlorpromazine |
|   Piperazine side chain | Fluphenazine |
| Thioxanthines | Flupenthixol |
| Butyrophenones | Haloperidol |
| Dibenzodiazepines | Clozapine, olanzapine |
| Benzisoxazole/piperidine | Risperidone |
| Substituted benzamides | Amisulpride |

**Table 7.5** Side-effects of conventional antipsychotics.

| Side-effects | Comments |
| --- | --- |
| *Common* | |
| Extrapyramidal (EPS) | See text. Related to $D_2$ receptor blockade in basal ganglia. |
|   Acute dystonia | |
|   Parkinsonism | |
|   Akathisia | |
|   Tardive dyskinesia | |
| Hyperprolactinaemia | Due to $D_2$ receptor blockade in the pituitary. May lead to osteoporosis in women. |
|   Galactorrhoea | |
|   Amenorrhoea | |
|   Sexual dysfunction | |
| Anticholinergic | As for TCAs. See Table 7.3. |
| Antiadrenergic | As for TCAs. See Table 7.3. |
| Weight gain | Due to histamine $H_1$ or $5\text{-}HT_{2C}$ receptor antagonism. |
| *Rare or idiosyncratic, but severe* | |
| Neuroleptic malignant syndrome | Dangerous. See text. |
| Photosensitivity | Especially chlorpromazine. |
| Cholestatic jaundice | Especially chlorpromazine. |
| Retinal pigmentation | |
| Blood dyscrasias | |
| Seizures | |
| Tachyarrhythmias | |
| Hypothermia | |

- *Individual TCAs.* *Lofepramine* is an effective TCA and generally well tolerated. *Amitriptyline* is very sedating and anxiolytic.
- *Overdose.* Dangerous in overdose, causing tachyarrhythmias, seizures, coma and death.
- *Cautions and contraindications.* Avoid in glaucoma, prostatism, recent myocardial infarction, cardiac failure, and porphyria. Increase seizure frequency, so caution in epilepsy. Avoid combining with MAOIs.

## Monoamine oxidase inhibitors (MAOIs)

MAOIs (e.g. *phenelzine* (15–90 mg/day), tranylcypromine (10–30 mg/day)) are third-line antidepressants; their use is limited by toxicity and by their lesser efficacy than TCAs or SSRIs.
- *Mode of action.* Prevent breakdown of monoamines in presynaptic terminals by the enzyme MAO, thereby increasing transmitter availability.
- *Uses of MAOIs.* The main indication is atypical depression (Chapter 9). Also used in depression unresponsive to other treatments, either alone or in combination.
- *Practical usage.* Ensure the patient is aware of the necessary dietary restrictions and drug interactions (see below). Wait 2 weeks after stopping a TCA and 5 weeks after an SSRI. Prescribe in divided doses.
- *Side-effects.* Postural hypotension, insomnia, ankle oedema, dry mouth, dizziness, agitation and headache.
- *Overdose.* Hypertension, delirium, coma and death.
- *Cautions and contraindications.* Prescribe with caution. MAO also metabolizes tyramine, so eating tyramine whilst on MAOIs can cause a hypertensive crisis ('*the cheese reaction*')—headache, palpitations, fever, convulsions and coma. Certain food and drinks must consequently be avoided—for example, cheese, red wine, broad beans, pickled herrings, game and Marmite. There are also dangerous interactions with many drugs, including opiates, insulin, cold remedies, antiepileptics, SSRIs and some TCAs. Avoid MAOIs in cardiac or hepatic failure or porphyria.
- *Reversible MAOIs.* Unlike classical MAOIs, *moclobemide* (300–900 mg/day) is virtually free

from the cheese reaction and associated risks (because it only inhibits one form of MAO, and does so reversibly), although its effectiveness may be less.

## Selective serotonin and noradrenaline reuptake inhibitors (SNRIs)

*Venlafaxine (75–375 mg/day)* and *duloxetine (60 mg/day)* are the only members of this group.
- *Mode of action.* Like TCAs, venlafaxine potently blocks 5-HT and NA reuptake. Unlike TCAs, it doesn't block cholinergic receptors.
- *Practical usage.* Venlafaxine (but not duloxetine) is slightly more effective than SSRIs. Its main indication is for SSRI non-response. Give twice daily, though a long-acting (once daily) form is available. Also has pain-relieving properties.
- *Side-effects.* Resemble those of SSRIs, but may be worse. At high doses, hypertension may occur and should be monitored. Not sedative. Avoid MAOIs.

## Other antidepressants

Various other antidepressants are available which do not fall readily into a specific class. None is more effective than SSRIs or TCAs, and they are not widely used.
- *Mirtazapine* and *trazodone* have complex pharmacologies. Both are very sedating. Low-dose trazodone (50–100 mg at night) is a useful (non-addictive) hypnotic, often used in conjunction with SSRIs in the early stages of treatment. Despite the sedation which leads to poorer tolerability than other antidepressants, mirtazapine is effective and the combination with an SSRI is a routine second-line treatment for depression.
- *Reboxetine* is a selective NA reuptake inhibitor. It is non-sedating and may improve social functioning. It appears to be less effective *and* less well tolerated than SSRIs.
- *Agomelatine* is a new antidepressant: a melatonin $MT_1$ and $MT_2$ receptor agonist and $5\text{-}HT_{2C}$ receptor antagonist. Initial efficacy and tolerability data are encouraging, but its position in clinical practice remains unclear.
- *St. John's Wort* is an extract of the plant *Hypericum perforatum*, available without prescription and

tried by many patients. It is an effective but weak antidepressant. Though a 'natural' remedy, it has side-effects, drug interactions and there are reports of toxicity.

## Mood stabilizers

Not a pharmacological class, *mood stabilizer* is a clinically useful term used to describe a drug used to prevent mood swings in bipolar disorder. Lithium was the first and remains the standard therapy. Other mood stabilizers include antiepileptic drugs (e.g. valproate, carbamazepine and lamotrigine) and antipsychotics (e.g. olanzapine and quetiapine).

## Lithium

- *Mode of action.* Uncertain, but probably acts on second messenger systems via the phosphatidylinositol and glycogen synthetase kinase 3 (GSK3) pathways.
- *Uses.* Usually given as lithium carbonate. The main indication is to prevent relapse in bipolar disorder; effective against both manic and depressive relapses; reduces risk of relapse by about 40%. Needs to be given for at least 18 months for the benefit to be clear. Also effective in acute mania (though antipsychotics work faster) and as an adjunctive treatment for depression (Chapter 9). It is sometimes used to treat behavioural disturbance in learning disability.
- *Side-effects.* At therapeutic levels (0.5–1.0 mmol/l): fine tremor, metallic taste, dry mouth, thirst, mild polyuria, nausea and weight gain. Hypothyroidism occurs in 20% of women; rarer in men. Renal impairment may occur after prolonged use, but rare.
- *Overdose.* Toxic symptoms occur above 1.5 mmol/l: coarse tremor, agitation, twitching, thirst and polyuria. Above 2.5 mmol/l: polyuric renal failure, seizures, coma and death. Toxic levels can result from even mild dehydration, or with low-salt diets. Fatalities after overdose are not uncommon; survivors may be left with renal failure or brain damage.

- *Practical usage.* Before prescribing, a detailed discussion about the commitment and potential dangers is necessary. Do a physical examination and measure electrolytes, creatinine clearance, thyroid function and also ECG if indicated. During treatment measure lithium levels regularly (weekly at first, then 3 monthly once stable). Titrate dose (usually 400–1200 mg/day) to keep the plasma level at 0.5–1.0 mmol/l. Test thyroid and renal function every 6 months. Withdraw gradually, in order to avoid rebound mania.
- *Cautions and contraindications.* Many. Avoid if adherence is likely to be variable or short lived. Avoid in renal failure and pregnancy. Do not combine with diuretics, angiotensin-converting enzyme inhibitors or high dose antipsychotics. Use cautiously with NSAIDs (non-steroidal anti-inflammatory drugs).

## Valproic acid

Valproic acid (prescribed as sodium valproate or valproate semisodium) is commonly used but is less effective, and has a weaker evidence base, than lithium. It has a place when lithium is not tolerated, contraindicated or ineffective. The combination of lithium plus valproate is more effective than valproate monotherapy and, possibly, than lithium monotherapy.

- *Mode of action.* In epilepsy, works by blocking sodium channels and increasing GABA (γ-aminobutyric acid) turnover.
- *Practical usage.* Dose depends on the drug formulation. Valproate semisodium is started at 250–500 mg/day and titrated upwards every few days, depending on adverse effects. The usual maintenance dose is 750–1250 mg/day. Plasma levels can be measured, but no therapeutic range for mood stabilization has been established.
- *Side-effects.* Sedation, tiredness, tremor and gastrointestinal disturbance may occur. Reversible hair loss occurs in 10% of patients. May cause thrombocytopenia.
- *Cautions and contraindications.* May increase plasma levels of other protein-bound drugs (e.g. other antiepileptics). Teratogenetic—avoid in

pregnancy, and use with caution in women of childbearing potential.

## Carbamazepine

Carbamazepine is probably less effective than lithium or valproic acid, but may be used when these are contraindicated, ineffective or not tolerated.

- *Mode of action.* In epilepsy, works by blocking sodium channels.
- *Practical usage.* Start at low dose [200 mg twice daily (bd)] and build up to 600 mg bd. Measure plasma levels if signs of toxicity (ataxia, confusion, blurred vision) emerge. Check white cell count after a week.
- *Side-effects.* If erythematous rash or leucopenia occur, stop the drug. Other side-effects are nausea, dizziness, drowsiness and hyponatraemia.
- *Cautions and contraindications.* Carbamazepine is a potent enzyme inducer, so other drugs will be metabolized faster—for example, the contraceptive pill. Avoid MAOIs or if there is evidence of hepatic failure, arrhythmias or pregnancy.

## Lamotrigine

Lamotrigine is also an antiepileptic drug. It prevents depressive episodes but not manic episodes. It is also probably effective in acute depressive episodes in bipolar disorder, although its use as monotherapy is limited because of the slow titration required.

- *Mode of action.* In epilepsy, blocks sodium and calcium channels, and decreases glutamate release.
- *Practical usage.* Start very gradually, initially 25 mg daily for 2 weeks then 50 mg daily for 2 weeks. The usual dose in bipolar disorder is 100–300 mg daily.
- *Side-effects.* A rash occurs in 3–5% of patients, requiring that the drug be stopped. The risk is reduced by a gradual increase in dose. Other side-effects include nausea, headache, tremor and dizziness.
- *Cautions and contraindications.* Plasma levels are increased by valproate (so use 50% of dose), and a combination of lamotrigine and carbamazepine may cause neurotoxicity.

## Anxiolytics

These drugs are also known as *hypnotics* and *sedatives* if being used to help sleep. Benzodiazepines are the main class and in the 1960s and 1970s were very widely prescribed. With the awareness of their potential for dependency and withdrawal problems (Chapter 14), SSRIs or TCAs have replaced benzodiazepines as the usual drugs for anxiety. However, anxiolytics still have a role for short-term use.

## Benzodiazepines

The former popularity of benzodiazepines is understandable: they are highly effective and relatively free of unpleasant side-effects.

- *Mode of action.* Potentiate inhibitory transmission via the benzodiazepine-binding site of the $GABA_A$ receptor.
- *Uses in psychiatry.* Relief of acute anxiety and treatment of panic disorder, phobic anxiety and insomnia. Also used for delirium tremens, and to augment antipsychotics for sedation in acute psychosis.
- *Practical usage.* Diazepam (2–5 mg once or twice daily) is the standard anxiolytic. For intramuscular or intravenous administration use lorazepam (1–4 mg 4 hourly). *Temazepam* (20 mg) is shorter acting and used for insomnia. In the USA, *alprazolam* (250 µg three times a day) is widely used for panic disorder.
- *Side-effects.* Drowsiness, 'hangover effects', headache, nausea, ataxia, dysarthria and delirium. Occasionally, disinhibition or aggression. Should not normally be prescribed for longer than 4 weeks, to prevent dependency. Withdrawal symptoms include rebound anxiety, insomnia, visual and auditory hallucinations and seizures. This is managed by switching from short-acting benzodiazepines to diazepam, and by tapering the dose over several weeks or longer.

- *Overdose*. Very rarely fatal in healthy people. *Flumazenil* can be used acutely to reverse the effects.
- *Cautions and contraindications*. The sedative effect may interfere with driving ability, especially if combined with alcohol.

## Other anxiolytics

- *Propranolol* reduces the somatic symptoms of anxiety (tachycardia, tremor) but has a limited role. Avoid in asthmatics as it can cause bronchospasm.
- *Buspirone* is a non-sedating anxiolytic, used in generalized anxiety disorder. It is said not to be addictive, and takes several days to work.
- *Chloral hydrate* is an older hypnotic, still used in the elderly.
- The 'z-drugs' (*zolpidem, zopiclone* and *zaleplon*) enhance GABA transmission and are used mainly as hypnotics, claimed to produce fewer hangover effects and less tolerance than benzodiazepines, although the evidence that there are any worthwhile clinical benefits is limited. Zaleplon has a particularly short half-life.
- Low-dose TCAs also have anxiolytic and hypnotic effects—for example, *amitriptyline* (25 mg) or *trazodone* (50 mg)—and are not addictive.

## Antipsychotics

Antipsychotics (also called *neuroleptics* or *major tranquillizers*) are the mainstay of treatment for schizophrenia and all other psychoses.

- Antipsychotics have a range of chemical structures—a common if tedious exam question (Table 7.4).

A more important classification is into two main groups: the older, *conventional* (typical) antipsychotics, and the newer *atypical* ones (Box 7.3). There are differences between them (see below) but the fundamental properties are the same for all antipsychotics:

- All antipsychotics work primarily by blocking $D_2$ dopamine receptors. This reverses the excessive dopamine activity in the mesolimbic system that is thought to cause the symptoms of psychosis.

---

**Box 7.3 Conventional and atypical antipsychotics**

The term 'atypical' was applied to *clozapine* (see below), the first antipsychotic that did not produce extrapyramidal side-effects (EPS). This is the correct usage of the term: an antipsychotic that does not produce EPS at clinical doses. Since clozapine, many other antipsychotics have been marketed as atypical. However, the terminology is confusing because:

- Atypical is sometimes wrongly thought to imply greater efficacy, because clozapine also proved to be more effective than other antipsychotics. This property is not shared by other atypical antipsychotics.
- Atypicality is a spectrum, with clozapine at one end and haloperidol at the other; many antipsychotics are in the middle (e.g. sulpiride). This means that the distinction is blurred—bear this in mind when reading this section.
- Alternative terms—which are also unsatisfactory—include '*second generation*' and '*novel*'.
- Several mechanisms have been proposed to explain 'atypicality'. One is that the drugs block $D_2$ receptors transiently and are sensitive to endogenous dopamine levels; another is that they also block 5-HT$_{2A}$ receptors.

---

$D_2$ receptor blockade also contributes, along with antagonism at other receptors, to their side-effects.

- Antipsychotics are effective against positive psychotic symptoms—that is, delusions, hallucinations and thought disorder—regardless of diagnosis, in about 70% of patients within 6 weeks. *Clozapine* is the only antipsychotic with a greater efficacy (see below). Their onset of action is gradual, over 1–2 weeks (but there is no delay in onset of effect, as previously believed). Antipsychotics are also used in prevention of relapse of psychosis, in delirium and in severe depression.
- There are several serious side-effects (see below). Knowing how and when to explain the potential side-effects is difficult if a patient is acutely psychotic. It should be done properly as soon as the mental state permits.
- Avoid the use of high doses (above recommended limits), either for non-response or to produce sedation. There is no evidence of greater efficacy, no pharmacological rationale and good evidence of harm.

## Side-effects of conventional antipsychotics

These are many and serious (Table 7.5). Their prevalence and severity vary from one drug to another, depending on their pharmacological profile. The main features of two widely used conventional antipsychotics, *haloperidol* and *chlorpromazine*, are summarized in Table 7.6.

*Extrapyramidal side-effects* (EPS) are a major problem. EPS are motor abnormalities related to the dopaminergic receptor blockade in the basal ganglia. There are four types:

- *Acute dystonia*—painful contractions of muscles in the neck, jaw or eyes. Young men given high doses are particularly vulnerable. Onset is within hours or days. They are treated with intramuscular or intravenous anticholinergic agents.
- *Parkinsonism*—decreased facial movements, shuffling gait, stiffness and sometimes tremor. Common in early weeks of treatment. Managed by reducing the dose or temporarily adding an anticholinergic. Easily mistaken for depression or negative symptoms in schizophrenia.
- *Akathisia*—a feeling of restlessness and a need to walk around. It is very unpleasant and occurs in the first months of treatment. May be mistaken for psychotic behaviour. Treat by lowering the dose or temporarily giving propranolol.
- *Tardive dyskinesia (TD)*—uncontrollable grimacing movements of face, tongue or upper body. This is both distressing and disabling. TD occurs in about 5% of patients taking long-term antipsychotics every year. There is no way of predicting

who will develop it. Neither is there any reliable treatment, and it can be irreversible. Vitamin E is ineffective.

Two other rare but life-threatening adverse effects to note are:

- *Neuroleptic malignant syndrome* (NMS). The features are pyrexia, stiffness, autonomic instability and seizures, leading to coma. Raised serum creatine kinase, metabolic acidosis and leucocytosis are characteristic. The incidence is about 1 in 500. It is fatal in about 10% of cases and requires urgent medical care. If a patient on an antipsychotic develops a fever without a clear cause, stop the drug temporarily and monitor. NMS can occur with any antipsychotic, especially the high-potency ones (e.g. haloperidol), and following a dose increase. After an episode of NMS, restart treatment gradually, using an atypical antipsychotic, and with careful monitoring.
- Prolongation of the QTc interval on the ECG, which predisposes to a serious arrhythmia called *torsade de pointes*, has been associated with some antipsychotics, probably related to inhibition of specific cardiac potassium channels. It may explain the low but increased incidence of sudden death reportedly associated with antipsychotics.

## Atypical antipsychotics

Atypical antipsychotics are widely used as first-line agents instead of the conventional drugs because of several advantages – some real, some perceived (Table 7.7). Side-effect profiles that differentiate

**Table 7.6** Side-effect profile of selected antipsychotics.

|  | Typical dose (mg/day) | EPS | Prolactin elevation | Anticholinergic side-effects | Sedation | Weight gain |
|---|---|---|---|---|---|---|
| *Conventional* | | | | | | |
| Haloperidol | 2–12 | +++ | +++ | + | + | − |
| Chlorpromazine | 50–400 | ++ | ++ | ++ | ++ | ++ |
| *Atypical* | | | | | | |
| Risperidone | 2–8 | + | ++ | − | − | ++ |
| Olanzapine | 5–20 | − | − | − | +++ | ı ı ı |
| Clozapine | 300–900 | − | − | + | +++ | +++ |

**Table 7.7** Atypical compared with conventional antipsychotics.

---

*Advantages of atypical antipsychotics*
  Fewer EPS (definite)
  Greater overall tolerability (probable)
  Lower risk of tardive dyskinesia (probable)
  Greater overall efficacy (unlikely)
  More efficacy against cognitive symptoms (possible)
  More efficacy against depressive symptoms (possible)
  More efficacy against negative symptoms (unlikely)

*Disadvantages of atypical antipsychotics*
  Metabolic syndrome more likely (probable)
  Weight gain more likely (probable)
  Type 2 diabetes mellitus more likely (possible)
  Stroke more likely in the elderly (possible)

*Specific advantages of clozapine*
  Efficacy in treatment-resistant schizophrenia
    (definite)
  Reduced risk of suicide in schizophrenia (probable)

*Specific disadvantages of clozapine*
  Risk of agranulocytosis
  Need for regular blood tests

---

EPS, extrapyramidal side-effects.

three widely used atypical antipsychotics are shown in Table 7.6.

- There is no good evidence that, as a group, atypical antipsychotics are meaningfully more effective than conventional antipsychotics.
- *Risperidone* has the best long-term evidence for efficacy and, unlike other atypical antipsychotics, is available as a depot injection.
- *Olanzapine* has the next largest body of evidence for its effectiveness and may be slightly more effective than atypical agents other than clozapine; its sedative effects can be useful. Equally, it probably has a greater propensity to cause metabolic syndrome (see below).
- *Amisulpride* may have some efficacy against negative symptoms.
- *Quetiapine* is very sedating.
- *Aripiprazole* has a different mode of action, it is a dopamine partial agonist. This means it 'stabilizes' dopamine—antagonizing it when levels are high and mimicking it when dopamine is low. It is not

yet clear whether this translates into tangible clinical benefits.

However, atypical antipsychotics also have potential disadvantages (Table 7.7):
- *Weight gain.* This varies between drugs, and also occurs with some typical antipsychotics. Clozapine and olanzapine are the worst culprits, with mean weight gains of about 5 kg over 6 months. A genetic polymorphism in the 5-HT$_{2C}$ receptor may contribute to individual vulnerability to weight gain.
- *Hyperglycaemia and type 2 diabetes.* There is an increased incidence of type 2 diabetes in patients with schizophrenia, and their relatives, and in people taking antipsychotics, and it is now known that atypical drugs (particularly olanzapine and clozapine) can induce hyperglycaemia and insulin resistance.
- The above two elements are part of *metabolic syndrome* which also comprises dyslipidaemia and hypertension. It markedly increases risk of death from cardiovascular disease, and should be screened for before and during treatment with any antipsychotic. Various monitoring guidelines have been produced; one is summarized in Table 7.8, along with the principles of management.
- *Stroke.* Atypical antipsychotics should not be used routinely in dementia because of some evidence that they increase the risk of stroke (Chapter 13). Caution should also be applied in all elderly patients.

## Clozapine

Clozapine is a unique antipsychotic, being effective in 30% of patients with schizophrenia resistant to, or intolerant of, all other antipsychotics. It may also reduce suicide risk in schizophrenia.
- It is not clear how clozapine achieves its greater efficacy. It may block dopamine receptors in a different way, or it may be the particular combination of additional receptors that it blocks.
- Clozapine does not have clearly greater efficacy against negative or cognitive symptoms.

Unfortunately, clozapine causes agranulocytosis. Although rare (1–2%), it means that:

**Table 7.8** Metabolic syndrome: monitoring and management in patients taking antipsychotics.

---

*Before treatment*
History of hypertension, cardiovascular disease, diabetes, obesity
Blood pressure and pulse
Weight and height (to calculate BMI)
Waist and hip circumference (and the ratio)
Glucose and lipid levels (does not need to be fasting)
Glycosylated haemoglobin
Agree responsibilities with GP (who will monitor, who will treat)

*Every clinic appointment*
Weight (calculate BMI)
Waist and hip circumference (and the ratio)
Blood pressure and pulse

*Every 3 months for first year, then annually*
Glucose and lipid profile

*Annually*
Glycosylated haemoglobin

*Management of abnormalities*
Advice and information, e.g. on dieting, exercise
Switch to antipsychotic with less propensity to metabolic syndrome
Treat diabetes, hypertension, hyperlipidaemias in usual way

---

- Clozapine is reserved for patients with schizophrenia who have not responded to, or are intolerant of, at least two other antipsychotics.
- Regular (weekly) blood tests are mandatory to monitor the white cell count, and patients must be registered with a monitoring service. This means the drug often needs to be (temporarily) stopped if the white cell count falls; it also makes the drug expensive.
- Other important side-effects of clozapine are weight gain, metabolic syndrome, hypersalivation and sedation. Seizures can occur at high dose. Plasma levels can be monitored.

## Anticholinergics

These drugs (e.g. procyclidine, benztropine) are used to counteract EPS resulting from the use of antipsychotics. They have no therapeutic role in themselves.

- *Mode of action.* They block muscarinic receptors. Their use may seem paradoxical given that other side-effects of antipsychotics are attributed to the same action (Table 7.5). The rationale is that they restore a dopaminergic–cholinergic balance in the basal ganglia.
- *Practical usage.* Procyclidine can also be given parenterally to reverse acute dystonias.
- *Side-effects.* Can exacerbate psychosis and cause delirium, memory impairment and euphoria. The anticholinergic side-effects of the antipsychotic may be worsened.
- *Cautions and contraindications.* Prophylactic and long-term use, though widespread, should be avoided for three reasons: (1) the efficacy of antipsychotics is maximal at a dose below that at which EPS occur, so reducing the dose is the logical response to these side-effects; (2) the long-term use of anticholinergics may increase the risk of tardive dyskinesia; and (3) anticholinergics may be misused because of the euphoric effect.

## Drugs for dementia

Several drugs are now licensed to treat Alzheimer's disease (Chapter 13). They have a small beneficial effect on cognition in the short to medium term, but do not modify the course of the disease.

## Cholinesterase inhibitors

*Acetylcholinesterase inhibitors* (e.g. donepezil, rivastigmine, galantamine) are used in the treatment of mild to moderate Alzheimer's disease.

- *Mode of action.* Inhibit the synaptic breakdown of acetylcholine, which is decreased in Alzheimer's disease and necessary for memory and cognitive functioning. Galantamine also stimulates nicotinic cholinergic receptors.
- *Uses.* Modestly improve cognitive function. Do not modify the disease process.
- *Practical usage.* Limited to specialist clinics and require formal assessments before and during treatment, including tests of cognitive, global and behavioural functioning, and activities of daily living.

- *Side-effects*. Anorexia, nausea, vomiting and diarrhoea can occur.

## N-Methyl-D-aspartate (NMDA) receptor antagonists

*Memantine* is licensed for moderate and severe Alzheimer's disease.
- *Mode of action*. Memantine blocks the effects of glutamate at the NMDA receptor, decreasing the potential neurotoxic effects of increased glutamate that may occur in Alzheimer's disease.
- *Practical usage*. As for cholinesterase inhibitors.
- *Side-effects*. Usually well tolerated but may cause dizziness, headache and hallucinations.

# Drugs for substance dependence

Drugs are available to help withdrawal, maintain abstinence or control intake of various substances. The beneficial effect of these drugs is relatively modest.

## Alcohol dependence

*Disulfiram (Antabuse)*:
- *Mode of action*. Interferes with alcohol metabolism by blocking one of the enzymes involved. If alcohol is consumed, acetaldehyde accumulates, leading to flushing, headache, choking sensations, tachycardia and anxiety.
- *Uses*. As a deterrent to drinking alcohol in people motivated to use the drug.
- *Practical usage*. Usually employed in specialist practice in combination with non-drug treatments.
- *Side-effects*. Sedation and nausea.
- *Cautions and contraindications*. Avoid in heart disease, suicide risk, psychosis or severe liver disease.
*Acamprosate*:
- *Mode of action*. Unknown, probably acts via GABA and glutamate receptors.
- *Uses*. Used to reduce craving in abstinent patients.
- *Practical usage*. Used in specialist practice, in combination with other non-drug treatments.
- *Side-effects*. Diarrhoea, nausea.

## Opiate dependence

*Opiate agonists*:
- *Mode of action*. *Methadone* is an opiate agonist and an effective substitute for other opiates such as heroin. *Buprenorphine* is a partial agonist, effective in patients with moderate dependence, but which may precipitate withdrawal in patients with severe dependence.
- *Uses*. To reduce craving and withdrawal symptoms.
- *Practical usage*. Used by specialists in combination with other medical and psychological treatments.
- *Side-effects*. Drowsiness, nausea and vomiting, constipation, respiratory depression.
- *Cautions and contraindications*. Acute respiratory depression or raised intracranial pressure.
*Opiate antagonists*:
- *Mode of action*. *Naltrexone* blocks the effects of opiates and precipitates withdrawal symptoms.
- *Uses*. To block the effect of opiates in patients after withdrawal.
- *Practical usage*. Used only in specialist clinics at a usual dose of 50 mg daily.
- *Side-effects*. Nausea and vomiting.
- *Cautions and contraindications*. Do not use in patients currently dependent on opiates or with acute hepatitis or liver failure.

## Nicotine dependence

*Nicotine replacement therapy* is usually considered to be the drug treatment of choice in managing smoking cessation.
- *Mode of action*. Replaces the nicotine provided by cigarettes (which is what makes them addictive).
- *Uses*. Reduces craving and withdrawal symptoms in patients after stopping smoking.
- *Practical usage*. No prescription needed. Available as patches, chewing gum, nasal spray or inhaler. Varies depending on preparation: up to 15 pieces of gum per day.
- *Side-effects*. Nausea, dizziness and flu-like symptoms.
- *Contraindications*. Seizure disorders or eating disorders.

*Bupropion*

- *Mode of action.* Weakly inhibits reuptake of dopamine, 5-HT and NA. Used in the USA as an antidepressant; unclear if this contributes to its (modest) efficacy in smoking cessation.
- *Uses.* Reduce craving and withdrawal symptoms in patients after stopping smoking
- *Practical usage.* Dose: 300 mg daily.
- *Side-effects.* Dry mouth, gastrointestinal upset and insomnia.
- *Contraindications.* Seizure disorders or eating disorders.

## Prescribing in specific groups

Special care is needed when prescribing for patients who are pregnant, breastfeeding, children or elderly. Many drugs are not approved for use in these groups, but nevertheless are widely used. As a rule:

- Choose a well-established drug, and the lowest possible dose.
- Consult the *British National Formulary* or other expert source first.
- Review the need for, and contraindications to, every drug.
- Ensure the patient (or carer) is aware of possible side-effects.
- Monitor closely. If in doubt, stop drug and review.

### Pregnancy

Strike a balance between the wish to avoid all drugs for the sake of the foetus, and the potential adverse effects on mother (and foetus) of leaving the psychiatric disorder untreated. Few drugs are established as completely safe in pregnancy (or when breastfeeding), so use all drugs cautiously and ensure that the mother is fully aware of the known risks and benefits, and also the uncertainties.

- *Antidepressants.* TCAs and SSRIs (and ECT) are not contraindicated. There is some evidence of an increase in the risk of congenital malformations on paroxetine, so it is best to avoid this drug where possible. The use of a TCA near term may result in

a 'twitchy' baby. The dose requirement increases in the third trimester. There is most evidence for the safety of amitriptyline and fluoxetine.

- *Mood stabilizers.* As a rule, avoid lithium and valproic acid, especially around conception and first trimester, due to a small but clear teratogenicity risk. Use of lithium near term may result in neonatal hypothyroidism.
- *Anxiolytics and hypnotics.* These are best avoided.
- *Antipsychotics.* EPS may occur in the baby if these are taken near term.

### Breastfeeding

Most drugs are excreted into the breast milk. Therefore, weigh up the need for medication against the mothers wishes to breastfeed and the risks of doing so. As in pregnancy, always proceed with caution and seek expert advice.

- *Antidepressants.* TCAs (especially amitriptyline, imipramine) and SSRIs are probably safe. MAOIs are not recommended.
- *Mood stabilizers.* If lithium is used, the baby should be monitored. Carbamazepine, valproate and lamotrigine are probably safe.
- *Anxiolytics and hypnotics.* Avoid benzodiazepines as they can make the baby lethargic and cause failure to thrive.
- *Antipsychotics.* These can sedate the baby and are not recommended.

### Children

The prescribing of psychotropic drugs for children is best left to child psychiatrists. See Chapter 16.

### The elderly

In general, prescribe at lower doses or increased intervals to compensate for the slower metabolism and excretion in the elderly. Always consider medication as a cause of delirium (Chapter 13).

- *Antidepressants.* TCAs may cause delirium (due to their anticholinergic effects) and falls (due to postural hypotension). SSRIs are therefore preferable if sedation is not needed.
- *Mood stabilizers.* These are not contraindicated.

- *Antipsychotics*. Best avoided in dementia (see above).
- *Anxiolytics and hypnotics*. Notorious for causing delirium and falls. Avoid.

## Other biological treatments

### Electroconvulsive therapy (ECT)

ECT is an effective and safe treatment for severe depression although it can have some negative effects on cognitive function, especially memory. Its bad press reflects understandable fears, misinformation and its past misuse. Current guidelines are intended to ensure its use is limited, and made as safe, effective and acceptable as possible.

- *Mode of action*. Unknown. ECT has many effects in the brain. It may act on monoamines, producing the same result as antidepressants.
- *Clinical indications*. ECT is mainly used for, and has the best evidence of effectiveness in, severe depression including depressive stupor and depressive psychosis. The response is often better than drug therapy and may be dramatic. It is also used for puerperal psychosis and treatment-resistant depression and mania.
- *Practical usage*. Obtain informed consent, or use the Mental Health Act (MHA). Always do a physical examination, and obtain an ECG and routine blood tests first. During a brief general anaesthetic with muscle relaxant, an electric charge (~300 mC) is passed across the head to produce a generalized seizure of 30–60 seconds. Treatment can be bilateral, with one electrode on each temple, or unilateral into the non-dominant hemisphere. Bilateral ECT is slightly more effective but causes more short-term memory impairment. ECT is usually given twice a week for 6–12 treatments. A good response is predicted by a greater severity of depression, and a past response to ECT.
- *Side-effects*. Anaesthetic effects—nausea, dry mouth and headache. Memory loss occurs for the hours surrounding the seizure. Significant long-term memory loss is sometimes reported by patients; objectively, subtle deficits in recall of personal memories may occur (but it is unclear if this is due to ECT or to the depressive disorder).

Nonetheless, it should be discussed when obtaining consent. No neuropathological effects of ECT have been found, even following multiple treatments.

- *Cautions and contraindications*. Few, and mainly related to anaesthetic risk. Avoid if the patient has a suspected intracranial lesion (as intracranial pressure rises during seizure). ECT can be given in conjunction with antidepressants and antipsychotics. ECT is extremely safe, with a mortality rate of 5 per 100 000 treatments.

### Psychosurgery

In the 1940s and 1950s—prior to the introduction of antidepressants and antipsychotics—thousands of patients each year were operated on to sever pathways between frontal lobes and limbic structures. Psychosurgery is still used very occasionally for intractable OCD and depressive disorder, but only after wide consultations under the MHA and never without informed consent. Modern stereotactic procedures avoid most of the earlier complications (haemorrhage, seizures and death).

- Recent case series suggest worthwhile improvement in one-third of patients—at the expense of some frontal lobe impairment, and with continuing ethical concerns about the principle.

## Psychological treatments (the psychotherapies)

All medical treatments require an interaction between doctor and patient. This interaction is a major determinant both of the patient's satisfaction with the consultation and of their subsequent adherence to the recommended treatment. 'Psychotherapy' in the sense of a helpful relationship is consequently a part of all medical practice, whether the doctor realizes it or not. However, the term is normally applied to specific psychological treatments, the main ones being psychodynamic psychotherapy, behavioural therapy, cognitive therapy and cognitive behavioural therapy (CBT). We first consider non-specific factors common to all psychotherapies, and then the specific characteristics of each one.

- Box 7.4 is a historical note on the position of psychotherapy in medicine.

## Factors common to all psychotherapies

All psychotherapy is based on general or non-specific therapeutic factors. The therapist:

- Is credible and has a plausible rationale for what they do.
- Behaves in an empathic and interested fashion.
- Instils hope of improvement in the patient.

Similarly, to be successful, all forms psychotherapy need attention to several practical issues:

- *Select the right therapy for the right patient.* Take account of factors predictive of good outcome to psychotherapy in general (e.g. motivation) as well as pros and cons of a specific therapy.

- *Prepare the patient for therapy.* Many people have either no idea, or the wrong idea, of what psychotherapy is and what it involves.
- *Ensure the therapy is available.* Many treatments are not widely available, or have long waiting lists.

## The evidence base for psychotherapy

Psychotherapies have been less well evaluated than drugs, partly due to the practical difficulties of doing so and partly because of the absence of pharmaceutical industry funding for trials. However, there have now been many good randomized trials and systematic reviews, and there is good quality evidence for specific psychotherapies, especially cognitive and behavioural therapies, in several disorders, as outlined below.

## Adverse effects of psychotherapy

Like all medical treatments, psychotherapy can have adverse as well as beneficial effects. These are more likely with poorly trained and unsupervised therapists and with therapists who are in a position to deliberately exploit the patient.

- Even well-delivered therapy can be ineffective or harmful. An example is requiring patients who have suffered a trauma to talk about it in great detail to a therapist (so-called *debriefing*).

## Simple forms of psychotherapy

Simple psychotherapies are formalized versions of the therapeutic component of all doctor–patient relationships, as mentioned in Chapter 1 and at the start of this section.

- *Psychoeducation* is the provision of information to people to help them to understand and cope with the illness. Psychoeducation may take place individually or in groups, and will usually take the person's own strengths and coping strategies into account.
- *Counselling* is a loosely defined activity whereby people are helped to overcome or cope with life's problems. The counsellor serves as a support, a facilitator of emotional expression, a source of information and as someone off whom ideas can

be bounced. Counselling is provided in many settings, mostly non-psychiatric. There is evidence for its short-term effectiveness in mild neuroses and stress-related disorders.

- *Supportive psychotherapy* is a formalized version of what a good friend might provide: listening, accepting and encouraging. All health professionals—as well as relatives and friends—provide supportive psychotherapy whether they realize it or not. It does not aim to produce change, but rather to help people cope with adversity or insoluble problems over a sustained period.
- *Problem-solving therapy* is a structured mix of counselling and CBT. It helps the patient learn to deal actively with life's problems—by specifying them, selecting an option for tackling each one, trying out solutions and reviewing the effect. It is effective in mild neurotic and depressive disorders and can be given effectively by GPs and nurses.

## The major types of specific psychotherapy

The major psychotherapies can be divided into two classes: those that are descendants of psychoa-nalysis (i.e. psychodynamic psychotherapy) and those which are based upon behavioural and cognitive theories. The key differences are highlighted in Table 7.9.

## Psychodynamic psychotherapy

Psychodynamic therapy is usually a time-intensive and lengthy process that may go on for months or even years. With the arrival of the more evidence-based, briefer (and more widely available) psychotherapies outlined below, psychodynamic psychotherapy now has a lesser role, and its provision on the NHS is very limited. Nevertheless it remains important to know about its principles and its contemporary indications. Several psychodynamic concepts also remain useful throughout medicine (Box 7.5).

The principles of psychodynamic psychotherapy are:

- Emotional and interpersonal problems result from unconscious processes, driven by psychological mechanisms and internal representations (of people and things) developed early in life.
- These processes can be revealed and resolved by gaining access to the unconscious mind. The thera-

Table 7.9 Comparison of the two major classes of psychotherapy.

|  | Psychodynamic psychotherapy | Other psychotherapies |
| --- | --- | --- |
| Examples | Psychoanalysis<br>Psychodynamic therapy | Behaviour therapy<br>Cognitive behavioural therapy |
| Focus | Unconscious phenomena | Observable phenomena and behaviour |
| Time focus | The past (as evidenced in the present) | The present |
| Aim | Insight and self-understanding, thence altered interpersonal behaviour | Direct, practice-driven change in behaviour and/or cognitions |
| Practical issues | Therapist listens and interprets<br>Sessions unstructured | Therapist explains<br>Sessions highly structured |
| Therapist | Extensive training (years)<br>Usually psychiatrists<br>Key is therapist's skills and attributes | Briefer training (months)<br>Psychologists, psychiatrists, nurses<br>Key is adherence to treatment manual |
| Duration | Unspecified, can be prolonged (years) | Agreed number of sessions (e.g. 8) |
| Efficacy | Largely unknown | Proven in trials |
| Main indications | Difficulties with relationships<br>Some personality disorders | Depressive disorders<br>Neuroses and somatoform disorders<br>Eating disorders |

**Box 7.5 Psychodynamic concepts of continuing value**

• *Transference*. The feelings and attitudes a patient develops toward their therapist. They are considered to have been transferred onto the therapist from another relationship, usually that with a parent. It is important to consider transference during any doctor–patient relationship if a patient starts to behave in an unexpected or unusual way (e.g. inappropriate signs of affection, or threatening self-harm if an extra appointment is not given).
• *Counter-transference*. The feelings the therapist may develop toward the patient (e.g. excessive involvement, attraction or dislike). Counter-transference is a response to the patient's transference but is also influenced by the therapist's own past experiences and relationships. It is important for all doctors to be aware of the emotions invoked in them by patients, to try and understand their origins and ensure they do not affect their ability to treat the patient effectively.
• Psychological *defence mechanisms* (see Table 6.2).

pist can do this in various ways (e.g. free association, hypnosis, dream analysis).

• The therapist is particularly interested in the patient's pattern of previous relationships, evidenced most directly by the way the patient interacts with the therapist (transference; Box 7.5).
• The therapist makes interpretations about what the patient says, and draws connections between events and feelings that he conveys to the patient.
• During therapy, the patient is expected to gain insight into their emotions and behaviour as a result of the interpretations.
• The therapeutic effect may emerge directly from greater self-understanding, and be promoted (reinforced) by new patterns of behaviour and relating which arise from it.

Psychodynamic therapy is now used mainly for people with 'personality difficulties', especially recurrent problems with relationships. It also has a role in chronic neuroses and depressive disorders resistant to other drug and psychological treatments. It should be avoided in people with paranoid or antisocial personality disorder, and in those with psychosis.

• *Brief psychodynamic psychotherapy* compresses psychodynamically oriented therapy into a more feasible 10–20 session course. The therapist takes a more active role than in traditional psychoanalysis and focuses on particular issues. There is evidence for its efficacy in depression.

## Behaviour therapy

Behaviour therapy arose from the behavioural theories of experimental psychology (Chapter 6). It is effective in anxiety disorders (especially phobias and OCD) and in behavioural problems in people with learning disability. The central idea is that adaptive behaviours can be learned and maladaptive behaviours unlearned.

*Exposure* is a key component of behavioural treatment. Either the patient is reintroduced (re-exposed) to a situation or behaviour he has come to avoid (e.g. an agoraphobic leaving the house), or he learns to stop an inappropriate, excessive response (e.g. recurrent hand washing in OCD). Exposure is usually graded (graded exposure).
• Sudden and prolonged exposure (*flooding*)—such as shutting a claustrophobic in a lift until the panic subsides—also works, but is too unpleasant for routine use.

The elements of graded exposure are:
• The therapist assesses the problem behaviour, its antecedents and consequences. He explains the nature of the treatment and its rationale to the patient.
• A step-by-step programme is developed jointly with the patient. Homework tasks are set which re-expose the patient to the situation to a degree that produces a tolerable level of anxiety. The patient finds that each extra exposure increases anxiety, but that it then subsides. In this way the patient is desensitized to the stimulus.
• Subsequent sessions review progress and problems, and set the next series of tasks.

*Mr Q had not been out of his house for 2 years, fearful he might faint in the street. His therapist elicited a detailed account of the problem, how it started and its effect on Mr Q. She explained what behavioural treatment was and how it worked. She agreed a plan with Mr Q to do a task* he felt he could just manage: to walk to his front gate and stand there for 20 minutes. He felt anxious doing so, but achieved this goal several times in homework sessions. He found that as he stood there the anxiety subsided. He was then encouraged to move to the next steps by walking increasing distances from his house. He was able to do the shopping again, which reinforced his feeling of success. During the agreed 12 sessions he made steady progress that was maintained thereafter.

Many other treatments and techniques are based on the premise that changing behaviour and other bodily functions, such as muscular tone and posture, helps mental well-being. They include relaxation training, assertiveness training, biofeedback and social skills training. They are available in occupational therapy and physiotherapy departments, from private therapists and by using self-help manuals.

## Cognitive therapy

The aim of cognitive therapy is to correct inaccurate or unhelpful ways of thinking, with the aim of improving mood, reducing anxiety and allowing return to normal behaviour. The main components are:
• The therapist obtains a detailed description of the problem, paying particular attention to the thoughts (cognitions) the patient has when experiencing the problem.
• The therapist provides an explanation (formulation) of the role of cognitions in perpetuating the problem to the patient.
• The patient is then taught how to become aware of and to challenge the negative and inaccurate cognitions and to practise thinking in more accurate and helpful ways.
• The therapeutic techniques include education about the role of cognitions and their consequences on emotion and behaviour; becoming more aware of the occurrence of particular thoughts and inferences using diaries; and doing 'experiments' to test cognitions against alternatives.

Ms R had a depressive disorder. Her therapist helped her identify a number of negative cognitions that made her feel depressed (including 'nobody likes me' and 'there's no point trying to change anything, it won't help'). The therapist formulated the depression as being maintained by the effect of these cognitions on her mood and behaviour. He helped Ms R become aware of the distorted and negative slant to her cognitions. Ms R was helped to make alternative cognitions ('not everybody likes me but I have evidence that some people do' and 'some things probably will help and if I don't try I won't find out') and practised challenging the thoughts and replacing them with more positive ones. She became skilled at doing this and her mood and activity improved. At follow-up a year later she remained well, and was using the techniques she had learned whenever she felt negative cognitions or low mood creeping back.

## Cognitive behavioural therapy (CBT)

In practice, cognitive and behavioural treatments are usually combined as CBT. In phobic anxiety, for example, this would involve working both on cognitions and on graded exposure. There is good evidence for the efficacy of CBT (with varying proportions of C and B) in many disorders:
• In mild to moderate depressive disorder, CBT is at least as effective as antidepressant drugs.
• In panic disorder and phobic anxiety, CBT is probably the most effective treatment; the benefits are more persistent than with anxiolytics, and avoid the problems of the latter.
• There is good evidence of efficacy in other neuroses, including somatoform disorders and OCD.
• A modified form of CBT is the most effective treatment in bulimia nervosa.
• CBT has some effect against psychotic symptoms in schizophrenia.
• There is inconsistent evidence that CBT prevents relapse in bipolar disorder.

### Other psychotherapies

#### Hybrid therapies

The distinction between the two major types of therapy in Table 7.9 is oversimplified and there are

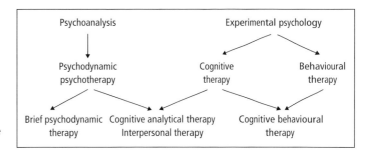

**Figures 7.2** Links between the psychotherapies.

several hybrid therapies (Figure 7.2), and other therapies that have additional components. None is widely available in the UK.

• *Cognitive analytical therapy* (CAT) combines a cognitive approach and psychoanalytic concepts. It is used in depression and other conditions.

• *Interpersonal therapy* (IPT) uses cognitive, behavioural and psychodynamic concepts and techniques to focus on the patient's relationships and the problems arising from them. Limited evidence suggests similar efficacy to CBT in depression and bulimia nervosa.

• *Dialectical behavioural therapy* (DBT) was developed specifically for people with borderline type personality disorder. It combines psychoeducation with behavioural skills training, creating a strong therapeutic relationship.

• *Eye movement desensitization and reprocessing* (EMDR) is used in people with post-traumatic stress disorder.

## Group therapy

Many of the psychotherapies have been adapted to treat several people at once. Group therapy originated from the view that it is therapeutic to share experiences and feelings, and to examine the relationships that form in a group.

• Most therapies including CBT can be given effectively in a group format for the same indications as individual therapy. Some patients like groups but others don't.

• A therapeutic community is a form of psychodynamic group therapy where the participants are resident for 6–12 months. It is mainly used in attempts to treat personality disorder.

## Family therapy

Family therapy is based upon the theory that the problem is located in the family rather than in the (child) patient. The family 'system' is therefore the therapeutic target. Psychodynamic, behavioural and other concepts are used. There is some evidence for its efficacy in children with conduct disorder, substance misuse, eating disorders, schizophrenia and bipolar disorder.

## Social treatments

Social factors have major roles in the aetiology and maintenance of many psychiatric disorders. Social factors also determine the environment in which therapy is given and affect its outcome. Equally, social treatments—intervening to change some aspect of the person's circumstances—are themselves important therapeutic interventions.

## Acute social interventions

• *Psychiatric admission* is a major social intervention. It may relieve a crisis at home which is exacerbating the psychiatric disorder, or represent the best means of ensuring a homeless person gets a decent assessment.

• *Crisis intervention* includes practical measures such as finding temporary accommodation, helping get emergency benefits, or daily home visits. Crisis intervention services are currently being introduced, in part to reduce acute admissions.

## Social interventions during psychiatric care

Practical social interventions are needed at some stage in most patients' care.

• Accommodation and financial problems are common. Help with practical matters such as housing, rescheduling debts, etc. can be therapeutic by reducing the stressors that are maintaining the disorder. Involvement of the patient in these processes gives them a sense of mastery over circumstances and improves their practical social skills.

• Family support and education can be an important part of care, even if specific family therapy is not being carried out.

• Social isolation is often a problem for people with psychiatric illness. This can be addressed by home visits, attendance at day centres, putting the person in touch with self-help groups, etc.

• In chronic psychiatric disorder, social and occupational skills and self-confidence are often damaged. Rehabilitation involves continuing support of the kinds outlined above, as well as more extensive interventions such as sheltered accommodation and supported employment.

## The wider social environment

Preventing domestic violence, child abuse and unemployment would no doubt improve the psychological well-being of the population. Whilst such utopian ('primary prevention') goals are not relevant for the management of individual patients, there are measures that can affect their prevalence or impact:

• *Public education.* To increase awareness of psychiatric disorders, and decrease the stigma attached to them and to their treatment.

• *Social policy.* Political decisions alter the social fabric and influence behaviours associated with psychiatric disorder. For example, taxation affects alcohol consumption, and legislation determines the extent of compulsory treatment. Some events are, however, beyond control—for example, the effect of national football results on rates of self-harm.

## Compulsory treatment

The nature of psychiatric disorders means that some people refuse help, even though to do so puts their health or that of others at risk. Psychiatrists in most countries thus sometimes treat people against their will.

• There is continuing debate about balancing the benefits of treatment against infringement of civil liberties.

• The laws relating to mental health differ markedly between countries. They even differ between England and Wales, Scotland and Northern Ireland.

However, before considering mental health law specifically, we raise the broader issue of how consent to treatment is determined, and the circumstances in which treatment may be given in the absence of informed consent: the key word is *capacity*.

• This applies to patients, and doctors, in all branches of medicine.

## Common law and capacity

Treatment without informed consent is technically an assault. However, in an emergency, a doctor may treat a patient without consent if rapid action is called for to save life—for example, to maintain an airway in a comatose patient, or to sedate an uncontrollably delirious patient. Such actions were, until recently, carried out under the *'common law'*, applying the principle that a doctor can and should do what the public would consider reasonable in that situation (and where failing to act would be considered unreasonable). Most such situations are now covered, in England and Wales, by the *Mental Capacity Act* (2005).

• The Mental Capacity Act (MCA) applies to all of medicine, but has particular relevance to psychiatry because capacity can be affected by psychiatric

### Box 7.6  Mental Capacity Act (2005)

**Five key principles**

**1.** Capacity is assumed until proven otherwise
**2.** The person must be helped to make decisions before capacity is judged to be absent (e.g. given time if capacity fluctuates; use of interpreters).
**3.** Patients are entitled to make unwise decisions. It is the process by which a decision is made, not the decision itself, which determines capacity.
**4.** Decisions made for people who lack capacity must be in their best interests.
**5.** Decisions must be the least restrictive option, in terms of their human rights.

**Other elements**

● Independent Mental Capacity Advocates—someone to advocate for those who lack capacity.
● Lasting power of attorney—a person can nominate someone authorized to make decisions for them if they ever lose capacity.
● Advance decisions (directives)—to specify interventions the person would not want if they lost capacity.
● Deprivation of liberty safeguards ('DOLS') introduced in 2009: designed to ensure that patients who lack capacity are not subject to undue restraints of their liberty. Particularly applies to patients in nursing homes with dementia.
● Expanded court of protection—to arbitrate on a wide range of capacity issues.
● Clinicians are expected to respect all the above elements.
● Failures to comply with the Act are potentially criminal offences.

**Figures 7.3** Assessing mental capacity. The starting assumption should always be that the person has capacity. If the assessment is being done under the Mental Capacity Act, demonstration of lack of capacity is followed by several steps before deciding on actions, following the principles of the Act (Box 7.6).

MCA jurisdiction or not, it is important to be able to assess capacity (see Figure 7.3).
● About 30% of in-patients on acute medical wards, and 45% on psychiatric wards, lack capacity.
● *Competency* is a concept closely related to capacity, and a widely used term (e.g. with regard to making a Will), but it is not defined legally in the present context.

disorders, and because psychiatrists may be seen as having particular expertise.
● The MCA is separate from the MHA, discussed below, and the two Acts use different criteria and standards. People detained under the MHA commonly but not always lack capacity.

## Mental Capacity Act (2005) and the assessment of capacity

Some people, some of the time, lack the *capacity* to consent to (or refuse) treatment. The MCA aims to identify and protect these people. It has five key principles (Box 7.6). Whether working under the

## Mental Health Act (1983, amended 2007)

Compulsory psychiatric admission and treatment in England and Wales is carried out under Sections of the 1983 MHA, amended in 2007 (Box 7.7 and Table 7.10).
● The 2007 Act is an amendment of the 1983 Act; many aspects remain unchanged.
● All doctors need to know about Section 5(2).
● GPs are involved in most Sections.
● Scotland has different regulations, and is covered by the Mental Health Care and Treatment Act (Scotland) 2003 (Table 7.11).
● In the MHA, 'mental disorder' is used instead of 'psychiatric disorder', and has a legal definition.

## Box 7.7 Key aspects of the Mental Health Act (1983/2007)

- The behaviour must be the result of a known or suspected 'mental disorder' (defined in the Act). Disruptive behaviour, intoxication, drug abuse and dependence are not of themselves grounds for detention.
- The person must be at acute, significant risk of self-harm, self-neglect or harming others.
- The person must have refused voluntary treatment.
- Other options have been considered but are not appropriate.
- There must be an appropriate medical treatment available to the patient.
- Implementing most Sections involves an application from one of two people. (1) An Approved Mental Health Professional (AHMP), usually a senior social worker. (A nearest relative can apply instead of an AMHP, but this is very rare.). (2) Based on two medical recommendations, one a Responsible Clinician (RC), usually a senior psychiatrist, approved under Section 12 of the Act; the other doctor is usually the GP or another doctor who knows the patient.
- Detained patients can appeal to hospital managers or to a Mental Health Review tribunal for the Section to be discharged. A Section is discharged by the RC once the patient's mental state no longer justifies it, and/or when he adheres consistently to treatment.
- There is an independent Mental Health Advocate scheme.
- There is a legal Code of Practice which all professionals must take note of.
- The Act only covers treatments for psychiatric disorder. It cannot be used if a patient refuses treatment for a medical problem—such as setting a fracture or providing dialysis.

## Section 2: admission for assessment

- *Uses*. Assessment of a suspected mental disorder. It would apply, for example, to a man who set fire to his car because he believed it was demonically possessed, or to a depressed woman who has tried to kill herself. Drug treatment can be given without consent, but use Section 3 once compulsory treatment becomes the main reason for in-patient care.
- *Applied for by*: AHMP (Box 7.7) in consultation with the nearest relative. Medical recommendation from an RC and another doctor (usually the GP). The AHMP must have seen the person within the past 14 days, the doctors within 5 days.
- *Duration*: 28 days.
- *Right of appeal*: in first 14 days, to the Mental Health Review Tribunal (MHRT).

**Table 7.10** Key Mental Health Act Sections and their uses.

| Situation | Section |
|---|---|
| Psychiatric admission, for assessment | 2 |
| Psychiatric admission, for treatment | 3 |
| Psychiatric admission, when no psychiatrist is available | 4 |
| Stopping an in-patient leaving a hospital | 5(2) |
| For police to find and take person to a safe place | 135 |
| For police to take person from a public place to a safe place | 136 |
| Psychiatric assessment or treatment of prisoners and those on remand | 35–38, 41 |

**Table 7.11** Key Sections of the Scottish Mental Health (Care and Treatment) Act 2003.

| Situation | Section | Duration | Applicants |
|---|---|---|---|
| Emergency detention | 36(1) | 72 hours | Registered doctor[a], plus MHO[b] if available |
| Nurses' holding power | 299 | 2 hours | Registered specialist nurse |
| Short-term detention | 44(1) | 28 days | Approved doctor[c] and MHO |
| Compulsory treatment order | 64(4) | 6 months | Two doctors, one approved, plus MHO, plus approval of mental health review tribunal |

[a]Registered doctor: any doctor registered with the General Medical Council.
[b]MHO: Mental Health Officer, a specially trained social worker.
[c]Approved doctor: a psychiatrist approved under the Act.

## Section 3: admission for treatment

- *Uses*. For an established mental disorder (in practice, often schizophrenia) where admission is intended to alleviate the condition or prevent deterioration.
- *Applied for by*: as for Section 2. Cannot normally proceed if the nearest relative objects.
- *Duration*: 6 months, renewable. Section 3 patients can go on leave for up to 6 months on a *Section 17*. Before discharge, a *Section 117 meeting* is held to discuss future management; there are statutory responsibilities for subsequent care.
- *Right of appeal*: one per 6 months to the MHRT. Reviews are instituted automatically if no appeal is made.

## Section 4: admission in an emergency

- *Uses*. For compulsory admission when it is urgent and a second medical recommendation cannot be obtained. Can't be used just because it is easier to organize than a Section 2.
- *Applied for by*: AHMP or nearest relative. Medical recommendation by any doctor, usually GP.
- *Duration*: 72 hours, during which a full assessment for a Section 2 or 3 is made.
- *Right of appeal*: none.

## Section 5(2): emergency detention of an in-patient

- *Uses*. A '5-2' prevents a patient leaving any hospital where to do so would put their health in jeopardy. For example, a patient on a medical ward who is confused post-operatively and tries to run off, drip stand in tow, can be stopped at first under the MCA but, if the attempt to leave persists, a Section 5(2) should be used. A Section 5(2) does not allow treatment to be enforced. [A Section 5(4) is used by psychiatric nurses to detain a psychiatric in-patient for 6 hours if no psychiatrist is to hand.]
- *Applied for by*: the doctor in charge of the treatment of the patient, or their nominee (in practice, a consultant or junior doctor in the team, but not a Foundation doctor). In a general hospital, this means the physicians managing the patient, ideally in consultation with a liaison psychiatrist.
- *Duration*: 72 hours, during which a full MHA assessment is carried out. Once completed, the Section 5 is converted to a Section 2, or a Section 3 is instituted, or it lapses.
- *Right of appeal*: none.

## Other Sections

- *Section 135* allows the police to enter private property and take a person to a nominated place of safety (e.g. a hospital or police station) for 72 hours. It is requested by an AMHP and granted by a magistrate.
- *Section 136* empowers the police to take someone in a public place who they suspect has a mental disorder (e.g. because of bizarre behaviour) to a safe place (police station, hospital). Lasts for 72 hours.
- *Sections 35–38* are used by a Court to send offenders to hospital for psychiatric assessment or treatment. *Sections 47* and *48* allow for transfer of a prisoner or other detainees to hospital.
- ECT may not be given without consent to detained patients, unless it is necessary to prevent death or deterioration. A second opinion must be obtained and Section 58 completed before the course of ECT proceeds.

## Supervised Community Treatment

The 2007 MHA amendment introduced *Community Treatment Orders (CTOs)*, allowing compulsory treatment in the community as well as in hospital —a controversial change. CTOs apply to a restricted set of patients and circumstances:

- The patient is currently detained under Section 3. Thus they have a severe and chronic psychiatric disorder, most commonly schizophrenia, which continues to meet the criteria for detention under the MHA.
- A CTO is designed for patients with cycles of relapse and readmission ('revolving door patients') associated with treatment non-compliance in the community, and for whom the structure and monitoring provided by a CTO may be valuable.

- A CTO is necessary for the patient's health or safety, or for the protection of others.
- The appropriate treatment does not require the patient to remain in hospital.
- A CTO lasts 6 months and is renewable.

Before initiating a CTO, a risk assessment is performed to assess the risk of relapse, and its consequences. The application is made by the RC, and an AHMP must agree. A CTO means that the patient must make themselves available for examination as requested by the RC (e.g. to attend clinic for review of their mental state, or to receive depot medication). The RC can also recall the person to hospital for treatment.

- A CTO does not include physical restraint to administer medication in the community without consent.
- It is unclear how many patients will be subject to CTOs, and their worth and ethics continue to be debated. Their use in practice is an alternative to the option for 6 months' hospital leave under Section 17 (see above).

## Other aspects of the law and psychiatry

Forensic psychiatrists specialize in the law, but all psychiatrists find themselves involved with the law from time to time. Not all issues are strictly related to treatment, but they are summarized here for convenience.

- *The law and child psychiatry.* Children under 16 are subject to different laws and conventions, and there are additional safeguards for 16 and 17 year olds. The main legislation is the Children's Act (1989). Consult a child psychiatric team or social services for advice.
- *Writing legal reports.* Psychiatrists may be asked to write a report on a patient who has been charged with an offence, usually to give an opinion as to whether psychiatric factors contributed to the offence or influence how it should be dealt with. They may also be asked to write a report concerning the psychiatric consequences of an accident as part of a compensation claim.

- *Fitness to enter into contracts.* Psychiatric opinion may be sought regarding the person's capacity (or competence) to make a will, get married, etc. These issues are now covered by the MCA.
- *Fitness to drive.* Psychiatric disorders and medications can impair driving by affecting judgement or concentration. Psychiatrists should warn patients of this and of their duty to inform the relevant authority. A person may not drive for 6 months after a psychotic episode. People with dementia (even mild cases) have an excess of accidents and should be discouraged from driving.
- *Confidentiality.* There are exceptional circumstances that over-ride the principle of medical confidentiality in psychiatry. For example, if a patient tells you he is going to murder his wife (perhaps because of morbid jealousy; Chapter 12), or if you suspect a colleague is unfit to practise, you have a duty to act. If unsure, always seek advice and keep notes.

### Key points

- Psychiatric disorders are treated with drugs (psychopharmacology) and/or psychological methods (psychotherapy). Social interventions are also important.
- The main classes of drugs are antidepressants, antipsychotics, mood stabilizers and anxiolytics. The most common form of psychological treatment in primary care is simple counselling, and in psychiatric services is CBT.
- The choice of treatment depends upon the diagnosis and on other contextual factors, including the patient's preference and history, and treatment availability.
- There is good evidence for the efficacy of most commonly used drugs, but all also have limitations and side-effects. CBT is of proven benefit for several disorders but has limited availability.
- Involve patients fully in treatment decisions.
- Always assess capacity, and act appropriately if capacity is lacking, using the principles of the Mental Capacity Act.
- A small minority of patients require compulsory treatment under the Mental Health Act.

# Chapter 8

# Psychiatric services and specialties

This chapter covers how psychiatric services are organized in the NHS. It is via these services that the treatments discussed in Chapter 7 are delivered. It then describes the main features of the various psychiatric specialties.

- Psychiatrists see only a small (and rather unrepresentative) fraction of all people suffering from psychiatric disorders, and the services provided are 'biased' accordingly. In particular, the perspective from general practice—where most patients with psychiatric needs are managed—is very different. This issue is covered in Chapter 18.
- Service organization and service delivery in psychiatry vary markedly from one health care system to another. As with mental health legislation (Chapter 7), there are also some differences within the NHS between England and Wales, Scotland and Northern Ireland.

## Organization of psychiatric services

### Trends in service delivery and organization

Over the past 30 years, psychiatric services have progressively moved out of psychiatric hospitals (asylums) to the other settings shown in Figure 8.1.

*Lecture Notes: Psychiatry*, 10e. By Paul Harrison, John Geddes and Michael Sharpe. Published 2010 by Blackwell Publishing Ltd.

The shift of psychiatry to the community has occurred for several reasons:
- The community is where psychiatric disorders present, and provides their context.
- Public preference and social attitudes.
- In-patient care is often unnecessary and sometimes harmful.
- Economic and political pressures.

Despite these trends, in-patient care remains an important component of psychiatry for several groups:
- Assessment of suspected severe psychiatric disorder.
- Those at significant risk of suicide.
- 'Asylum' for those in crisis.
- Those who may be dangerous to others as a result of psychiatric disorder.
- Treatment of acute schizophrenia, mania and severe depression.
- Longer term care of some patients with dementia, chronic schizophrenia and mental retardation.

As the number of psychiatric hospital beds has fallen, the threshold for admission has risen and an increasing percentage of in-patients are psychotic, disturbed and detained compulsorily. This is especially true in inner cities, and has stimulated efforts to ease the pressure on in-patient facilities. Research suggests that admission can be avoided in approximately 40% of cases by using day hospitals or 'crisis teams'.

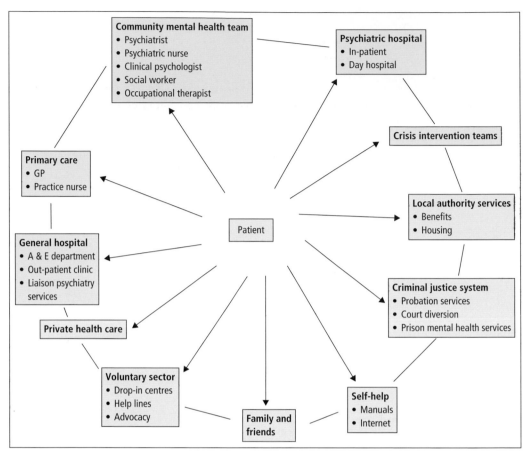

**Figure 8.1** Psychiatric services.

• Crisis intervention services are currently being set up in many areas.

Making the move from hospital to community-based care has posed problems and has led to a gap between the intention and reality of community care:

• Hospital services have been removed before community services are fully in place.

• Community care is not in fact a cheap option, and has been under-resourced.

• A considerable burden is placed upon relatives and carers.

• It is difficult to provide care for some groups of people—the homeless, those with complex psychiatric and social problems, and those whose illness interferes with adherence to treatment.

## Community care

Logically, this term should refer to the management of all psychiatric problems outside a hospital setting; numerically this would mainly comprise the neuroses looked after by GPs. Usually, however, community care means care *within psychiatric services*—patients who tend to be more severely and chronically ill, especially with schizophrenia, severe mood disorder and comorbid conditions.

The main features of contemporary community care in psychiatry are:

• Psychiatric problems are managed at the patient's home, in GP surgeries or in local mental health centres. To facilitate this, the psychiatrists usually divide their responsibility into geographical sectors.

- Care is provided by a *community mental health team* (CMHT; see below).
- Management includes social interventions as well as drug and psychological treatments.
- Admission is reserved for severe episodes of illness and crises.
- Most patients are treated with their consent. A few need some form of legal coercion, under the Mental Health Act (Chapter 7).

## Multidisciplinary teams

As psychiatry has moved into the community, it has also become less medically dominated. Most psychiatrists now work as member of multidisciplinary CMHTs, as one amongst many 'mental health professionals'. The psychiatrist may or may not be the team 'leader'. The psychiatrist's particular roles in the team generally centre on:
- Making diagnoses.
- Prescribing medication.
- Use of the Mental Health Act (although psychiatrists are no longer necessarily the 'responsible' clinician under the Act).
- Taking medico-legal responsibility.

The other members of multidisciplinary teams usually comprise:
- *Community psychiatric nurses* (CPNs). CPNs perform much of the day-to-day psychiatric work of the CMHT. CPNs are often the designated *key worker* (see below), they do many of the initial and follow-up assessments and they give medication. Some have additional therapeutic skills (e.g. in CBT) and are called *nurse practitioners*.
- Social services departments have statutory responsibilities affecting psychiatric patients which *social workers* attached to the team fulfil. For example, the social worker takes the lead role in assessing social circumstances and arranging accommodation, helping with benefits, etc. Some social workers are Approved Mental Health Professionals, with particular roles in the Mental Health Act (Chapter 7).
- *Secretary/administrator.* Teams generate a lot of paperwork and its members are often out and about. A central person who handles the adminis-

tration, takes messages and arranges meetings is therefore a key figure.
- *Clinical psychologist.* Many teams have a clinical psychologist, who helps in assessments and in providing psychological treatments.
- *Other team members* may include occupational therapists, accommodation officers, befrienders, etc.
- *Voluntary organizations* and *self-help groups*, though not formally part of the CMHT, provide important additional sources of support and help for many people—including those with needs but who are not receiving formal psychiatric care.

## The key worker

Every patient under the care of more than one member of a multidisciplinary team has a *key worker* (the actual term used may vary) who:
- Is usually a CPN or social worker.
- Coordinates and administers treatment.
- Knows about local resources and how to access them.
- Liaises with the GP and other agencies.
- Assists in planning and monitoring of the care package, usually as part of the *care programme approach* (CPA; see below).
- Informs others of changes in the patient's state or needs.

## The care programme approach (CPA)

The way in which adult mental health services are delivered in the community varies markedly between countries, due to differences in the structure of health and social care services, and the relationship between them. It is also subject to rapid changes in policy, emphasis and terminology.

Since 1991 the specified model for community psychiatric care in the UK has been the CPA. The aim of the CPA was to improve and standardize the planning and provision of care for psychiatric patients. The key aspects of CPA are that:
- It starts with a detailed assessment. This covers psychiatric, medical and social needs, and assessment of risk to self and others.
- A key worker is assigned.

- A *care plan* records the identified needs, how they will be tackled and by whom. The care plan is drawn up in consultation with the patient and nearest relative. Both get a copy, as do all the professionals involved.
- Progress of the case is monitored by the key worker, who reports regularly back to the CMHT.
- Formal 'CPA meetings' are held to review and plan care. The meetings involve all people/agencies involved in the case, together with the patient, and carers or significant others who the patient wishes to be present. The record of the meeting, and decisions made is then sent to all parties.
- All patients have a right to refuse CPA, unless detained under the Mental Health Act.

Until 2008, CPA applied to all patients. Now it has been restricted to those with a wide range of needs from a number of services, or who are at most risk. What difference this makes in practice remains to be seen.

- Regardless of whether the CPA 'badge' is in use, the principles of good communication within the CMHT, inclusion of the patient and their significant others in care decisions and careful assessment of the patient's medical and social needs, should always be applied.

*Assertive outreach* is another form of community care 'package', with smaller caseloads per staff member and more intensive support than the usual CPA. It has not been shown to be superior to good community care in the UK.

*Ms D is 27 and has been admitted informally with schizophrenia. At the ward round, Rob, a CPN from the CMHT, agrees to be her key worker. Ms D has been made homeless and unemployed, and she remains vulnerable to abuse and neglect. Rob liaises with the social worker and sorts out financial arrangements and accommodation in a group home, and contacts Ms D's parents with whom she had lost touch. A pre-discharge CPA meeting is held, at which all professionals, Ms D and her parents are present. After discharge, Rob visits weekly, giving Ms D her depot and monitoring her mental state. The psychiatrist sees Ms D every 3 months or whenever there is cause for concern. An exacerbation of her illness is managed at home with support and increased medication. Rob begins therapy with Ms D's family, who are supportive but have become*

*overinvolved. However, Ms D relapses and is found wandering the street in a state of neglect. She is detained under Section 3 of the Mental Health Act. When almost ready for discharge, a Section 117 meeting plans her future care.*

## Psychiatric specialties

Psychiatric subspecialties are delineated by the patients' age, and/or the type of disorder they treat:
- General adult psychiatry.
- Psychiatry of old age (psychogeriatrics).
- Child and adolescent psychiatry.
- Liaison psychiatry (psychological medicine).
- Substance abuse.
- Forensic psychiatry.
- Learning disability.

The main elements and distinguishing features of each specialty (except learning disability, covered in Chapter 17) are now described.

- Most of the main features of service organization noted above (e.g. move to community care, CMHTs, etc.) are common across the various specialties.

### General adult psychiatry

Adults with psychiatric disorders are looked after by general adult psychiatrists unless their problems come into the domain of another subspecialty, and their care is transferred to it. The precise boundaries of general psychiatry will depend on the availability of specialist services. Schizophrenia and other psychoses have traditionally been the focus of most general psychiatry services. Although this remains the case, general adult psychiatrists increasingly work in partnership with primary care, and assist GPs in the management of patients with the more common psychiatric disorders.

### Psychiatry of old age (psychogeriatrics)

Most old-age psychiatrists deal with the whole range of psychiatric disorder in the elderly and not just dementia.

- Concurrent medical problems and medications affect the presentation and management of psychiatric disorders. For example, constipation is common in the elderly and is therefore a less useful diagnostic sign for depression; it may also produce delirium and may limit the dose of antidepressant which can be given.

• Psychiatry of old age CMHTs have close ties with both geriatrics and social services. This is necessary given the prevalence and nature of dementia, and the frequency of associated physical and social problems of the elderly mentally ill.

*Mr A is 75 and has become forgetful. He lives with his healthy wife. A domiciliary visit revealed cognitive impairment and depressive symptoms. A trial of antidepressants did not help, and his cognitive impairment has got worse. Routine investigations were negative and you diagnose probable Alzheimer's disease. An occupational therapist visits to assess his daily living skills. His wife can care for him with help from 'meals on wheels' and visits from a CPN. You liaise with the GP regarding Mr A's leg ulcers (which make him delirious when infected); the GP prescribes antibiotics and contacts a district nurse. Two years later Mr A has become severely demented and aggressive, seemingly in response to hallucinations. His wife is not coping. The psychologist gives advice about managing his behaviour, which settles with this. You help his wife by organizing day care and a 2 week respite admission for him. The next year she dies. Mr A is admitted to a nursing home. A social worker sorts out the finances. Six months later Mr A breaks his hip. After discussion with his son, conservative management is agreed on. Mr A is kept comfortable in the nursing home and dies the next day.*

## Child and adolescent psychiatry

Children's psychiatric problems differ in important respects from those of adults, and the approach to their assessment and management is also different (Chapter 16).

• A child psychiatrist requires a detailed understanding of physical and psychological development. Some are also trained in paediatrics.

• The first contact with child psychiatric services may come from the GP, paediatrician or school educational psychologist.

• A child psychiatry team includes specialized social workers, nurses and psychologists. Some

of the team may concentrate upon family therapy.

• On the rare occasions when in-patient care is needed, other members of the family may be admitted too, to help in evaluation. The in-patient team includes teachers who assess the child's problems in an educational setting, as well as continuing the child's education whilst in hospital.

## Liaison psychiatry (psychological medicine)

Liaison means link, and liaison psychiatrists provide an important link between psychiatric services and medical and surgical services. Such linking services are often referred to as departments of psychological medicine. They are based in general hospitals and are principally concerned with three patient groups:

• People who present to A&E having self-harmed. Some hospitals have trained counsellors to carry out screening of all self-harm patients; elsewhere it is left to the medical or nursing staff to decide when to refer to a psychiatrist.

• Patients whose doctors suspect they have a psychiatric problem (such as delirium, depression or substance misuse) contributing to, arising from or complicating their medical disorder.

• Patients whose somatic symptoms are unexplained by demonstrable medical disease.

Liaison psychiatrists offer specialist opinions on these patient groups; they may then offer treatment themselves, or refer on to other local psychiatric services.

*You are asked to see Mr B in A&E. He is 49 and has taken an overdose. He is not suicidal but does have depressive and anxiety symptoms. You suspect he has an adjustment reaction after recent life events. You offer him an appointment next week, give him a number to call if he feels the urge to self-harm again, and phone his GP. On review, the severity of depression becomes clearer. He starts antidepressants. You discuss the case with the local CMHT who take over his care. Six months later you are called to see him on a surgical ward where he is awaiting a cholecystectomy. The houseman discovers his psychiatric history and wants your opinion on his mental state. Mr B is fine, but you note that his antidepressant (a monoamine oxidase inhibitor) may interact with analgesics. You alert the anaesthetist.*

## Substance abuse psychiatry

Abuse of alcohol and drugs leads to a wide range of psychiatric disorders and related problems (Chapter 14), which are dealt with by this subspecialty (also known as *community addictions service*). The workload comprises:

• Management of psychiatric disorder resulting from alcohol or drug abuse.

• Management of the psychological and social consequences of substance misuse. Many people have complex and multiple needs that both cause and result from their substance abuse.

• In-patient care for detoxification (in some units).

• Advice and support for people wanting to stop abusing drugs or alcohol.

• Advice to other doctors managing patients in whom substance abuse may be a factor.

• Public education and local health initiatives about the dangers of drug and alcohol abuse.

Counsellors and outreach workers play important roles in this specialty in addition to the CPNs and social workers. Considerable efforts are made to make contact with people with drug or alcohol problems who are unwilling to attend a medical setting. Cooperation with physicians is important because of the medical problems that often coexist.

*Mr C had delirium tremens. After his recovery, a liaison psychiatrist referred him to the drug and alcohol clinic. You take a history and discuss his medical condition with his GP. He is given information about alcohol and introduced to a CPN who will visit regularly to review progress and give support. A social worker investigates his benefit problems and contacts his ex-wife about access to his children. Mr C does not want medication to help him abstain. Things go well until he loses his job. He starts to drink heavily and drops out of care. He turns up later wanting admission for detoxification. Needle marks are noticed. He admits to injecting heroin and is found to be hepatitis B positive. He again cuts down his alcohol and denies taking other drugs thereafter. He gets a new job*

*and his wife returns to him. He has had no relapse when seen a year later.*

## Forensic psychiatry

Forensic means 'of the courts'. All psychiatrists become involved in forensic issues for various reasons:

• Writing psychiatric court reports or attending court on behalf of a patient.

• Assessment of local offenders/prisoners with suspected psychiatric disorder. Court diversion schemes are being developed to reduce the delay such people experience before receiving psychiatric help.

• A forensic history (e.g. of assault) may affect management decisions even if not directly related to current psychiatric problems.

Forensic psychiatrists concentrate on work in three areas:

• Psychiatric assessment of persons charged with serious crimes, especially murder.

• Providing treatment for convicted prisoners with a psychiatric disorder. This includes running psychiatric care in Regional Secure Units and the Special Hospitals (e.g. Broadmoor).

• Giving advice to other psychiatrists encountering forensic issues—for example, when assessing dangerousness.

In practice, the decision as to when a patient with a 'forensic history' should be transferred to the forensic psychiatric services depends on the crime, the likelihood of recurrence and the availability of resources.

## Groups with special psychiatric needs

Because of their circumstances, several groups have particular psychiatric needs, or are more likely to have needs unmet by the services.

## The homeless

*Difficulties:*

• Multiple social and medical needs.

• High prevalence of psychiatric disorder, especially schizophrenia and substance misuse.

- Lack of a supportive network—family, friends, GP.
- Hard to engage in treatment and follow-up.

*Solutions:*
- Flexible CMHT care packages.
- Outreach workers.
- Realistic goals.

## Ethnic minorities

*Difficulties:*
- Psychiatric disorder harder to diagnose because of cultural differences in presentation.
- Language barrier.
- Concerns about racial prejudice and stigmatization.
- Increased rates of some psychiatric disorders.

*Solutions:*
- Awareness of cultural differences in how psychiatric disorders present.
- Trained interpreters.
- Staff reflect the ethnic make up of the community.

## People with psychiatric comorbidity (multiple psychiatric diagnoses)

*Difficulties:*
- Worsens prognosis.
- Hampers management.
- Increases risk of violence (especially the combination of psychosis, substance misuse and personality disorder).

*Solutions:*
- Recognition.
- Extra resources.
- Prioritize management plans—target major and soluble problems.

## Health care workers

*Difficulties:*
- Reluctance to admit to psychiatric problems.
- May knowingly mislead or conceal symptoms.
- Increased risk of alcohol abuse and suicide.
- Hard to maintain confidentiality.
- Blurring of boundaries between being a colleague and being a patient.

*Solutions:*
- Confidential, publicized, accessible local arrangements.
- For UK doctors, the National Counselling Service for Sick Doctors (0870 241 0535).

---

### Key points

- Most psychiatric patients are treated in the community. Care is delivered by a community mental health team (CMHT).
- In a CMHT, the psychiatrist works with psychiatric nurses, social workers and other disciplines.
- Psychiatric admission is reserved for cases where there is known or suspected severe psychiatric disorder coupled with a significant risk of harm to self or others.
- A variety of subspecialty services address specific aspects of psychiatric need.
- Most psychiatric disorders are managed not in specialist care, but in general practice.

---

# Chapter 9

# Mood disorders

In mood disorders there is a persistent disturbance of mood sufficiently severe to cause impairment in the activities of daily living. This alteration in mood is beyond the fluctuations we all experience. Normal mood (*euthymia*) can become lowered (*depression*) or elevated (*mania*). Figure 9.1 shows the spectrum of mood.

- The term depression, in a clinical sense, may refer either to someone's current mood, or to their underlying diagnosis. This can cause confusion, so the former is sometimes called *depressive episode* and the latter *depressive disorder*. The same applies to *mania* and *manic episode*.
- Mood is also called *affect*, hence the alternative term *affective disorders*.
- Review the relevant parts of the core assessment (Chapter 2) and the mood modules (pp. 22 and 24) for fuller description of the key features of mood disorders and how they are elicited.

## Clinical features of a depressive episode

The core features are:
- Low mood. The subjective feeling of being depressed. It may be described as feeling down, fed up or sad.

*Lecture Notes: Psychiatry*, 10e. By Paul Harrison, John Geddes and Michael Sharpe. Published 2010 by Blackwell Publishing Ltd.

- Lack of energy (*anergia*). May be experienced as fatigue or tiredness.
- Decreased pleasure and interest in life—*anhedonia*.
- The symptoms must have been present for at least 2 weeks to meet the diagnostic criteria.

Depending on the severity of the episode, additional symptoms may also be present, described below. They include somatic (bodily) symptoms, summarized in Table 9.1.

## Mild depression

The main complaint is often of feeling stressed or tired. Anxiety symptoms frequently coexist, leading to the term *mixed anxiety–depression* (Chapter 10). Suicidal thoughts can occur but serious self-harm is unusual. The mood generally remains responsive, so that the person is cheered up by good news and pleasurable events. The patient may be able to work, but will become more tired than usual and concentration may be impaired.

- Though mild, the term is reserved for people who are more than just unhappy, based on the key features outlined above.
- Mild depression is the most common form of depressive episode.

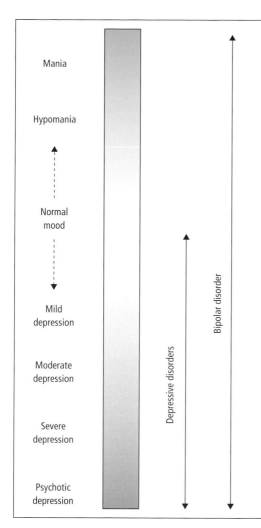

**Figure 9.1** The spectrum of mood and its disorders.

**Table 9.1** Somatic symptoms of depression.

Psychomotor retardation
Poor sleep with early morning waking
Diurnal variation of mood (worse in morning)
Lack of energy or tiredness
Loss of appetite
Loss of weight
Loss of libido
Constipation
Amenorrhoea

## Moderate depression

The 'textbook' form of depressive episode seen by psychiatrists. The key features are:
● Mood is objectively as well as subjectively depressed.
● Somatic symptoms such as sleep and appetite disturbance are usually present (Table 9.1).
● Anhedonia and lack of motivation.
● Anergia.
● Poor concentration.
● Negative cognitions—focus on unpleasant memories, perceived failings, disappointments and a bleak future.
● Psychomotor retardation is common, though some patients become agitated with whatever's on their mind.
● A sense of hopelessness and helplessness.
● Suicidal thoughts and intent, driven by the low mood, negative cognitions and sense of hopelessness—these should always be asked about and taken seriously (Chapter 4).
● Social anxiety and withdrawal.
● Dysfunction becomes prominent (e.g. inability to work properly or marked social withdrawal).

## Severe depression

In severe depression, the symptoms of a moderate depressive episode are magnified. A deep and pervasive sense of gloom is evident. The person no longer experiences nor is interested in the normal pleasures of life. There are many somatic symptoms. Suicidal thoughts and intentions become prominent.

## Psychotic depression

Depression at its most severe becomes *psychotic depression* (also called *depressive psychosis*). Worries and perceived misdemeanours become delusional in intensity. The patient may believe she, or a part of her, is dead (*Cotard's syndrome*); she may experience *auditory hallucinations* with voices cursing her or telling her that she is worthless. Suicidal risk is high.

**Table 9.2** Ways depression presents.

| Example | Depressive explanation |
| --- | --- |
| An old man who's become forgetful | Poor concentration |
| A mother unable to cope with her child | Lack of motivation and anhedonia |
| A student with weight loss and fatigue | Somatic symptoms |
| A woman worrying about having AIDS | Ruminations |
| A man with panic attacks | Anxiety secondary to depression |
| Marital conflict | About sex, due to husband's loss of libido |
| In A&E after failed hanging attempt | Delusions of worthlessness |

**Table 9.3** Symptoms of mania.

*Core features*
Elevation of mood
'Infectious gaiety' or irritability
Distractable
Poor concentration
Flight of ideas
Pressure of speech
Expansive or grandiose ideas
Disinhibited behaviour (e.g. financial, sexual)
Increased energy
Decreased need for sleep

| *Features of hypomania* | *Features of mania* |
| --- | --- |
| Present for at least 4 days | Present for at least 7 days |
| Core features mild or moderate | Core features marked |
| Mild or moderate dysfunction | Substantial dysfunction |
| Partial insight preserved | Minimal or absent insight |
| No psychotic features | Psychotic symptoms may occur |

- Psychomotor retardation can increase to the point where the person sits motionless and mute—*depressive stupor*. This often used to be fatal (from dehydration); it now calls for emergency ECT.
- Psychotic depression must be distinguished from other psychoses (Chapter 12). This is based on the presence of other depressive symptoms, and the *mood congruity* of the delusions and hallucinations.

## How depression presents

Not all depressed patients complain of or admit to low mood. Rather, they present with the associated cognitive, behavioural or somatic symptoms (Table 9.2). Consequently, depression often surfaces in non-psychiatric settings (Chapter 18), and all doctors must be alert to its various guises.

- Somatic presentations of depression are particularly common in Asian cultures.

## Clinical features of a manic episode

As with a depressive episode, there is a spectrum of severity from mild to moderate to severe (Figure 9.1). Sometimes *mania* refers to all pathological elevations of mood, but sometimes *hypomania* is used to refer to the milder or shorter lived form. Features of mania and hypomania are compared in Table 9.3.

## Mild mania (hypomania)

*Hypomania* is a happiness and zest for life in excess of that which is normal. The degree of functional impairment is variable. A daily routine may be just about maintained, though with less need for sleep and more nocturnal activities (e.g. spring cleaning, writing a novel). Though subjectively productivity may be increased, tasks are rarely done well or completed. *Concentration* is impaired and *distractibility* is usual. The infectious gaiety easily switches to irritability.

- Hypomania often progresses to a full manic episode, especially in those with a past history of mania.
- Note that there is no satisfactory category or term for manic symptoms lasting less than 4 days (Table 9.3).

## Moderate and severe mania

In moderate and severe mania the symptoms cause substantial impairment of occupational and social functioning. Thought processes become disordered and jumpy (*flight of ideas*), accompanied by *pressure of speech* (p. 25). Psychotic symptoms may emerge. These are mood congruent and *grandiose*: a patient may believe themselves blessed with special powers (e.g. that they can fly or have been sent to save the world). They may hear voices supporting these beliefs. Unfortunately, reality or gravity supervene, and people with mania do things they later regret. For example, they may suffer consequences of promiscuity or generate huge debts.

## Mixed affective states

In *mixed affective states*, manic and depressive symptoms coexist within the course of a day. The disorder is not rare, but it is difficult to diagnose. It may be triggered by antidepressant treatment in a patient with a tendency to bipolar disorder. The treatment of mixed states usually focuses initially on the manic symptoms.

## Classification of mood disorders

Recognition of a depressive or manic episode is only the first part of diagnosing a mood disorder. The diagnosis also depends on the nature, severity and course of the episodes. The classification of mood disorders is confusing; a simplified approach is shown in Figure 9.2.

First, consider the unlikely but important possibility of an organic mood disorder (i.e. one attributable directly to a medical disorder or a consequence of substance misuse; see Chapters 13 and 14).

The vast majority of cases of mood disorder do not come into this category and organic factors are more commonly just one component of a multifactorial aetiology (Chapter 6). In all these cases, the next diagnostic decision is between *bipolar disorder* and (unipolar) *depressive disorder* (Figures 9.1–9.3). This distinction is based upon the presence or absence of a history of mania. Bipolar and depressive disorders are in turn subdivided by *course* and *severity*.

## Depressive disorder

ICD-10 divides depressive disorders into those with discrete episodes with recovery in between (*recurrent depressive disorder*) and those with persistent, mild symptoms (*dysthymia*). In reality, this is not always a clear-cut distinction.

- If only one episode has been experienced, the ICD-10 label is just '*depressive episode*' (though in practice the terms 'depressive disorder' or just 'depression' are used loosely).

Recurrent depressive disorder is then described in terms of the severity of the episode, using the features outlined above.

- Dysthymia is longstanding but mild depression, often experienced as a lack of pleasure in life and of things being an effort; symptoms worsen at times of stress.

- Dysthymia used to be considered as depressive personality disorder. Its reclassification as a form of depressive disorder is supported by some genetic evidence, and it encourages dysthymia to be seen as treatable, which to a degree it is.

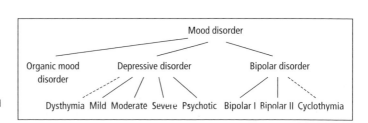

**Figure 9.2** Classification of mood disorders.

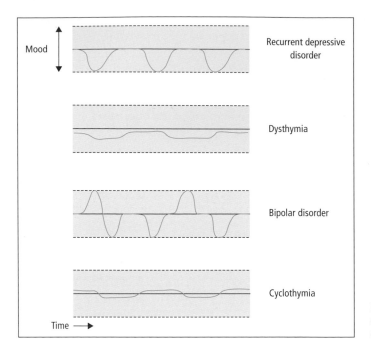

**Figure 9.3** Course of mood disorders. (NB the actual course of mood disorders is rarely as regular as this.)

*Mrs J has a 6-week history of low mood, anhedonia, tearfulness and early morning waking. She is off her food and has lost weight. Every day is a struggle and she finds it hard to concentrate or motivate herself to go to work or look after her children. However, she is just about coping and has no suicidal ideation. She had a similar episode 3 years ago. There is no evidence of an organic mood disorder. Your provisional diagnosis is that she has a recurrent depressive disorder and is currently in a depressive episode of moderate severity.*

## Bipolar disorder

The key feature of *bipolar disorder* is that normal mood is interspersed with both depressive and manic episodes. The frequency and magnitude of the shifts is very variable, as is the proportion of depressive to manic mood swings, although sooner or later depression almost always occurs.

- Bipolar disorder is synonymous with the older terms *manic depression* or *manic depressive psychosis*.
- Bipolar disorder in which only hypomania but not mania has ever occurred (Table 9.3) is some-

times called *bipolar II disorder*; bipolar disorder with true mania is *bipolar I disorder*.

- For people who have only had one episode of mania and none of depression, the (temporary) diagnosis is *manic episode*.
- *Cyclothymia* is a mild, chronic bipolar variation of mood. Like dysthymia, it is sometimes viewed as a personality trait. Psychiatric help is rarely sought since the mild mood elevations are pleasant and associated with a sense of productivity and creativity.
- A history of cyclothymia or a family history of bipolar disorder are significant in someone presenting with a depressive episode; they increase the chances that the patient will actually turn out to have bipolar disorder. They may also increase the risk that antidepressants induce a manic episode.

*Mrs J then informs you that she recalls two periods several years ago when she felt elated, slept little, became unusually gregarious and spent money uncharacteristically. After each episode she was embarrassed and distressed by her actions, but she had not sought treatment. Your diagnosis now becomes one of bipolar (II) disorder, currently in a moderate depressive episode.*

## Other terms and types of mood disorder

We have already mentioned an array of mood disorder terms and types. Table 9.4 summarizes a few more which are sometimes used.

## Epidemiology of mood disorders

Mood disorders are common. The risk is higher in women, and increased by a positive family history. Table 9.5 shows figures from recent population surveys. The finding of more depression in women than men is robust. Possible explanations include:

- Genetic predisposition.
- Sex hormone influences.
- Social pressures.
- Greater willingness to admit to depressive symptoms.
- Depressed men are given other diagnoses, such as alcohol abuse.

Mood disorders seem to be getting more common and are now the fourth leading cause of worldwide disability. This rise in incidence is unexplained.

**Table 9.4** Other mood disorder terms and types.

| | |
|---|---|
| *Atypical depression* | Depression with increased sleep, increased appetite and phobic anxiety. Some evidence it responds better to MAOIs than other antidepressants. |
| *Agitated depression* | Depression with prominent anxiety, agitation, restlessness. Contrasted with *retarded depression*, a distinction of value when deciding whether to use a sedative antidepressant. |
| *Double depression* | Depressive disorder on top of dysthymia. Poor prognosis. |
| *Endogenous depression* | Depression attributed to genetic and biochemical factors. Prominent somatic symptoms, hence the term *biological depression* was applied to similar cases. Contrasted with *reactive depression*. |
| *Melancholia* | Depressive disorder with anhedonia and somatic symptoms. Term used in DSM-IV. |
| *Mixed affective state* | Simultaneous manic and depressive symptoms during the same episode of illness, even simultaneously. May respond better to valproic acid than lithium. |
| *Rapid cycling* | Bipolar disorder with >4 episodes a year. Women affected more than men. Hypothyroidism common. Poor response to lithium. |
| *Reactive depression* | Depression where the mood remains reactive to circumstances. Lacks somatic symptoms. |
| *Retarded depression* | See Agitated depression. |
| *Seasonal affective disorder* | Depression which recurs in autumn or winter, associated with increased sleep and carbohydrate craving. May respond to bright light therapy. |

**Table 9.5** Occurrence of mood disorders.

| | Bipolar disorder | Depressive disorder |
|---|---|---|
| Lifetime risk | 1% | 15% |
| 1 month prevalence | 0.4% | 5% |
| Sex ratio (M : F) | 1 : 1 | 1 : 2 |
| Mean age of onset | Early 20s | Late 20s |
| Risk in first-degree relatives: | | |
| of bipolar disorder | 10% | 2% |
| of depressive disorder | 15% | 15% |

## Management of depressive disorders

The first requirement is an ability to recognize depression in all its guises (Table 9.2). Depression frequently goes undiagnosed and untreated.

- Psychiatrists only see a small percentage of people with depressive disorder, highlighting the need for GPs and all doctors to be confident about its diagnosis and first-line treatment.

Treatment depends largely on severity. In the absence of previous episodes, mild depressive episodes are often self-limiting and antidepressant drug treatment may not be indicated. Information, advice and simple measures such as self-help guides to problem solving may be adequate. There is evidence that increased physical exercise and activity helps. On the other hand, if there have been previous episodes of at least moderate severity that have responded to treatment, then treatment should be started while symptoms are still mild.

### Drug treatment

The first-line treatment for a depressive episode of at least moderate severity is usually an antidepressant drug. However, before prescribing, consider several factors (Table 9.6). Over 70% of depressive episodes respond to an antidepressant, either an SSRI or a TCA, although only as few as a third of patients may respond to first-line therapy (Chapter 7). The chances of successful treatment can be increased if simple measures are taken (Table 9.7; see also Table 7.2).

- In practice, SSRIs are now prescribed much more commonly than TCAs, based mainly on tolerability and safety.
- There are small differences in efficacy and tolerability between SSRIs and, while the likelihood of specific adverse events should be discussed with the patient, a good first-line choice is sertraline.
- It is important to *monitor for emergent suicidal ideation* as this may occur as the patient improves, and may actually be increased by SSRIs, especially in younger people. However, there is no evidence

**Table 9.6** Factors affecting management decisions in depression.

| Question | Implication |
|---|---|
| Is there a serious suicide risk? | May need admission. Use SSRI not TCA as less toxic in overdose |
| Are there psychotic symptoms? | Add an antipsychotic to the antidepressant, or use ECT |
| What are the main symptoms? | Affects choice of drug, e.g. use sedative antidepressant if insomnia |
| Is there a past history of response? | Use the treatment which worked last time |
| Is there a past history of mania? | Caution with antidepressants; consider mood stabilizer |
| Are there medical problems? | Avoid TCAs after recent myocardial infarction |
| What does the patient want? | May have a preference for drug or psychological therapy |

**Table 9.7** Prescribing antidepressants effectively.

| Principle | Examples |
|---|---|
| Educate patient | About efficacy, onset of effects and side-effects, and non-addictiveness |
| Attend to the psychosocial aspects | Restore hope; education about depression; give practical advice |
| Give an adequate dose | Know dose ranges for specific SSRIs and TCAs |
| Check drug being taken | Non-adherence is common reason for non-response |
| Give the drug for long enough | Therapeutic trial should be 6–8 weeks, at adequate dose |

that SSRIs are associated with an increase in suicidal acts.

*Mr S has a moderate depressive episode. He is married and unemployed. He initially doesn't accept he's depressed and blames his problems on his own inadequacies. You explain that he has a depressive disorder which would benefit from treatment. You summarize what depression is and how antidepressants work, including their possible side-effects and delayed onset of action, but also emphasize that they will help him sleep and reduce his anxiety. You recommend he takes 50 mg sertraline. His wife is present and agrees to supervise his tablets. You will see him in a week to review progress. You gradually increase the dose of sertraline to 150 mg.*

After recovery, continue treatment at the same dose for at least 6 months. The dose is then tapered off over several weeks. Continuing treatment in this way reduces the high risk of relapse in the months after a depressive episode and tapering off reduces the risk of 'withdrawal' symptoms.

- There is no good evidence that long-term use of antidepressants is harmful.

*Mr S took his tablets as prescribed. His sleep and agitation improved rapidly. The depressive symptoms responded over the next few weeks, though it was necessary to increase amitriptyline to 200 mg/day for a full response. He became constipated but this improved with laxatives. He subsequently accepted that he had been ill, and conceptualized the amitriptyline as correcting a chemical imbalance which helped him solve life's problems more effectively. He no longer blamed himself for his redundancy and found a new job. His wife confirmed the improvement. On your advice, he remained on medication for a further 9 months.*

## Psychological treatment

CBT, IPT and probably other psychological treatments, such as problem-solving therapy (Chapter 7) or brief psychodynamic therapy, are effective alternatives to antidepressants in mild and moderate depressive disorder, especially for patients who prefer psychological therapies to drug treatment.

- CBT is much the most widely available psychological treatment, but is nevertheless of restricted availability due to a shortage of trained therapists. New NHS initiatives using internet- and phone-based CBT appear promising and mean that the treatments can be provided to more patients.
- Combining an antidepressant with CBT is a bit more effective than either alone and should be considered when CBT is available.

There are no established predictors of who will benefit from psychological rather than pharmacological treatment of depression. A few pointers suggesting good psychotherapeutic response are:

- Depression not severe (as defined in Table 9.1).
- 'Psychological mindedness' (the ability and willingness to think about psychological matters).
- Willingness to engage in therapy and carry out homework tasks.
- Preference for psychological treatment or reluctance to take medication.

## Non-response to first-line treatment

In up to two-thirds of cases, a depressive episode does not respond to a first-line antidepressant (or to a psychological treatment). If so:

- Check the antidepressant has been taken as prescribed. Measuring plasma levels can sometimes be useful.
- Increase to the maximum tolerated and recommended dose.
- Review the case. Is the diagnosis right? Could there be powerful perpetuating factors, such as an endocrine disorder, marital strife or alcohol misuse? Can their impact be reduced?

If the patient has still not improved, there are various options to consider. The most common option is to switch from one class of antidepressant to another (e.g. SSRI to SNRI) or to try a second drug from the same class (SSRI to SSRI). There is limited evidence in favour of either strategy. Alternative options, with at least some evidence of efficacy, are:

- Add lithium, if depression is severe. This has a good evidence base but the risks and drawbacks of lithium limit its popularity.
- Add mirtazapine to an SSRI; the sedative effect of mirtazapine is useful if insomnia or agitation is a problem.
- Add a second-generation antipsychotic, such as olanzapine, aripiprazole or quetiapine, especially if there are psychotic symptoms, or agitation and insomnia.
- Add CBT or other psychological treatment.

- Add tri-iodothyronine (T3).
- Switch to an MAOI, especially in atypical depression (Table 9.4). Remember MAOI cautions (Chapter 7).
- Psychiatric referral, if this has not already occurred (see below).
- Consider ECT for severe and drug-resistant depression.

## Psychiatric referral for depression

Referral for psychiatric assessment or ongoing care of depressive disorder is appropriate when:
- The patients has not responded.
- There is a substantial risk of harm to self or others.
- A second opinion on diagnosis or treatment is required.
- Combinations of drugs or rarely used agents are being considered.
- To access specialized psychological treatments, occupational therapy, etc.
- The patient is severely unwell and hospital admission or ECT may be required.

## Prevention of relapse

Continuation of an antidepressant after recovery cuts relapse rates by at least 50% in patients with recurrent depressive disorder and should be recommended to all appropriate patients. Psychological treatments such as CBT may also be effective, by a long-term reduction in negative cognitions or by teaching strategies for recognizing and treating re-emergent symptoms.
- In people who do relapse, reinstitute the treatment that worked the first time but continue it for longer. Some patients appear to benefit from prolonged antidepressant treatment.

## Management of bipolar disorder

## Treatment of mania and mixed episodes

Patients with mild manic symptoms can be successfully treated as out-patients, if the patient has insight that they need treatment. More severe mania, especially if psychotic, usually requires admission, often compulsorily.
- Antipsychotics (e.g. risperidone, olanzapine) or valproate and lithium are effective antimanics. Antipsychotics are probably slightly more effective, but cause more sedation and weight gain. Benzodiazepines are used, as required, for sedation.
- The choice of drug is influenced by the patient's existing medication—they may already be on a mood stabilizer. If they are on an antidepressant, stop it. If the patient is on lithium, check the blood level to assess recent adherence.
- Some patients learn to recognize prodromal symptoms of mania (e.g. initial insomnia, increased energy). If so, a short course of antipsychotic or valproate may successfully treat the episode.
- ECT can be highly effective in patients with severe mania that does not respond to drug treatment.

Mania can last for months if untreated. Death from 'manic exhaustion' was well recognized before treatments became available.

## Treatment of depressive episodes

Depressive episodes and symptoms in bipolar disorder ('*bipolar depression*') can cause severe dysfunction and can be difficult to treat. There is increasing evidence that optimal drug treatment of bipolar depression is quite different from that described for unipolar depression.
- Quetiapine, an atypical antipsychotic, is the treatment with the best evidence and can be highly effective, with a rapid onset of action. Sedation and weight gain may limit longer term acceptability.
- Antidepressants may be less effective than in unipolar depression and they should be used in combination with an effective antimanic drug (see above) because antidepressants used alone can precipitate mood destabilization or mania.
- Lamotrigine, an antiepileptic drug, is probably also effective, although it needs to be started slowly.
- For severe depression, antipsychotics, ECT and psychiatric admission may all be necessary.

## Prevention of relapse

- The guiding principle should be that the patient needs to understand their own illness and learn to recognize signs of mood instability.
- Long-term mood monitoring by the patient can be extremely helpful.
- Relapses in bipolar disorder are often heralded by non-specific symptoms (e.g. deteriorating sleep), as mentioned above. Some patients become adept at recognizing and responding to these warning signs.
- Conventionally, long-term drug treatment is not offered until a patient has had at least two manic episodes, or one manic and one depressive episode. However, the effective early treatment of bipolar disorder may improve its long-term outcome, and increasingly the trend is to start long-term treatment after one serious episode, especially when there is a family history of bipolar disorder. The decision is an important one and the patient should be given sufficient information and time to make a properly informed choice.
- Long-term lithium treatment is the standard prophylaxis for bipolar disorder and is supported by the most robust evidence. Lithium reduces the risk of both manic and depressive relapse by 40–50%. Long-term lithium treatment should not be initiated unless both patient and doctor intend to continue it for at least 2 years. Valproate and olanzapine also reduce the risk of manic relapse. Lamotrigine reduces the risk of depressive relapse. Other drugs such as carbamazepine may also be used, although the evidence is limited.
- Psychological approaches such as CBT or family therapy may also help in preventing relapses.

## Prognosis of mood disorders

### Depressive disorders

Over 50% of people who have had one depressive episode will have another. The more severe the depression, the worse the prognosis; most people with psychotic depression suffer multiple episodes, and 10% never recover fully.

- The proportion with severe, recurrent and chronic illness is higher in psychiatric care than in general practice.
- The risk of suicide is increased at least 10-fold in people with depressive disorder. About 4% of patients who have had depression will die by suicide, rising to 15% in those ill enough to have required psychiatric admission at some stage.
- Mortality is also increased from natural causes, notably cardiovascular disease, accidents and substance misuse.

### Bipolar disorder

Bipolar disorder runs a remitting and relapsing course in 90%. After one episode, the annual average risk of relapse is about 20%. After more than three episodes, the annual average risk of relapse is about 40%. The prognosis is worse in young-onset cases, rapid cycling bipolar disorder (Table 9.4) and women.

- Suicide and mortality rates are similar to those of depressive disorder.
- The disruption caused by the illness, especially the manic phases, often leads to problems maintaining relationships, employment and accommodation.
- Over time, it is the depressive episodes rather than the manic episodes that cause most disability for most patients.

## Aetiology of mood disorders

### Organic mood disorders

Mood disorders which have a known physical cause are termed organic mood disorder. Recognized causes of organic mood disorder are summarized in Table 9.8. See also Chapter 13.

- Even when an organic diagnosis is made, psychological and social factors may still be relevant to course and treatment.

*A 65-year-old man presented with insomnia, anorexia, back pain and weight loss. He also felt fed up and irritable. The provisional diagnosis was depression with somatic symptoms. However, physical examination*

**Table 9.8** Causes of organic mood disorder.

| Usually depression | Usually mania |
|---|---|
| Cushing's disease | Hyperthyroidism |
| Addison's disease | Steroids |
| Hypothyroidism | Amphetamine (acute) |
| Hypercalcaemia | L-DOPA |
| Diabetes mellitus | Antidepressants |
| Carcinomas | Bromocriptine |
| β-Blockers | Isoniazid |
| Digoxin | |
| Amfetamine (chronic) | |

| Either depression or mania |
|---|
| Multiple sclerosis |
| Cerebrovascular disease |
| Systemic lupus erythematosus |
| Epilepsy |
| Brain tumours |

**Table 9.9** Aetiological factors in depressive disorders.

Biological
  Genes
  Medical conditions (organic mood disorder)
  Neurochemical changes
    Monoamine abnormalities
    Altered HPA axis function

Psychological
  Childhood environment
    Emotional deprivation
    Parental loss
  Abnormal cognitions
  Learned helplessness
  Personality factors—neuroticism

Social
  Life events
  Unemployment

*revealed bony tenderness over his lumbar spine and a hard nodular prostate. Blood tests showed hypercalcaemia and anaemia. He had metastatic carcinoma of the prostate. His depressive symptoms resolved as the hypercalcaemia was treated, along with an antidepressant.*

## Depressive disorders

For all other mood disorders, a mixture of genetic, biological, psychological and social factors contribute to varying degrees (as in the rolling vignette in Chapter 6). There is a moderate genetic predisposition to depression (heritability 40–50%), more so in early-onset cases. The predisposition is shared between the various types of depressive disorder and overlaps with those associated with anxiety disorders, but not bipolar disorder. The number and identity of genes are unknown.

Environmental influences contribute substantially to depressive disorders (Table 9.9) and are discussed in Chapter 6.

• Hypofunction of monoamine neurotransmitter systems (5-HT and NA) in conjunction with altered HPA regulation is implicated. However, though these systems are all altered in depression, their causal role and inter-relationships remain unclear.

• Psychological models have centred on the role of abnormal ways of thinking with a tendency to think negatively about the self, the future and the world (the cognitive theory of depression). The personality attributes of 'neuroticism' (anxiety, obsessionality, poor coping with stress) and low self-esteem are also associated with depressive disorder.

• Current approaches to understanding mood disorders integrate findings from neuropsychology, psychopharmacology and neuroimaging. People who become depressed have negative biases in emotional processing which may involve a failure in the frontoparietal regulation of processes in the amygdala. These biases can be reversed by antidepressant drugs.

• Adverse experiences in childhood, recent life events and lack of social support are major risk factors.

• Focal lesions of the subcortical white matter, visible on MRI scans, are a risk factor for late-onset depressive disorder and are associated with a poor prognosis.

• Other structural brain changes reported in depressive disorder include a reduction of glial cells in the prefrontal cortex, and hippocampal atrophy. It is not known if these changes are cause, consequence or coincidental.

## Bipolar disorder

Bipolar disorder is strongly heritable (80%). MZ:DZ twin concordance is 75%:25%. Relatives of someone with bipolar disorder have an increased incidence of both bipolar and unipolar depressive disorder (Table 9.5).

- Many chromosomal loci and genes are implicated, and overlap with those for schizophrenia (Chapter 13). Current leading bipolar disorder candidate genes include the HLA (human leucocyte antigen) complex, ANK3 and CACN1C. There is some evidence for inheritance down the maternal line.

No childhood risk factors are known. Life events can precipitate the initial episodes; once the disorder is established, its course is increasingly immune to environmental circumstances.

- Most of the neurobiological abnormalities described for depressive disorder (Table 9.9) are also implicated in bipolar disorder, although there may be differences in the abnormalities in emotional processing.

- Always consider drug-induced mania (an example of organic mood disorder) in young people with no family history of bipolar disorder. In someone first presenting in middle age, exclude cerebrovascular disease, tumours and medication side-effects (Table 9.8).

## Other aspects of mood disorders

### Puerperal (postpartum) disorders

The postnatal period (puerperium) is a hormonally, and often psychologically, turbulent time. It is traditional to group psychiatric disorders that occur at this time together as puerperal disorders, partly because their clinical picture and management differ somewhat from similar disorders occurring at other times.

### Maternity blues

The 'blues' refer to a tearful, irritable labile mood that affects over 50% of mothers on the third or fourth postnatal day. Symptoms resolve within days without treatment, though explanation and reassurance are appropriate. There is no association of the blues with mood disorder.

- Maternity blues may be due to the precipitous fall in sex steroids after delivery, as well as to the impact of childbirth and concerns about mothering.

### Postnatal depression

Postnatal depression tends to start within a month of delivery; 1 in 7 mothers are affected. The symptoms are unremarkable, with the negative thoughts tending to focus on the woman's perceived failings as a mother or on her baby's well-being. Physical exhaustion exacerbates matters.

- As well as the standard mood and risk assessments, remember to consider the mother–baby relationship. Postnatal depression may put the baby at short-term risk and, if untreated, may lead to problems with bonding and child development.

- Most cases are managed at home. Use supportive measures, including explanation and reassurance. Mobilize resources (e.g. the local mothers' group), and liaise with the GP, midwife and health visitor. Many cases resolve within a few weeks, but antidepressants or psychological treatment should be considered if the disorder is moderate or severe. If admission is necessary, it should ideally be to a mother-and-baby unit, to maintain and observe their relationship.

- Before prescribing antidepressants, check whether the mother is breastfeeding (Chapter 7).

- Postnatal depression is more common in women with a history of psychiatric disorder and in those lacking support. A postnatal change in sensitivity of the dopaminergic system is implicated.

### Puerperal psychosis

Puerperal psychosis was formerly due mainly to sepsis—that is, it was an organic disorder. Now, it is more often a psychotic mood disorder or schizoaffective disorder. The disorder can be severe. Perplexity and a delirium-like state are characteristic. Onset is usually in the second postnatal week. About 1 in 500 women are affected.

- Risk factors include a past or family history of psychosis and being a primigravida.
- The baby is at potential risk because of the mother's delusions, or because she is so preoccupied by her symptoms that he is neglected. The assessment should specifically address these issues.
- Admission to hospital is usually necessary. Treatment is with antipsychotics and antidepressants, and with a low threshold for ECT—which often produces a dramatic response. Full recovery is usual, but there is a 25% relapse rate after the next delivery and a 50% lifetime risk.

## Premenstrual syndrome

Up to 80% of women suffer from symptoms in the days before their period: irritability, depression, abdominal bloating and breast tenderness. However, a specific premenstrual syndrome has proved difficult to validate (and is not included in ICD-10). The term *premenstrual dysphoric disorder* is sometimes used for women with prominent psychological premenstrual symptoms.

- If a woman complains of premenstrual syndrome, establish the symptoms and their relationship with the menstrual cycle. Ask her to keep a diary—it may transpire that the symptoms are present at other times too.
- There is some evidence for the efficacy of SSRIs, oestrogens, gonadotrophin agonists, danazol and CBT. There is no good evidence for progestogens or primrose oil. There is a high placebo response rate.

## Other psychiatric issues specific to women

Abortion, sterilization, hysterectomy and the menopause have all been said to cause psychiatric distress, especially mood and anxiety disorders. There is no good evidence for any of these claims. Each of these events may, however, act as stressors that are relevant to the understanding, presentation or treatment of a disorder occurring soon afterwards.

## Grief

If you know you are dying, or you have been bereaved, emotional pain and turmoil are to be expected. Many of the features overlap with those of depression. Psychiatrists and other doctors are asked to assess or support people during these times, so it is necessary to know:

- The characteristic psychological reactions to impending death and to bereavement.
- The features which distinguish these from depressive disorder.

## Normal grief

People may grieve a death (*bereavement*) or other major loss, or may grieve an impending event (*anticipatory grief*). The responses are forms of adjustment reaction (Chapter 10). Three stages have been described:

- *Shock and disbelief.* On being told of the event there is an initial numbness that usually lasts a day or two. Behaviour may be acutely disturbed.
- *Preoccupation.* This central phase involves a preoccupation with the deceased. In the early stages anger is common, and may be directed at doctors, God or other target of blame. Uncontrollable crying, low mood, social withdrawal and somatic symptoms akin to those of depression may be pronounced. The voice or image of the deceased may be vividly perceived, though usually with an 'as if' quality rather than being truly hallucinatory.
- *Acceptance and resolution.* With time, the person comes to term with the event, symptoms subside and life begins to return to normal. This phase may take several months to start, and several more to be completed. Recurrence of grief is common around anniversaries.

In uncomplicated grief, *bereavement counselling* and support (e.g. from Cruse) may be useful. Such grief should not be labelled as a disorder but viewed as a natural, if painful, process. The therapist should, however, be on the look out for signs of abnormal grief or depressive disorder.

**Table 9.10** A comparison of depression and grief.

|  | Depression | Grief |
|---|---|---|
| Suicidal thoughts | Common, driven by low mood | Transient, driven by wish to be with the deceased |
| Blame for situation | Self | Other people or fate |
| Psychomotor retardation | Yes | No |
| Psychotic features | If severe; mood congruent | No, but may 'see' or 'hear' the deceased |
| Symptom course | Pervasive | Fluctuating |

## Abnormal (pathological) grief

Grief can be abnormal in three ways:

- *Absent or delayed grief.* There may appear to be no outward signs of grief despite an event of grief-inducing proportions (absent grief). Grief usually begins a few weeks later (delayed grief).
- *Prolonged grief.* A term used if there are prominent symptoms more than 6–12 months later. At this time, actively consider a developing depressive disorder and the need for treatment.
- *Excessive grief.* The intensity of grief is unusually great—this may reflect the person's closeness to the deceased, their personality or a depressive disorder.

## Grief and depression

A depressive disorder occurs in 1 in 3 grieving people, and is severe in 1 in 5. As the foregoing sections show, it is not easy to decide when the threshold from grief to depression is crossed. The distinction is made largely on the basis of excessive intensity or duration of symptoms, but other features may also help (Table 9.10). The person may need persuading that their suffering is no longer just the pain of normal grief but is now a depressive disorder meriting treatment.

### Key points

- Mood disorders involve excessive deviations or fluctuations of mood. They affect 1 in 6 people at some stage in their lives. Unipolar depressive disorders are much more common than bipolar disorder.
- The core features of depression are low mood, lack of energy, and anhedonia. Many other psychological and somatic symptoms also occur.
- Depression may present with somatic symptoms such as fatigue and weight loss, and should always be considered in the differential diagnosis of these symptoms.
- Suicidal risk needs detailed and regular assessment in everyone with mood disorder.
- Antidepressants are the usual first-line treatment for depressive disorder. Give an adequate dose and continue for at least 6 months after recovery. CBT is as effective as antidepressants for mild and moderate depression: availability is increasing but there can still be long waits. ECT is reserved for severe cases.
- Mania is treated with antipsychotics and/or mood stabilizers. Long-term treatment with the latter reduces the risk of relapse.

## Chapter 10

# Neurotic, stress-related and somatoform disorders

## General characteristics of neurosis

### Neurotic symptoms and syndromes

We all experience anxiety and worries. Sometimes these become so persistent and inappropriate that they can be regarded as an illness. *Neurosis* ('to do with the nerves') or *neurotic disorders* are the traditional terms for those symptoms when they are not due to an organic brain disease, psychosis or personality disorder. The symptoms of neurosis are emotional, cognitive, behavioural and somatic. Neuroses are often but not always associated with an external stressor.

- Anxiety is the primary emotion in all these disorders, although depressed mood is often present.
- The cognitions are worries, fears and concerns that are inappropriate or excessive but (by definition) not delusional.
- Behaviours include avoidance and other strategies intended to reduce anxiety, such as repeated checking.
- Somatic ('physical') symptoms, not explained by a medical disease but associated with tension, autonomic arousal and hyperventilation (such as aches and pains, bowel disturbance and breathlessness), are common.

---

*Lecture Notes: Psychiatry*, 10e. By Paul Harrison, John Geddes and Michael Sharpe. Published 2010 by Blackwell Publishing Ltd.

Neurotic disorders may present with the emotion of anxiety (e.g. attacks of panic) but may also present with one of the other symptoms such as cognitions (e.g. recurrent worries about having a serious medical condition), behaviour (e.g. the agoraphobic unable to leave her house) or somatic symptoms (e.g. palpitations).

- Neuroses are common in primary care and also in medical clinics where the diagnosis is easily missed (Chapter 18).
- Neuroses are not necessarily 'minor' illnesses; they can be chronic and disabling.
- For the clinical features of neurosis, review the module (p. 27).

The individual *neurotic disorders* are listed in Table 10.1. Mild cases can sometimes not be placed into any one of these specific categories and are best described as *undifferentiated neurosis* or *minor emotional disorder*.

- Depressive symptoms are common in patients with neurosis, and neurotic symptoms are very common in patients with depressive disorders. Indeed, in many patients seen in primary care, anxiety and depressive symptoms coexist in similar proportions. A diagnosis of *mixed anxiety–depression* is appropriate for such cases.
- Culture-specific variants of neurosis occur. These include *amok* (dissociative disorder in Indonesia), *koro* (severe anxiety about penis shrinkage in Chinese men) and *dhat* (semen-loss anxiety in Asian men).

**Table 10.1** Classification of neurotic, stress-related and somatoform disorders.

| |
|---|
| *Neurotic disorders (neuroses)* |
|     Anxiety disorders |
|         Phobic anxiety |
|         Panic disorder |
|         Generalized anxiety |
|     Obsessive–compulsive disorder (OCD) |
|     Dissociative disorders |
|     Neurasthenia (chronic fatigue syndrome) |
|     Depersonalization–derealization syndrome |
| |
| *Stress-related disorders* |
|     Acute stress reaction |
|     Adjustment disorders |
|     Post-traumatic stress disorder |
| |
| *Somatoform disorders* |
|     Hypochondriasis |
|     Dysmorphophobia |
|     Somatization disorder |
|     Other somatoform disorders |

## Stress-related and somatoform disorders

The term 'neurosis' has been used to describe patients with predominantly somatic symptoms and also for symptoms clearly caused by stress. In the current classification (Table 10.1) these types of neurosis have each been given their own category; somatoform and stress-related disorders, respectively.

• If somatic symptoms (e.g. palpitations, pain) are unexplained by a medical disease or other psychiatric diagnosis the diagnosis is *somatoform disorder*. This diagnosis is controversial (see below) because of its assumption that such medically unexplained symptoms are better regarded as a psychiatric than as a medical condition.

• If there is a major external stressor that appears to explain the symptoms a *stress-related disorder* may be diagnosed.

## Diagnosing neuroses

If a patient presents with symptoms suggestive of a neurotic disorder, ask two questions:

*First, do the patient's symptoms warrant any diagnosis?*

• Gauge whether the symptoms are diagnostically significant from their intensity, number and pervasiveness, and from the resulting *dysfunction*—are they interfering with the person's life?—and do they need treatment (e.g. see social phobia)?

*Second, is an alternative diagnosis more appropriate?*

• Neurotic symptoms can occur as part of another psychiatric or medical condition, especially depression, but also substance misuse, psychosis, eating disorders and certain organic conditions (e.g. anxiety due to thyrotoxicosis). Life-long symptoms may be better regarded as a personality disorder.

## Epidemiology of neurosis

Neurosis is very common indeed, afflicting about 15% of the population at any one time (Chapter 18). Most neurotic disorders are about twice as common in women. The onset is generally between early adulthood and middle age, though children may have neuroses (Chapter 16).

## Management of neurosis

Management should consider biological, psychological and social factors. Neuroses all respond to certain drugs and psychological treatments. However, some neurotic disorders respond better to certain types of treatment than others:

• Antidepressants and anxiolytic drugs are both effective, though anxiolytics are less commonly used because of concerns about dependence. Antidepressants are effective even when there are few, if any, depressive symptoms—they could also be called 'antineurotics'.

• Simple psychological interventions such as reassurance and explanation are important. Specific psychological therapies, especially CBT, are at least as effective as medication for most neuroses and especially effective for some (e.g. panic disorder). The specific type of CBT used differs between neurotic disorders.

● Social interventions such as removal of stressors and improvement of social support where possible can also be helpful.

## Prognosis of neurosis

The majority of cases of neuroses in primary care are acute and transient. Psychiatrists tend to see the small proportion of cases that are severe, chronic or disabling. The prognosis is better when there is no personality disorder, the patient is strongly motivated to get better and the duration of the illness is short.

## Aetiology of neurosis

Neuroses have a multifactorial aetiology that is best considered from a combination of biological psychological and social perspectives:
● Biologically, neuroses are moderately heritable, are associated with alterations in the 5-HT, noradrenergic and associated brain systems. Neuroimaging studies have demonstrated altered brain function and even altered brain structure (e.g. hippocampal atrophy in post-traumatic stress disorder).
● Psychologically, cognitive factors and behavioural conditioning (Chapter 6) are important, especially in phobias and panic disorder.
● Socially, relevant factors include life stressors, unhelpful responses by the medical system and lack of social support.

The precise combination of these factors in an individual patient in predisposing, precipitating and perpetuating a neurosis can be described in an aetiological formulation (Chapter 5).

## The specific disorders

So far, this chapter has considered the factors common to neurotic syndromes. The rest of the chapter considers factors specific to the individual disorders listed in Table 10.1.

## Anxiety disorders

These neuroses are dominated by the emotion of anxiety together with the anxious thoughts, avoid-

**Table 10.2** Common symptoms of anxiety.

| Component | Prominent features |
|---|---|
| Emotion/mood | Anxiety, irritability |
| Cognitions | Exaggerated worries and fears |
| Behaviour | Avoidance of feared situations<br>Checking<br>Seeking reassurance |
| Somatic symptoms | Tight chest<br>Short of breath<br>Palpitations<br>'Butterflies'<br>Tremor<br>Tingling of fingers (due to hyperventilation)<br>Aches and pains<br>Poor sleep<br>Frequent desire to pass urine and defecate |

ance behaviour and the somatic symptoms of sympathetic arousal that accompany it (Table 10.2). Anxiety disorders are divided into three main subtypes: *phobic, paroxysmal (panic) and generalized* (Table 10.3).
● Somatic symptoms of anxiety (e.g. chest pain) may cause the patient to present initially to general medical services (Chapter 18).

## Phobic anxiety

Phobic anxiety occurs in relation to something. The anxiety is said to be *situational*, and is largely restricted to the experience or anticipation of that situation. This situation may be a specific concern (e.g. heights, spiders) or a more general one (e.g. agoraphobia). As a result of this anxiety the person tends to *avoid* those situations (e.g. a severe mouse phobic may avoid old houses or nature programmes). Although avoidance produces immediate relief from anxiety, it is ultimately counter-productive because it reinforces the fear. Overcoming avoidance is therefore a key part of psychological treatment for phobia.
● The main differential diagnosis is from the other anxiety disorders. Occasionally, phobic anxiety

**Table 10.3** Features distinguishing the three types of anxiety disorder.

|  | Phobic anxiety | Panic disorder | Generalized anxiety |
|---|---|---|---|
| Occurrence of anxiety | Situational | Paroxysmal | Persistent |
| Associated behaviour | Avoidance | Escape | Agitation |
| Associated cognitions | Fear of situation | Fear of symptoms | Worry |
| Somatic symptoms | With exposure | Episodic | Persistent |

**Table 10.4** Symptoms of agoraphobia.

| Component | Prominent features |
|---|---|
| Emotion | Situational anxiety—in shops, crowded large places |
| Cognition | Thoughts of collapsing and being left helpless in public |
| Behaviour | Avoidance of panic-provoking situations |
| Somatic symptoms | Physical sensations of panic |
| Associations | Strong association with panic disorder |

**Table 10.5** Symptoms of social phobia.

| Component | Prominent features |
|---|---|
| Emotion | Situational anxiety in social gatherings |
| Cognition | Being judged negatively by others |
| Behaviour | Avoidance of social occasions |
| Somatic symptoms | Blushing, trembling |
| Associations | Secondary alcohol misuse |

may arise from delusions in a psychosis (e.g. fear of others because they are believed to be aliens). Phobia of having a serious disease is classified separately, as hypochondriasis (see below).

• Behavioural treatment for phobia is based on graded exposure to the situation (either in reality or in imagination), a form of behavioural therapy. In CBT, a cognitive component is added to help the patient more accurately evaluate the dangerousness of the stimulus (e.g. a flight phobic may be encouraged to find out the actual statistical risk of dying in a plane crash).

• Antidepressants and anxiolytic drugs have a role, but exposure therapy may also be required to overcome avoidance.

## Agoraphobia

One of the most common phobias is *agoraphobia* (literally 'fear of the market place') (Table 10.4). Intense anxiety is provoked either by open spaces, or large spaces which are crowded and difficult to escape from (e.g. supermarket queues). Panic attacks are commonly associated, and having a panic attack may itself become the feared situa-

tion. The appropriate diagnosis is then *panic disorder with agoraphobia*.

• The associated cognitions commonly concern fainting, dying or other catastrophe, rather than a fear of shops or spaces *per se*.

• The condition can be severe, and the avoidance can lead the person to become housebound.

• On average symptoms have been present for over 2 years before help is sought. It is most common in young women.

• For a vignette of agoraphobia and its psychological treatment, see pp. 77–8.

## Social phobia

Social phobia is a fear of other people associated with anticipation of negative evaluation by them (Table 10.5). It must be distinguished from normal shyness, and from social withdrawal due to depression. In social phobia there is often a history of low self-esteem and a triggering incident when the person feels they made a fool of themselves. The anxiety may lead to shaking or blushing which becomes a focus for further anxiety.

• Treatment is with CBT and antidepressant drugs, particularly SSRIs.

• Alcohol misuse may develop as a result of self-medication.

● There has been controversy about the boundary between normal shyness and social phobia, reflecting the debate over the degree of 'medicalization of life' and the sometimes arbitrary boundary between neurosis and 'problems of living'.

## Panic disorder

*Panic attacks* are episodes of severe paroxysmal anxiety. They are associated with somatic symptoms and unpleasant feelings of depersonalization or derealization (Table 10.6). In *panic disorder*, the attacks are recurrent over a period of at least 1 month. The somatic symptoms may be severe and lead to a misdiagnosis of angina, epilepsy or other medical disorders.

● The differential diagnosis is from panic attacks occurring only as part of a phobia or occasional panic occurring as part of other neuroses and depressive disorder. Also certain medical conditions can occasionally be a cause of paroxysmal anxiety (Chapter 13).

● CBT is very effective for panic. It is aimed at helping the patient to see their symptoms as the result of anxiety and not as indicators of an impending catastrophe (such as a heart attack). Antidepressants are also effective, although patients with panic disorder may find them hard to tolerate as they may exacerbate panic before reducing it.

● Aetiologically, patients with panic disorder appear to have a low biological threshold for anxiety. Cognitive factors such as a tendency to catastrophically misinterpret somatic symptoms (e.g. the chest pain means that I am having a heart attack) are also important (Chapter 6). Panic attacks may start during a period of stress.

## Generalized anxiety disorder

Generalized anxiety is persistent anxiety associated with chronic uncontrollable and excessive worry (Table 10.7). It may fluctuate in severity but is not paroxysmal (as with panic), situational (as with phobia), life-long (as with a personality disorder) or clearly stress related (as with a stress-related disorder).

● Chronic somatic symptoms such as aches and pains and bowel symptoms may lead to medical presentations.

● Treatment is based on the same pharmacological, psychological and stress-reducing methods used in other anxiety disorders, but their efficacy may be lower.

## Obsessive–compulsive disorder (OCD)

Obsessions and compulsions were defined in Chapter 2. In OCD they are the most prominent and persistent symptoms (Table 10.8). The main differential diagnosis is from depressive disorder (in which obsessional symptoms are common), psychotic disorder (obsessions are usually regarded as untrue, unlike delusions) and obsessional (anankastic) personality disorder.

● Reassure the patient that their condition is one that does not progress to 'madness'.

**Table 10.6** Symptoms of a panic attack.

| Component | Prominent features |
|---|---|
| Emotion | Severe, incapacitating anxiety |
| Cognition | Of dying, going mad or otherwise losing control |
| Behaviour | Escape |
| Somatic symptoms | Prominent symptoms of sympathetic arousal (Table 10.2) |
| Associations | Agoraphobia, depression |

**Table 10.7** Symptoms of generalized anxiety disorder.

| Component | Prominent features |
|---|---|
| Emotion | Anxiety |
| Cognition | Excessive, disproportionate, uncontrollable worry |
| Behaviour | Easily startled, on edge |
| Somatic symptoms | Multiple chronic aches, headache, tension, sweating |
| Associations | Depression |

**Table 10.8** Symptoms of obsessive–compulsive disorder (OCD).

| Component | Predominant features |
|---|---|
| Emotion | Anxiety about the topic of the obsessional thought |
| Cognition | Preoccupation with obsession(s) |
| Behaviour | Compulsions |
| Somatic symptoms | Tension, especially if prevented from doing compulsive act |
| Associations | Depression, anankastic personality disorder, Tourette syndrome |

**Table 10.9** Symptoms of acute stress reaction.

| Component | Predominant features |
|---|---|
| Emotion | 'Dazed' |
| Cognition | Amnesia or denial of event |
| Behaviour | Overactivity or withdrawal |
| Somatic symptoms | Many autonomic symptoms |
| Association | Acute stressor |

- 5-HT-predominant antidepressants (SSRIs, clomipramine) are effective, as is behavioural therapy. A higher dose of antidepressant than in depression is often needed.
- The prognosis untreated is poor. Because of the chronicity of the condition, patients with OCD are frequently used as cases in psychiatry exams.
- Aetiological factors include genetic vulnerability, an anankastic personality and social stressors. The condition is perpetuated by the avoidance of situations that trigger the obsessions, and by the performance of the compulsions; both of which stop the anxiety habituating.
- OCD is unusual amongst neuroses in being equally common in men and women.

## Stress-related disorders

In some cases presenting with neurotic symptoms, the stressor appears to be of such overwhelming importance in causing the symptoms that they are classified as 'reactions to stress'. The whole range of neurotic symptoms may occur, commonly in a diffuse picture of distress, anxiety and depression. The subtypes of stress-related disorders are:
- *Acute stress reaction*—beginning and ending within hours or days of the stressor.
- *Adjustment disorder*—beginning less acutely and lasting several months.
- *Post-traumatic stress disorder (PTSD)*—a delayed response to an extreme stress associated with particular symptoms and especially the re-experiencing of the trauma in dreams or imagination.

## Acute stress reactions

These are transient, but severe, emotional reactions immediately following an exceptional stressor (e.g. rape) and are colloquially referred to as 'nervous shock' (Table 10.9). The differential diagnosis includes the initial stages of other neuroses, acute psychosis (behaviour can be very odd and out of character) and delirium. Management is by removal of the stressor (if possible), reassurance and the provision of support. A short course of benzodiazepines may sometimes be used to reduce arousal.
- Trials show that early 'debriefing' (requiring that the patient tells a therapist about the stressful incident in detail soon after it has occurred) is unhelpful and may even worsen outcome for some patients.

## Adjustment disorders

Also called *adjustment reactions*, these are reactions to stress that are more prolonged than acute stress reactions. The symptoms typically begin within a month of the stress and do not last longer than 6 months (Table 10.10).
- Grief reactions (Chapter 9) and psychological reactions to medical conditions (Chapter 18) are types of adjustment reaction.

  Management includes helping the patient to address a continuing stressor more effectively (perhaps by problem-solving therapy), discouraging unhelpful coping strategies such as substance misuse and treating depressive or anxiety symptoms as necessary.

**Table 10.10** Symptoms of adjustment disorders.

| Component | Prominent features |
|---|---|
| Emotion | Depression, anxiety, poor concentration, irritability |
| Cognition | Preoccupation with event |
| Behaviour | Angry outbursts |
| Somatic symptoms | Moderate autonomic symptoms |
| Associations | Chronic stressor |

**Table 10.12** Symptoms of dissociative disorder.

| Component | Prominent features |
|---|---|
| Emotion | May be suppressed, with denial of anxiety |
| Cognition | Denial of psychological impact of stressors |
| Behaviour | Loss of function |
| Somatic symptoms | Loss of function, e.g. paralysis |
| Associations | Acute stressors, depression |

**Table 10.11** Symptoms of post-traumatic stress disorder (PTSD).

| Component | Prominent features |
|---|---|
| Emotion | Anxiety and irritability, numbness and detachment |
| Cognition | Repeated reliving of the event in images ('flashbacks') and nightmares |
| Behaviour | Avoidance of situations associated with the trauma |
| Somatic symptoms | Exaggerated startle response |
| Associations | Substance misuse, depression, severe previous stressor |

## Post-traumatic stress disorder (PTSD)

PTSD is a delayed response to an exceptionally severe traumatic event (e.g. serious road accident, major disaster, severe assault). It was initially described in Vietnam War veterans and more recently it has been recognized in UK law as a basis for personal compensation claims such as those following road traffic accidents. The onset may be months or years after the original trauma. A central feature is an involuntary re-experiencing of the traumatic event in nocturnal dreams or as intrusive 'day dreams', often triggered by reminders of the trauma (Table 10.11).

Management includes treating comorbid psychiatric disorder or substance misuse, and encouraging a return to normal activities. Antidepressant drugs are modestly effective. There is also good evidence for the effectiveness of CBT.

- A treatment called eye movement desensitization and reprocessing (EMDR) in which the patients is asked to think about an image of the traumatic event whilst moving their eyes from side to side is moderately effective, although there is controversy about how it works.
- The prognosis for PTSD is generally good, with a gradual resolution in most cases, although a minority of cases become chronic; associated alcohol misuse and depression is very common.

## Dissociative and conversion disorders

In dissociative disorders, also called *conversion disorder*, there is a loss of function, either psychological or physical, that is not explained by organic disease (Table 10.12).

- These disorders were called *dissociative* because they were thought to represent a loss of the normal association between different mental processes such as personal identity and memories, sensory and motor function.
- The term *conversion* was used for loss of physical function because of the unsubstantiated theory that psychological conflicts got converted into physical symptoms, thereby resolving the mental conflict (so-called *primary gain*) and often providing practical benefits such as the attention of others (so-called *secondary gain*) (see Chapter 6).
- Dissociative disorders were previously known as *hysterical*; this archaic term (suggesting causation by a wandering uterus) has now been abandoned. Presentations include loss of psychological function such as memory (psychogenic amnesia), wandering in a trance (fugue), loss of motor function

(paralysis, pseudoseizures) or loss of sensory function (glove and stocking anaesthesia).

- When the possibility of a dissociative disorder is raised, organic causes for the loss of function must be excluded. This may require extensive medical investigation.

- Dissociative disorders (which are regarded as originating in unconscious processes) must be distinguished from the consciously motivated symptoms. The latter in turn are divided into *factitious disorder*, in which symptoms are produced deliberately to obtain medical care, and *malingering* which is behaviour that is designed to achieve personal gain (see below). Deciding if someone is feigning illness is difficult and requires evidence of marked inconsistency (e.g. limping into the consulting room and then running for a bus).

- The current diagnostic criteria require that there should be a plausible 'psychogenic' explanation for the symptoms, in terms of severe internal conflicts or a traumatic life event; this is, however, often difficult to establish in practice.

- There have been very few randomized treatment trials. Clinical experience suggests that important components of management are: (a) to accept the reality of the patient's symptoms but to explain that they are potentially reversible; (b) to encourage a gradual return to normal function; (c) to treat coexisting depression; (d) to refer for psychotherapy in some cases; and (e) to refer for physical rehabilitation for chronic disorders that impair motor function.

## Somatoform disorders

The somatoform disorders category was created to accommodate those patients who present with predominantly somatic complaints where neither depression and anxiety nor a medical condition provides a better explanation (Table 10.13). It includes many subcategories. There are two main groups:

- Conditions in which the main feature is concern about having disease (*hypochondriasis*) or deformity (*dysmorphophobia*).

- Conditions in which the main feature is concern about somatic symptoms (*somatization disorder*,

**Table 10.13** Symptoms of somatoform disorders.

| Component | Prominent features |
|---|---|
| Emotion | Anxiety and depression usually present (but not predominant) |
| Cognition | Concern with physical symptoms, disease or deformity |
| Behaviour | Medical help seeking |
| Bodily symptoms | Prominent, defining |
| Associations | Depressive and anxiety disorders, iatrogenic harm from inappropriate medical care (e.g. surgery) |

*persistent autonomic dysfunction, persistent somatoform pain disorder* and *undifferentiated somatoform disorder*).

To make the diagnosis of a somatoform disorder (see module in Chapter 3):

- The concerns and/or symptoms must be unexplained by or disproportionate to any organic disease, severe enough to cause distress and have persisted for at least 6 months.

- Depressive and anxiety symptoms are insufficient to justify a diagnosis of depressive or anxiety disorder.

- The symptoms are not delusional (e.g. distinguish from a psychotic disorder with somatic hallucinations).

- The symptoms are not deliberately manufactured (cf. factitious disorder, malingering), nor is there prominent loss of a specific function (cf. dissociative and conversion disorder).

- Aetiologically, childhood deprivation and abuse are risk factors. A predisposition to health anxiety and serious (and perhaps mismanaged) illness in a relative are also common.

A complementary perspective on the diagnosis of unexplained medical symptoms is discussed in Chapter 18 and shown in Figure 18.2.

## Assessment and management of somatoform disorders

The principles of managing neuroses also apply to somatoform disorders. However, since such patients (and sometimes their doctors) often believe these somatic symptoms indicate medical disease rather than a psychiatric condition, the patients may seek and receive medical rather than psychiatric care. Patients are often hostile to the idea that their symptoms are 'psychogenic' or that they will benefit from psychiatric treatment. The effective management of somatoform disorder therefore requires a close liaison between GP, physician and psychiatrist. The principles are:

• Take the patient's somatic concerns seriously. Neither dismiss them as 'just psychological', nor collude with unfounded beliefs about unproven medical causes.

• Medical investigations should be determined by the doctor's interpretation of the symptoms, not by the patient's demands. People with somatoform disorder are no more likely to die of undiagnosed organic disease than the general population, although they are at risk of harm from unnecessary medical tests and treatments. It is worth remembering that (perhaps counter-intuitively) the more somatic symptoms a patient has, the less likely they are to have a medical disease.

• Ensure a clear and consistent explanation for the symptoms is given that, if possible, is agreed on by all doctors involved.

• Treat coexisting depression and anxiety in the usual way.

• Antidepressants are beneficial in most somatoform disorders, even when there is no good evidence of depression. However, their use needs careful explanation if they are not to be rejected as inappropriately 'psychiatric'.

• CBT is of proven value but must be adapted to be consistent with the patient's predominantly somatic concerns.

• Encourage a return to normal functioning and a decrease in illness behaviour.

## Hypochondriasis and dysmorphophobia

The characteristic feature of these somatoform disorders is a preoccupation with the possibility of having a serious physical disease or deformity.

• The main differential diagnoses are depressive disorder (in which hypochondriacal worries and concerns about appearance are common) and psy-

chotic disorders (with hypochondriacal delusions or somatic hallucinations).

## Hypochondriasis

Patients with hypochondriasis are preoccupied with the idea that they have a serious medical condition when they do not. Hypochondriasis has also been considered a form of anxiety disorder or of OCD. Patients repeatedly seek medical reassurance and investigation, but are not reassured by either.

• Repeated requests for investigation to exclude a serious disease may be the presenting feature.

• Both antidepressants and CBT can be effective. It may be necessary to help the patients to restrict their tendency to seek reassurance or check their bodies as these behaviours tend to perpetuate the condition.

• The prognosis is variable: transient hypochondriasis is common (e.g. in medical students), but once established the condition can last many years and lead to extensive medical investigations.

## Dysmorphophobia

Also called *body dysmorphic disorder*, in this disorder the preoccupation is with a subjectively abnormal physical appearance (e.g. perceived ugliness or deformity) that is not objectively present and often associated with avoidance of social interaction.

• Management follows the principles described for somatoform disorders in general. Patients often request cosmetic surgery which may sometimes be helpful but which can also lead to further dissatisfaction. Specialist assessment is advisable before surgery is performed.

## Somatic symptom disorders (somatization disorder and associated diagnoses)

Somatic symptoms such as fatigue and pain that are not adequately explained by medical disease are very common. When these are persistent and associated with disability and or distress they may appropriately be regarded as illnesses and consequently require a diagnosis. Such patients comprise about a third of all attenders in medical out-patient clinics, and so are clinically important (Chapter 18).

- Confusingly, medicine and psychiatry have developed parallel diagnostic systems for these problems. Medicine uses diagnoses of so-called 'functional disorders' describing the symptoms in terms of the bodily system they relate to (see below). Psychiatry uses somatoform diagnoses based mainly on the number of symptoms and their duration. The current psychiatric classification is as given below.

## Somatization disorder (Briquet's syndrome)

These patients, almost always women, present with multiple different medically unexplained symptoms that have occurred over many years. They have often had normal abdominal organs surgically removed, an observation which highlights the risk of iatrogenic harm. They have been described as adopting 'illness as a way of life'. Recurrent major depression and personality disorder are common associations—indeed some regard the condition as a personality disorder.

- Management is based on 'damage limitation' and containment by long-term follow-up. There is no specific treatment, but active treatment of associated recurrent depression and anxiety may be helpful.
- The prognosis is very poor. Iatrogenic problems, such as drug reactions and abdominal adhesions, may result from unnecessary medical and surgical interventions.

## Undifferentiated somatoform disorder

This is the diagnosis used instead of somatization disorder when the patient has few symptoms.

## Persistent somatoform pain disorder

This diagnosis is used when the main symptom is pain that is inadequately explained by a medical disease. Antidepressants are useful; TCAs and SNRIs (Chapter 7) are more effective than SSRIs. CBT may be helpful.

## Somatoform autonomic dysfunction

This is a rarely used diagnosis for cases where the symptoms are thought to be clearly explicable in terms of autonomic arousal and associated overbreathing (e.g. breathlessness, chest pain, flushing, diarrhoea and tremor).

## Functional somatic syndromes and their relationship to somatoform disorders

The medical classification of functional somatic symptoms (Table 10.14) is a parallel one to the psychiatric classification of somatoform disorders. Functional somatic syndrome diagnoses are commonly made in most medical specialities and account for a very substantial number of the patients seen. For example, irritable bowel syndrome is the most common diagnosis made in many gastroenterological clinics; the majority of cases of acute chest pain are 'non-cardiac', and often associated with panic disorder. Similarly, numbness, weakness and tingling are frequent symptoms in neurology clinics, yet are often 'functional'. It should also be noted that more than half of patients with a functional somatic syndrome satisfy criteria for depressive or anxiety disorder rather than a somatoform disorder (see Figure 18.2). This is important for treatment. Because the diagnostic systems overlap, but emphasize different aspects of the presentation, a combined medical and psychiatric diagnosis may be preferred—for example, irritable bowel syndrome and generalized anxiety disorder

**Table 10.14** Common functional somatic syndrome diagnoses.

| Medically unexplained pain syndromes |
| --- |
| Non-cardiac chest pain |
| Facial pain |
| Pelvic pain |
| Back pain |
| Irritable bowel syndrome |
| Muscular pain and fibromyalgia |
| Medically unexplained chronic fatigue |
| Chronic fatigue syndrome |

or chronic fatigue syndrome and somatization disorder.

- See the vignettes in Chapter 18.

## Neurasthenia (chronic fatigue syndrome, CFS)

The term neurasthenia is now rarely used in the UK or the USA but remains in common usage in China and some other countries. There is substantial overlap with the functional syndrome of *chronic fatigue syndrome* (CFS). Although classified separately, neurasthenia has much in common with somatoform disorders, in that physical complaints predominate, no definite medical disease has been identified and the presentation is usually to non-psychiatric services. The main feature is persistent, disabling mental and physical fatigue, often accompanied by pain and other symptoms (Table 10.15).

The differential diagnosis is from fatigue associated with medical conditions and from depressive and anxiety disorders. A simple explanation that the symptoms are real and not imagined but reversible rather than fixed can be helpful.

- There is good evidence for the efficacy of CBT and graded increases in activity, but less for antidepressants.
- The prognosis is often poor, with a tendency to chronicity. Avoidance of physical activity and belief in a physical cause are associated with a worse outcome.

**Table 10.15** Symptoms of neurasthenia (chronic fatigue syndrome).

| Component | Prominent features |
| --- | --- |
| Emotion | Exhaustion, tiredness, irritability |
| Cognitions | Concern about fatigue and its causes, poor concentration |
| Behaviour | Avoids physical exertion |
| Bodily symptoms | Physical and/or mental fatigue after minor exertion, muscular pain (myalgia), headache, patchy sleep |
| Associations | Depression |

- The aetiology is very controversial. Biological, psychological and social factors are involved. Biologically, there is evidence for disturbed cerebral 5-HT function and reduced cortisol. Although many patients report onset after a viral infection, and patients with documented Epstein–Barr virus (EBV) infection can develop a fatigue syndrome, the aetiological role of viruses (or retroviruses) overall remains uncertain. Psychologically, depression, anxiety and excessive concern with symptoms leading to inactivity is common. Socially, a fear of a stigmatizing psychiatric diagnosis and widely available misinformation may shape patients' illness beliefs and help-seeking behaviour.
- A similar constellation of symptoms is also referred to as *myalgic encephalomyelitis (ME)*. This condition is thought by some to be better regarded as a neurological disorder and distinct from CFS, although this is also controversial.

## Factitious disorders and malingering

The relationship between bodily symptoms and psychiatric disorder is complicated further by patients who consciously elaborate or even deliberately make up symptoms. These are not neuroses but are included here because of their importance in the differential diagnosis of patients presenting with somatic symptoms.

- If the behaviour appears to be aimed at receiving medical treatment it is called *factitious disorder*. People with persistent, severe factitious disorder who travel from one hospital to another have been described as having *Munchausen's syndrome* (after Baron von Munchausen, who told stories of fantastic exploits). The degree of conscious manipulation is often unclear. Little is known about the condition, which is usually viewed as a personality disorder.
- If the behaviour is for fraudulent purposes (e.g. to avoid legal proceedings or military conscription) it is referred to as *malingering*. Factitious disorder is a psychiatric disorder; malingering is not.

If there is suspicion that symptoms are being manufactured, discrete but determined efforts to verify the person's details and history should be made. Once a factitious disorder has been confirmed, the patient should be gently confronted with the evidence. However sympathetically handled, self-discharge commonly results. People with factitious disorder make doctors feel angry and manipulated—most doctors have been 'fooled' by a patient with Munchausen's syndrome. Take care not to generalize these negative feelings to the larger group of patients who have medical problems you cannot explain by a disease diagnosis.

## Depersonalization–derealization syndrome

Depersonalization and derealization (Chapter 3) are symptoms that can occur in all neuroses. Occasionally they are the predominant feature, in which case this rarely used diagnostic category applies. The differential diagnosis is from a depressive or anxiety disorder, or psychosis, and from organic causes, especially complex partial epilepsy. The usual guidelines for managing neurosis apply.

Antidepressants may help, but the prognosis for established cases is poor.

### Key points

- Neuroses are syndromes of emotional, cognitive, behavioural and somatic symptoms that are not secondary to another disorder. Neurotic symptoms occur commonly in other psychiatric disorders.
- Neuroses afflict 15% of the population, women more than men. They may become chronic and disabling. The main subtypes are anxiety disorders and somatoform disorders.
- Stress-related disorders are neuroses in which there is a clear relationship to a major psychological stressor.
- Somatoform disorders encompass medically unexplained symptoms (somatization) and fears about having physical disease (hypochondriasis), and are closely related to other neuroses. They are usually seen in non-psychiatric medical settings.
- Neuroses, stress-related disorders, and somatoform disorders can all be treated psychologically (especially with CBT) or with antidepressants. Anxiolytics can also be useful in the short term.

# Chapter 11

# Eating, sleep and sexual disorders

Disorders of eating, sleeping and sex are grouped together as they are syndromes associated with a disturbance in basic desires and behaviours.

- Assessment of eating disorders was covered in a module (Chapter 3); assessment of sexual functioning is dealt with later in this chapter.

## Eating disorders

All eating disorders share the same core features:

- A preoccupation with, and overemphasis on, body shape and weight. These thoughts are overvalued ideas, rather than delusions or obsessions.
- The use of extreme dietary restriction, often with other weight control behaviours (e.g. exercise, vomiting, laxatives).
- There is a significant impairment of physical health or psychosocial functioning.
- The problems are not secondary to a general medical disorder or other psychiatric condition.
- They occur mainly in young women.

  Eating disorders are conventionally separated into *anorexia nervosa* and *bulimia nervosa*, as described below. However, bear two clinical realities in mind when reading the following sections:

- Many patients—maybe the majority—do not meet all the criteria for either disorder, or have

some features of both. They are labelled *atypical eating disorder* [or *eating disorder not otherwise specified (NOS)*] (Figure 11.1). This does not mean their disorder is any less severe.

- Many patients move from one category to another over time (Figure 11.2).

## Anorexia nervosa

### Clinical features

As well as the core features above, the key elements of anorexia nervosa are:

- *Deliberate weight loss*, induced primarily by restriction of food intake.
- *Weight ≥15% below normal* (BMI <17.5).
- *Amenorrhoea* (if post-menarche and not using hormonal contraceptive). Part of a wider endocrine disturbance that includes elevated cortisol and growth hormone levels.

  Additional features include:

- A range of bodily symptoms and signs, which get more pronounced as weight loss progresses (Table 11.1). The medical complications can be serious and life threatening, especially if the effects of starvation are exacerbated by the metabolic consequences of vomiting, or diuretic or laxative abuse.
- The core psychological features (e.g. 'fear of fatness') become paradoxically worse as weight is lost (maybe because it increases the 5-HT dysfunction which is thought to contribute to the

*Lecture Notes: Psychiatry*, 10e. By Paul Harrison, John Geddes and Michael Sharpe. Published 2010 by Blackwell Publishing Ltd.

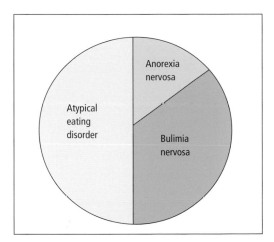

**Figure 11.1** Relative prevalence of eating disorders in community samples.

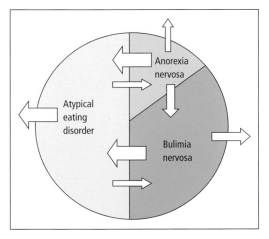

**Figure 11.2** Patients move with time from one eating disorder to another. The size of the arrows shows the likelihood of movement; arrows outside the circle indicate recovery.

disturbance). The disorder thus tends to be self-perpetuating—reinforced by the fact that achieving a lower weight has certain rewards: it may enhance feelings of self-control, result in perceived approval from peers, avoid sexual development or gain parental attention.
- Depressive and obsessional symptoms.
- If the onset is before puberty, secondary sexual development is delayed.

**Table 11.1** Physical features and medical complications of anorexia nervosa.

*Physical symptoms*
Sensitivity to cold
Gastrointestinal symptoms—constipation, bloating
Dizziness
Amenorrhea
Poor sleep

*Physical signs*
Emaciation
Cold extremities
Dry skin, sometimes orange (hypercarotinaemia)
Downy hair ('*lanugo*') on back, forearms and cheeks
Poorly developed or atrophic secondary sexual
    characteristics
Bradycardia, postural hypotension, arrythmias
Peripheral oedema
Proximal myopathy

*Abnormalities on investigation*
Low LH, FSH, oestradiol, $T_3$
Increased cortisol, growth hormone
Hypoglycaemia
Hypokalaemia, hyponatraemia, metabolic alkalosis
ECG: prolonged QT interval (serious)
Hypercholesterolaemia
Osteopenia and osteoporosis
Delayed gastric emptying
Acute gastric dilatation (due to over-rapid refeeding)

- Depression, fatigue and irritability, especially as weight loss becomes pronounced.
- Social withdrawal and narrowing of interests.
- Use of diuretics, laxatives, excess exercise or self-induced vomiting to enhance weight loss.

*Miss T, 14, was noticed to be losing weight although this was partially disguised by baggy clothing. She enjoyed cooking for the family and took up regular aerobics. She became vegetarian and avoided all fattening foods. When the issue of her weight was raised, Miss T became upset, insisting that she was fat. She had a history of obesity. The GP found she was underweight (BMI = 15) and suspected anorexia nervosa.*

## Epidemiology and aetiology

Anorexia mainly affects females (sex ratio 10:1). The average age of onset is 15–16 years. The

**Table 11.2** Risk factors for eating disorders.

| |
|---|
| *General factors* |
| Female (sex ratio ~10 : 1) |
| Adolescence and early adulthood |
| Living in a Western society |
| |
| *Family history* |
| Eating disorder |
| Depression |
| Substance misuse (bulimia nervosa) |
| Obesity (bulimia nervosa) |
| |
| *Premorbid experiences* |
| Adverse parenting—low contact, high expectations, arguments |
| Sexual abuse |
| Family dieting |
| Critical comments about eating, weight or shape |
| Pressure to be slim |
| |
| *Premorbid characteristics* |
| Low self-esteem |
| Perfectionism (anorexia nervosa) |
| Anxiety |
| Obesity (bulimia nervosa) |
| Early menarche (bulimia nervosa) |

prevalence in Western societies, including the UK, is about 1% in females aged 12–18. Social pressure to be thin has been blamed. The other risk factors are summarized in Table 11.2.

- Note that most risk factors are shared with bulimia nervosa.
- The familial risk of anorexia nervosa does not seem to be genetic in origin (in contrast to most other psychiatric disorders).

## Differential diagnosis

The classic picture of anorexia nervosa is unmistakeable. In the early stages it must be distinguished from other causes of weight loss. The psychiatric differential diagnosis includes depressive disorder, substance misuse, OCD and body dysmorphic disorder. The medical disorders include inflammatory bowel disease, malabsorption syndromes, hypopituitarism and cancer. The distinction is made by:

- Detecting the core psychological symptoms of anorexia nervosa.
- Excluding physical and other psychiatric causes of weight loss.

## Management

The objectives of treatment of anorexia nervosa are:

- Altering the person's attitude to weight and body shape via psychological treatments.
- Helping them increase weight.
- Detecting and treating medical complications.

The second and third components can be achieved reasonably successfully, at least in the short term; the first component is difficult as the core beliefs are often resistant to treatment. Some principles of management are:

- Establish a good therapeutic relationship—many patients are reluctant to accept treatment. Help them to see they need help, and maintain motivation thereafter. Agree some goals: what weight is the person prepared to work towards? At what rate? How much exercise is appropriate?
- Encourage early weight gain to break the cycle and to overcome the problem that starvation interferes with psychological treatments. Weight gain is promoted by behavioural strategies—for example, contingent rewards.
- The key element of therapy is to change attitudes towards weight and shape, and the person's preoccupation with them. There are no firmly evidence-based treatments for adults, although a modified type of CBT ('transdiagnostic CBT') shows promise. Most adolescent patients respond well to a specific form of family therapy.
- Drugs (antidepressants or antipsychotics) do not have an established role in management, though they are sometimes used to promote or maintain weight gain, or treat depressive symptoms.
- Monitor physical condition. Serum potassium should be checked regularly. Multivitamins and supplements may be used.

### In-patient treatment

In-patient care is indicated if weight loss is intractable and severe (e.g. BMI <14), or if there is a serious risk of death from suicide or medical complications. Admission is preferably to a specialist unit. It usually lasts 8–12 weeks. The purposes are to:

- Manage medical complications.
- Actively encourage re-feeding—ensuring a balanced diet of 3000 calories per day.
- Allow intensive psychological treatments.
- Compulsory admission is rarely used, and considered only if life is in immediate danger. Forced re-feeding is also used occasionally and controversially.

*Miss T is now 15 and has collapsed. For the past year, despite denials to her parents, she had dieted and exercised excessively. She weighed 29 kg (BMI = 12.5), was hypothermic and had a low blood potassium. After medical stabilization she passively accepted admission to an eating disorder unit. She began a behavioural programme with a target to gain 0.5 kg/week for 2 months. A psychiatrist and nurse therapist explored eating and weight issues in individual and family sessions. Her potassium was monitored regularly. Ten weeks later her BMI was 15 and she became an out-patient.*

## Prognosis

The outcome of anorexia nervosa is variable. About 20% have a good outcome, with a short-lived disorder and full recovery. Another 10–20% develop a chronic and intractable disorder. The rest progress to another eating disorder, have a relapsing illness or have residual features (Figure 11.2).

- The mortality rate is increased 10-fold in the first 10 years of illness, with a 10–20% death rate in long-term follow-up studies. Death is usually from complications of starvation, sometimes from suicide.
- Poor outcome is associated with: long duration prior to presentation; onset in adulthood; severe weight loss; vomiting.

*Miss T is now 27 and a beautician. She has a BMI of 16 and has occasional scanty menstrual periods. She continues to be preoccupied with her appearance, and gains self-esteem from her control over eating and weight. She diets continually and works out twice a day. Now and then she has a large binge followed by self-induced vomiting and extra gym sessions. She avoids doctors.*

## Bulimia nervosa

*Bulimia* refers to uncontrolled eating binges. Many people binge and feel bad about it, but in bulimia nervosa it is excessive, repetitive and associated with self-induced vomiting and other means to negate the calorific effect of the binges. It punctuates an otherwise anorexia nervosa-like pattern of dietary restriction.

## Clinical features

In addition to the core features of eating disorders, bulimia nervosa is characterized by:

- Recurrent binge eating (more than twice a week); 1000–4000 kcal (4–8 MJ) are typically consumed in a binge.
- 'Loss of control' during binges.
- Attempts to counteract the binges by vomiting, or by using other means such as laxatives, enemas, diuretics or excessive exercise.
- Does not meet diagnostic criteria for anorexia nervosa.
- The combination of dieting and bingeing means body weight is usually unremarkable—the most obvious difference from anorexia nervosa.
- A small proportion of bulimia nervosa occurs in women with borderline personality disorder who self-harm (often by cutting) and misuse alcohol or drugs. This is a much rarer combination than sometimes believed.

If body weight is decreased, some of the physical features and complications of anorexia nervosa may be present (Table 11.1). Otherwise, fewer abnormalities are seen in bulimia nervosa. Those which are reflect the self-induced vomiting, or abuse of laxatives or diuretics:

- Repeated vomiting may produce pitted teeth (eroded by gastric acid), calluses on the knuckles ('Russell's sign', from putting fingers down throat), hoarse voice, salivary gland enlargement, metabolic disturbances (Table 11.1).
- Diuretic use: electrolyte disturbances and renal dysfunction.

• Laxatives: electrolyte disturbances and colonic motility problems.

## Epidemiology and aetiology

Bulimia nervosa occurs in 2% of women aged 16–35 years but is otherwise rare. Based on community services, only 10% of cases ever present for help. Many of the risk factors are shared with anorexia nervosa (Table 11.2). There is a genetic predisposition, which overlaps with that for anxiety disorders.

• The genetic contribution to bulimia nervosa is controversial. Some studies suggest a surprisingly large heritability—over 80%.

> Miss V is 23. She has several episodes of bingeing and vomiting each week. In an hour she can eat 10 packets of crisps, 10 chocolate bars and a couple of loaves of bread washed down with a bottle of wine. She then makes herself sick. She is preoccupied with her weight and shape and feels fat (though her BMI is normal). She has a history of taking overdoses when particularly distressed. She was obese as a child, and sexually abused by an uncle. There is a family history of obesity and depression.

## Differential diagnosis

• Anorexia nervosa with bulimic features (anorexia trumps bulimia, diagnostically, although in reality a better term would be 'eating disorder NOS', as explained above).
• Sporadic bingeing in other psychiatric disorders (e.g. atypical depression).
• Medical causes of vomiting.
• Binge eating disorder—a controversial (American) category. Recurrent binges occur but without extreme weight control behaviour. Strongly associated with obesity. Compared with bulimia nervosa, it is more common in men (a third of cases) and in middle age.

## Management

Treatments are markedly more effective (and better evaluated) than in anorexia nervosa. Take a 'stepped care' approach, depending on the severity of the problem and the patient's wishes.

Self-help manuals are a cost-effective and increasingly used first-line treatment.
• A modified form of CBT is effective in 60–70% of patients, with the majority remaining well 5 years later. CBT aims to help the patient: (a) understand the links between bingeing, vomiting and dieting; (b) regulate their diet and break the vicious cycle between the three behaviours; and (c) decrease their preoccupation with body shape.
• Interpersonal therapy (IPT) also works, but takes longer. IPT emphasizes the role of relationship problems in the disorder.
• Antidepressants reduce the frequency of bingeing and vomiting. The best evidence is for fluoxetine. High doses (60–80 mg/day) may be required, and the disorder often relapses on stopping.

## Prognosis

The prognosis of bulimia nervosa is probably better than that of anorexia nervosa (the mortality rate is certainly lower), though there are few good data.
• People have had bulimia nervosa for an average of 5 years at presentation; 30–50% still have an eating disorder (bulimia nervosa or atypical eating disorder) 5–10 years later.
• Poor prognostic factors include: premorbid childhood obesity, low self-esteem and personality disturbance.

## Sleep disorders

Sleep problems are usually secondary to a psychiatric or medical disorder, but sometimes a sleep disorder is the primary diagnosis.

## Insomnia

### Assessment

Insomnia describes a persistently unsatisfactory quantity or quality of sleep. A third of adults complain of it. It causes much distress and is a risk factor for premature death; 80% of cases of insomnia are related to anxiety and depressive disorders.

Most of the rest are secondary to medical disease (e.g. it is common in Parkinson's disease), chronic pain and substance misuse. The remaining fraction (<10%) are *primary insomnia*. To distinguish these cases, exclude the presence of an underlying psychiatric or medical disorder (e.g. restless legs syndrome, lymphoma). Ask about other factors that affect sleep such as shift working, medication, alcohol, caffeine, etc. A sleep diary and corroboration from the sleeping partner are helpful.

## Treatment

Treat any associated disorder (e.g. use a sedative antidepressant if insomnia is due to depression). Interventions for insomnia include:

- *Stimulus control.* An effective method to restore a good sleep routine. The person should go to bed only when sleepy, put the light out straight away, get up if awake for more than 20 minutes, get up at a regular time and avoid daytime naps.
- *Sleep hygiene*—this approach pays attention to health practices (e.g. use of caffeine and alcohol) and stimuli (e.g. noise, light) that affect sleep.
- *Relaxation therapy*—behavioural, cognitive and biofeedback routines to reduce arousal. The person should wind down 90 minutes before bedtime and practise relaxation when in bed.
- *Hypnotics*—short-acting benzodiazepines and related drugs (Chapter 7). Effective in the short term and widely used, but may cause daytime drowsiness, and long-term use should be avoided because of dependence.

## Hypersomnia

*Hypersomnia* is excessive daytime sleepiness, or having a prolonged time in the twilight zone between sleep and wakefulness. The term excludes cases secondary to insomnia or where there are clear reasons for such behaviour (e.g. shift working). Causes are shown in Table 11.3.

- In *narcolepsy* there are repeated attacks of daytime somnolence usually leading irresistibly to sleep. It usually begins in the second decade and is associated with *cataplexy* (abrupt loss of muscle tone), *hypnagogic hallucinations* (Chapter 2) and

**Table 11.3** Causes of hypersomnia.

| |
|---|
| *Psychiatric disorders* |
|    Depressive disorder |
|    Neuraesthenia (chronic fatigue syndrome) |
| *Medical disorders* |
|    Narcolepsy |
|    Klein–Levin syndrome |
|    Sleep apnoea syndrome |
|    Chronic physical disease |
| *Other* |
|    Side-effects of drugs (prescribed or illicit) |

*sleep paralysis* (the patient wakes but is unable to move). An autoimmune origin is suspected as 98% have the DR15 variant of HLA-DR2. Pathologically, there is a loss of hypothalamic hypocretin-producing neurons. Stimulants (amphetamines or modafinil) are the main treatment; clomipramine is also used for the cataplexy.

## Parasomnias

Parasomnias are abnormal episodic events during sleep—sleepwalking, nightmares, etc. They are part of normal development in children; in adults they usually reflect emotional stress.

- Distinguish parasomnias from other causes of odd nocturnal behaviour, such as epilepsy.

## Sexual problems

Psychiatrists are sometimes portrayed as being obsessed with sex—a relic of Freudian theories, and perhaps by media portrayals. The reality is rather different and more mundane. Nevertheless, an understanding of sexual problems and how to assess them is important in psychiatry because:

- Sexual dysfunction is a common consequence of psychiatric disorders or their treatment. For example, loss of libido in depression; ejaculatory failure due to antipsychotics.
- Sexual dysfunction may contribute to psychiatric disorder. For example, an anxiety disorder may be exacerbated by a man worrying about his impotence.

**Table 11.4** Types of sexual dysfunction.

| |
|---|
| *Sexual desire disorders* |
|     Lack of |
|     Excess |
| |
| *Failure of genital response* |
|     Erectile dysfunction (impotence) |
|     Vaginal dryness |
| |
| *Orgasmic dysfunction* |
|     Premature ejaculation |
|     Anorgasmia |
| |
| *Other* |
|     Vaginismus (involuntary spasm of vaginal |
|       musculature) |
|     Dyspareunia |

- Disorders of sexual function, preference and identity are specific mental disorders.

## Sexual dysfunction

Each of the components of sex—desire, physiological arousal and orgasm—can go awry (Table 11.4). Each type of dysfunction may be due to psychological or medical causes, or both.
- Painful intercourse, loss of sexual desire and impaired orgasm are more common in women; the main problems for men are impotence and premature ejaculation.
- Sexual dysfunction is associated with sexual inexperience, anxiety and relationship problems.

## Assessment of sexual dysfunction

Asking about sex is the topic, along with suicide, which most health professionals feel least confident and most embarrassed about. This is unnecessary. Many patients are glad to be asked, since sexual problems are common and it may be their first opportunity to seek reassurance or treatment.
- Know when to introduce the subject—try and respond to cues. For example, if a depressed patient tells you he gets no pleasure from life, it is a good moment to ask whether this has also affected his interest in sex. If no cue presents itself, preface the assessment with a comment such as: 'I need to ask you some questions about your sex life, to help me understand your problem. Is this alright?'.
- Use terminology appropriate to the person's age and culture.

Assessment of sexual function covers several areas (Table 11.5). Some of the questions will be used regularly, others rarely. Below are further details of two common sexual disorders to illustrate the general approaches to assessment and treatment of sexual dysfunction.

## Erectile dysfunction

Erectile dysfunction is the inability to reach erection or to sustain an erection long enough for intercourse. Most erectile dysfunction is secondary—that is, full erection was possible at one time, but is now difficult to achieve. Primary erectile dysfunction is rare and usually has a neurological or circulatory basis.

Common causes of impotence include:
- Anxiety about sexual performance.
- Alcohol.
- Unwanted effects of prescription medicines.
- Diabetes.
- Vascular disease.

Treatment is usually with combined psychological and physical approaches. Underlying disorders should be treated. Psychological treatment is outlined below. Drug treatment with phosphodiesterase type V inhibitors (e.g. sildenafil) is now widespread and has largely replaced injections and devices.
- Prescribing of sildenafil for 'psychological' impotence is possible on the NHS, but restricted to specialist centres and for those 'suffering severe distress as a result of impotence'.

## Dyspareunia

Dyspareunia is pain on intercourse. It may result from impaired lubrication with vaginal secretions (due to anxiety or inadequate arousal) or from physical scarring (e.g. after childbirth). Pain on penetration may be due to pelvic pathology.

**Table 11.5** Assessment of sexual function.

| Questions | Comments |
|---|---|
| **Current sexual functioning** | |
| *What is the nature and frequency of sex?* | |
| Is there a particular problem? | Get a history of each difficulty |
| How much interest do you have in sex? Has this changed recently? | Increased libido is rarely complained of. A feature of mania |
| **In men** | |
| *Erectile function:* | |
| Any problems getting or keeping an erection? | |
| Do you get erections in the morning? | Loss of morning erections or when masturbating suggests organic cause |
| Do you worry about your sexual performance? | Impotence related to performance anxiety |
| *Ejaculatory function:* | |
| Do you come too quickly? | Common in inexperienced, anxious men |
| How long after penetration? | |
| Do you feel anxious about this? | |
| **In women** | |
| Do you have pain on intercourse? When? Where? | Dyspareunia and vaginal dryness have psychological and gynaecological causes |
| Do you feel anxious or tense about sex? | Extreme anxiety can lead to vaginismus |
| **Sexual development** | |
| *Estimate age of puberty* | |
| When did your voice break? Periods start? | Problems or delays in sexual development may lead to psychological effects or indicate an abnormality (e.g. Turner's syndrome) |
| When did you first masturbate? First intercourse? | Affected by cultural and individual differences |
| **Sexual orientation and preferences** | |
| *What is their sexual orientation?* | |
| Any particular sexual preferences or fetishes? | Detailed questioning indicated if the patient views it as a problem, or in a forensic context |
| If so, what? | |
| Have they ever got you into trouble? | |
| **Other issues** | |
| *Current psychiatric disorder?* | Most psychiatric disorders, especially depression, are associated with sexual dysfunction |
| *General health?* | Medical disorders (e.g. diabetes, vascular disease) affect sexual functioning; do a physical examination |
| *Current medication?* | Many drugs have sexual side-effects (e.g. thiazide diuretics, $H_2$ antagonists, antihypertensives—as well as antidepressants and antipsychotics) |

● When dyspareunia is secondary to psychological factors, sexual therapy techniques can be used (see below).

## Psychological treatment of sexual dysfunction

Sexual problems may respond to reassurance or use of self-help manuals. Others require sex therapy, which is provided by some psychiatrists and by private therapists. Sex therapy uses behavioural methods, and is effective (assuming no underlying medical cause for the dysfunction). The principles are:

● Treat the couple together.

● Educate about sex and the factors affecting it.

● Encourage open discussion of feelings and decrease anxiety and embarrassment.

● Use graded exposure (Chapter 7). The couple gradually rebuild their sexual relationship, setting aside time and commitment to follow a series of steps—starting with non-genital 'sensate focus', then moving on via genital focus before finally returning to full intercourse. Additional methods are used for specific forms of dysfunction. For example, dilators for vaginismus or the squeeze technique for premature ejaculation.

● Lack of sexual desire has the worst prognosis.

## Other sexual disorders

In these disorders the problem is not sex itself but the object of sexual desire—at least to the extent that it conflicts the law, societal views or causes harm. The person may or may not agree with this view. In ICD-10, these disorders are grouped with personality disorders.

● Forensic psychiatrists may be asked to report on the psychiatric status of sex offenders.

● Homosexuality used to be classified as a psychiatric disorder.

## Gender identity disorders

● In *trans-sexualism* the person, usually male, wishes to live as a member of the opposite sex. They seek hormonal or surgical treatment to match their body to their subjective gender. Sexual orientation is variable and sexual desire often low. Trans-sexuals may suffer great distress, and depression is common.

● *Transvestism* is the urge to dress in clothes of the opposite sex. If accompanied by sexual arousal it is called *fetishistic* transvestism. There is no desire to change sex. Transvestites are often married and cross-dress secretly. There is no specific treatment.

## Disorders of sexual preference (paraphilias)

Sexual desire can centre on a wide range of animate and inanimate objects. Such pleasures only constitute a disorder if the activity is illegal (e.g. paedophilia) or if sex becomes dysfunctional and overdependent on an object such as shoes (e.g. fetishism). Paraphilia is usually but not always a male disorder.

● In *paedophilia*, sexual interest or activity centres on prepubescent children. The prevalence is unknown, though there is a considerable demand for child pornography. Psychological treatments have been used to reduce reoffending rates; cyproterone acetate, an antiandrogen, has been used to suppress libido. The effectiveness of these treatments is uncertain.

● *Exhibitionism* is the exposing of the genitals to strangers. Two groups are recognized: (1) inhibited men who struggle against the urge, feel guilty and expose a flaccid penis (type 1); (2) aggressive men who expose an erect penis and masturbate then or later (type 2). The latter shows an association with actual sexual assaults. Behavioural treatments may be beneficial.

## Key points

- The core psychopathology of all eating disorders is a preoccupation with body shape and weight, with extreme methods to control weight—notably dietary restriction. They occur mainly but not exclusively in young women.
- Anorexia nervosa is characterized additionally by a low body weight (BMI <17.5), extreme dietary restriction, and amenorrhea in women.
- Bulimia nervosa is distinguished by recurrent binge eating and self-induced vomiting.
- Half of patients with an eating disorder do not meet criteria for anorexia or bulimia nervosa.
- Bulimia nervosa responds well to CBT. No effective treatments are proven for anorexia nervosa.
- Sleep disorders comprise insomnia, hypersomnia and parasomnias (disturbances during sleep). Many are secondary to other psychiatric or medical disorders. They may be treated psychologically or pharmacologically.
- Sexual dysfunction is common and can affect the desire, the mechanics or the orgasm. Assessment of sexual function is important. Sex therapy is effective for many of the problems.

# Chapter 12

# Schizophrenia

Historically, schizophrenia has been at the heart of psychiatry and is closest to the public conception of madness. Although by no means the most common disorder, it accounts for a significant proportion of psychiatric morbidity and the workload of psychiatric services.

- Patients with schizophrenia occupy over 25% of psychiatric beds, and account for 50% of admissions.
- Direct and indirect health costs of schizophrenia in England in 2004–5 were £6.7 billion.
- It is in the top 10 causes of worldwide disability.

## Clinical features

Schizophrenia is a psychosis, typically presenting in young adults. It is distinguished from other psychoses by:

- The presence of specific types of delusions, hallucinations and thought disorder.
- The absence of a mood disorder or organic psychosis.
- The clinical course.

The clinical picture of schizophrenia is complex. Here, the acute and the chronic stages of the disorders are described in turn—though in practice there is a continuum of features.

*Lecture Notes: Psychiatry*, 10e. By Paul Harrison, John Geddes and Michael Sharpe. Published 2010 by Blackwell Publishing Ltd.

- Before proceeding, review the relevant parts of the core assessment (Chapter 2) and the psychosis module (Chapter 3). These earlier sections include definitions of the cardinal symptoms.

## Clinical features of acute schizophrenia

The diagnostic features are shown in Table 12.1. Particular weight is placed on the presence of the first-rank symptoms (see also Table 3.2). The diagnosis does not require a certain number of features being present, but the more there are, the more likely schizophrenia becomes.

- The predominant features vary from case to case. At one extreme, a person may present with bizarre behaviour, a full house of first-rank symptoms and florid thought disorder. At the other, the most notable symptoms may be insidious social withdrawal and academic decline, with psychotic symptoms only becoming apparent after direct questioning or observation.
- The duration criterion is to exclude transient schizophrenia-like syndromes that have a better prognosis, and maybe a different aetiology. If the features of schizophrenia are present but for less than a month, the (temporary) label is *schizophreniform disorder*.
- Schizophrenia beginning after age 45 used to be considered a separate disorder, *paraphrenia*.
- Delusions, hallucinations and thought disorder in schizophrenia are grouped together as *positive*

*symptoms* (in contrast to *negative symptoms*, described below).
• Many patients have non-localizing ('soft') signs on neurological examination.

## Clinical subtypes of schizophrenia

Because of the clinical heterogeneity, schizophrenia has classically been divided into several subsyndromes, based upon the pattern of symptoms (Table 12.2).
• The catatonic subtype is much rarer than it used to be. This could reflect a change in the nature or treatment of the disease, or the past occurrence of organic disorders mistaken for schizophrenia (particularly a postviral condition called encephalitis lethargica).
• The disorganized subtype is also called *hebephrenic schizophrenia*.

**Table 12.1** Clinical features of acute schizophrenia.

*Characteristic symptoms*
First-rank symptoms
Thought insertion, echo, withdrawal or broadcasting
Third person auditory hallucinations
Running commentary
Passivity of thought, feelings or action
Delusional perception
Bizarre delusions
Odd behaviour
Thought disorder
Lack of insight (reality distortion)
Prodromal period of decline in performance and social withdrawal

*Duration criterion*
Symptoms present for at least 1 month

*Major exclusion criteria*
Not secondary to mood disorder
No demonstrable organic cause (e.g. amphetamines, temporal lobe epilepsy)

*Mr J is a 20-year-old student found having a conversation with imaginary demons. His room was covered in black paper to stop them interfering with his thoughts. His work had deteriorated markedly in the past term, and he had isolated himself. He was convinced he was part of a sinister plot and was being told what to do by unknown people whom he could hear talking about him. There was no evidence of substance misuse or mood disorder. A provisional diagnosis of paranoid schizophrenia was made.*

## Clinical features of chronic schizophrenia

In patients who progress to chronic schizophrenia, the acute symptoms have often largely resolved (with or without treatment). The characteristic picture becomes one of a 'burnt out' disease (Table 12.3). These features are called *negative symptoms*.
• The positive–acute/negative–chronic distinction is not absolute. Positive symptoms regularly persist or re-emerge in chronic cases, and some patients have negative symptoms in their first episode.

**Table 12.2** Subtypes of acute schizophrenia.

| Subtype | Predominant symptoms | Other features |
|---|---|---|
| Paranoid | Persecutory, systematized delusions<br>Hallucinations, usually auditory | Most common form<br>Personality relatively preserved |
| Disorganized | Thought disorder<br>Odd behaviour<br>Fleeting, bizarre delusions<br>Labile or inappropriate mood | Early onset<br>Poor prognosis<br>Premorbid schizoid or schizotypal personality |
| Catatonic | Motor signs | Now rare |
| Undifferentiated | A mixture of the above | |

**Table 12.3** Features of chronic schizophrenia.

*Negative symptoms*
  Flattened (blunted) mood
  Apathy and loss of drive (avolition)
  Social isolation
  Poverty of speech
  Poor self-care

*Other features*
  Positive symptoms persist or recur at times of stress
  Mild cognitive impairment is common

- Prominent, enduring negative symptoms are sometimes called *deficit syndrome*.
- *Residual schizophrenia* is a transitional state between acute and chronic schizophrenia. It describes patients with positive symptoms within the past year who have also developed negative symptoms.
- Research has shown that the symptoms of chronic schizophrenia fall more clearly into three clusters, rather than the two implied by the positive–negative distinction. The three are *reality distortion* (delusions and hallucinations), *disorganization* (thought disorder) and *psychomotor poverty* (similar to negative symptoms).

> Mr J is now 45. He has had multiple admissions. Between episodes, he never regained his previous level of functioning; by 35 he was living in a group home. He spends most of his time in his room or walking the streets, often mumbling to himself. He has no specific complaints or desires. His last admission was a year ago when hallucinations recurred following a fellow resident's suicide.

## Cognitive impairment in schizophrenia

Problems with memory and attention are a neglected aspect of schizophrenia. The profile is, as with everything about schizophrenia, complex.

- The most affected domains are attention, working memory and semantic memory. These deficits are superimposed on a generalized intellectual deficit averaging about one standard deviation—though there is a wide range, and many patients score above normal.

- The impairments are, like the negative symptoms, basically stable and independent of the positive symptoms. However, the details are controversial. Some decline probably occurs well before the onset of illness, with a further decline around the first episode. There is then a long period of stability, before deterioration in later life such that a significant minority of elderly patients with schizophrenia have moderate to severe dementia (which is not explained by any known neuropathological process).

The neuropsychological deficits of schizophrenia are thought to be central to the syndrome, and important for three reasons:

- They are the major determinant of poor functional outcome, along with negative symptoms.
- They may underlie the psychotic symptoms. By this view, psychosis is the 'fever' of schizophrenia—a problem which requires treatment, but which is non-specific and downstream of the disease process.
- They are potential targets for treatment, separate from the psychotic symptoms.

## Differential diagnosis

### Acute schizophrenia

Acute schizophrenia must be distinguished from other psychotic disorders (Table 12.4).

- Drug-induced psychoses (Chapter 14) pose a particular problem. At least a third of people with schizophrenia misuse alcohol or drugs, and it can be difficult, and sometimes arbitrary, deciding whether these constitute the 'cause' of their symptoms. Judgement is based on the timing, quantity and type of substances taken.
- The organic disorders which can produce an acute schizophrenic picture (sometimes called *symptomatic schizophrenia*) are collectively common enough—about 1 in 20 cases—to require a high index of suspicion, especially if aspects of the case are atypical.

### Chronic schizophrenia

In chronic schizophrenia the diagnosis itself is rarely in doubt, though occasionally neurological

**Table 12.4** Differential diagnosis of acute schizophrenia.

| Category of disorder | Distinguishing features/examples |
|---|---|
| *Other non-organic disorders* | |
| Delusional disorders | Absence of specific features of schizophrenia; preserved personality |
| Psychotic depression | Prominent depressive symptoms |
| Manic episode | Prominent manic symptoms |
| Schizoaffective disorder | Mood and schizophrenia symptoms both prominent |
| Schizotypal disorder | Nature of symptoms; chronic history |
| Puerperal psychosis | Acute onset after childbirth |
| *Organic disorders* | |
| Drug-induced psychosis | History of drug or alcohol misuse |
| Iatrogenic | Levodopa, methyldopa, steroids, antimalarials |
| Complex partial epilepsy | Other evidence of seizures |
| Delirium | Acute onset; clouding of consciousness |
| Dementia | Age; established cognitive impairment |
| Huntington's disease | Family history; choreiform movements; dementia |
| Systemic lupus erythematosus | Skin and renal involvement |
| Syphilis | Other evidence of infection |

**Table 12.5** Components in the management of acute schizophrenia.

| Intervention | Rationale |
|---|---|
| Admission | For diagnosis, investigation and starting treatment |
| Antipsychotic drugs | Treatment of positive symptoms |
| Benzodiazepines | For sedation |
| Establish context of disorder | |
| Evaluate current personal circumstances | To guide management—accommodation, work, etc. |
| Assessment of needs and of risk | |
| Education of patient and family | Improve understanding and treatment adherence |

syndromes (e.g. a leukodystrophy) can mimic the clinical picture.

• A more common problem is to distinguish negative symptoms from depression or from the sedative and parkinsonian effects of antipsychotics.

## Investigations

Schizophrenia is a clinical diagnosis. Physical investigations are mainly used to rule out the organic disorders in Table 12.4, and are chosen according to the features elicited in the history and examination.

• Brain imaging is not part of the routine assessment. It should be considered if there are neurological symptoms or signs.

## Management

The management of schizophrenia is considered according to the stage of the illness (acute vs chronic) and then by the intervention (physical, psychological, social).

## Management of acute schizophrenia

The key elements are summarized in Table 12.5.
• Admission for assessment is usual but not invariable. Compulsory admission may be needed, since patients are at risk from neglect or dangerous acts. Ideally, there should be several days of drug-free observation; this is rarely feasible due to shortage of beds or because the behaviour is too disturbed.

- Antipsychotics are effective against positive symptoms in a majority of patients over 2–3 weeks. Their onset is gradual; in the early stages, if behaviour is difficult to manage or the patient is very distressed, add a benzodiazepine.
- Investigate the context of the disorder, as it may give clues as to its development and prognosis. For example, comorbid substance misuse worsens outcome and may require intervention.
- Involve the family. Relatives need support and explanation, and they may be directly involved in therapy.
- First admissions can last many weeks depending on progress and external factors (e.g. finding accommodation). Future management is planned at predischarge CPA meetings (Chapter 8).
- Following an acute episode, *post-schizophrenic depression* is common, and may require treatment with antidepressants.

## Early intervention

There is a trend to try and intervene earlier in schizophrenia—before symptoms become established, and even during the prodrome before unequivocal psychotic symptoms have emerged. Early intervention services have been set up to identify, engage and treat these individuals.
- The rationale is that longer duration of untreated psychosis predicts poor outcome, and thus earlier intervention may improve it.

- Though preliminary, there is some evidence that early intervention, with either cognitive therapy, antipsychotics or antidepressants, may delay, if not prevent, the transition to 'full' psychosis.
- Early intervention is not without its risks. Some prodromes recover spontaneously, whereas labelling and treating it may produce side-effects and stigma.

## Management of chronic schizophrenia

After a first episode of schizophrenia, the aims are to prevent relapse, and to optimize the level of functioning. To do this, a combination of pharmacological, psychological and social methods is used (Table 12.6).
- The amount of support and treatments needed varies markedly depending on the course and severity of the disorder—and, in practice, whether the intervention is available. The emphasis here is on cases where full recovery has not occurred after the first episode.
- The most important specific intervention is antipsychotic medication, which reduces the rate of relapse in the 2 years after an episode from 70% to 50%. Even the benefits of psychological and family interventions operate partly by improving treatment adherence. Equally, however, a sustained relationship must be established with the patient and due attention paid to their 'problems of living'. Without this commitment, the patient is

**Table 12.6** Components in the management of chronic schizophrenia.

| Intervention | Rationale |
| --- | --- |
| Coordinated community care | Ensure medical and social needs are met |
| Continue antipsychotic drug | Prevent relapse |
| Readmission during relapse | Stabilize mental state and review management |
| Family therapy | Lower expressed emotion and prevent relapse |
| Social skills training | Improve social functioning |
| CBT | Reduce residual symptoms |
| Compliance therapy | Improve medication adherence |
| Cognitive remediation | Improve cognitive functioning |
| Supported employment | Financial, social and self-esteem benefits |
| Deal with drug or alcohol use | Improve outcome |
| Illness management skills training | Help coping with chronic illness |
| General medical care | High risk of poor physical health |

unlikely to adhere to the management plan—bear in mind that over 50% of patients do not take their antipsychotics regularly.

- The value of a multidisciplinary approach is apparent from the range of patients' needs—benefits, accommodation, employment, physical health, etc. The nature of the disorder, especially the effect of negative symptoms, makes people with chronic schizophrenia vulnerable in all these areas.
- Some patients with schizophrenia remain under the Mental Health Act [in hospital or in the community (Chapter 7)] for many years.
- Patients with schizophrenia have high risks of type 2 diabetes and cardiovascular disease, contributing to their excess mortality. Some of this is attributable to side-effects of antipsychotic medication. The other reasons are unclear, but probably include genetic predisposition, poor diet and lack of exercise. Regular medical review and investigations (e.g. for diabetes, lipids, blood pressure) should be an integral part of management.

## Modes of treatment

### Antipsychotic drugs

After a single episode of schizophrenia, antipsychotic medication is continued for 12–24 months. If the person remains well it should then be tailed off because there is little evidence that further medication is beneficial and because of the risk of tardive dyskinesia and other long-term side-effects. Patients who have had multiple episodes or persistent symptoms usually remain on medication for many years, though the need for it (and the effect of cautious reductions in dose) should remain under regular review. Medication is often given in depot form because of the poor adherence.

- See Chapter 7 for detailed coverage of antipsychotics.
- Clozapine has an important role in patients poorly responsive to, or intolerant of, other antipsychotics. It also decreases the risk of suicide.
- Avoid routine coadministration of anticholinergic agents, or of combinations of antipsychotics.

- Persistent negative symptoms are not improved by antipsychotics, even clozapine. Conversely, it is a myth that the drugs cause them. Similarly, medication has little overall effect, for better or worse, on the cognitive symptoms, although atypical antipsychotics may produce small improvements.

## Other physical treatments

- Benzodiazepines are useful for short-term sedation.
- Antidepressants should be used in the normal fashion for depression occurring in schizophrenia.
- ECT is not effective, except for catatonic stupor.

## Psychological treatments

Table 12.6 includes a range of psychological treatments. The two most widely used specific interventions are a form of family therapy, and CBT for residual symptoms. In addition to these specific interventions, remember that a supportive psychotherapeutic relationship is an integral part of management (as with every chronic illness).

The family approach arose from the finding that patients living with families who have *high expressed emotion* (EE) had a much higher chance of relapse than those exposed to low EE. EE is the intensity and amount of emotional involvement by the family with the patient. It was then found that high EE families could be taught to lower EE, and relapse rates fell. Family therapy focuses on education about the illness and changing the behaviour of the family. A recent systematic review confirms its (modest) effectiveness, but it has been difficult to implement widely because of practical and financial constraints (e.g. relatives are often out at work).

- The converse of high EE—a lack of stimulation—is also harmful as it exacerbates the apathy and withdrawal of chronic schizophrenia. This was first documented in institutionalized patients (and contributed to the drive to close the asylums).

CBT has some efficacy against auditory hallucinations and delusions, and is being adopted as an integral component of schizophrenia management, especially for the treatment of residual symptoms. However, it effect is rather small, the proven benefits are only short-term, and not all patients are able or willing to engage in treatment.

• Hallucinations can also benefit from simple practical manoeuvres—for example, use of ear plugs or personal stereos.

In a further recent development, *cognitive remediation therapy* and related psychological treatments, are showing some promise to improve the memory deficits of schizophrenia.

## Social interventions

The nature of chronic schizophrenia means that many patients have problems with daily living. These needs should be identified and met by the multidisciplinary team working through the care programme approach (Table 12.6). Assertive outreach teams (Chapter 8) are intended to maintain close contact with patients. The reality is, however, that some patients slip through the net, with occasionally tragic consequences.

• Some patients cannot live alone or with their family. *Group homes* are houses where several patients live together, supported by their key worker and the group homes organization.

*Ms C is a 28-year-old factory worker who has had one episode of schizophrenia. She was discharged home under the care of her CMHT on a depot. A CPN visited to monitor progress, give medication and advise the parents about how best to interact with Ms C. After discussion with her employers, Ms C returned to work part-time but 3 months later she refused medication and began smoking cannabis. She relapsed, lost her job and her behaviour became unmanageable. She was readmitted. Once her condition had settled, a meeting was held between Ms C, her parents and the CMHT. Ms C was offered a place in a group home. She agreed to take medication regularly. She was found sheltered employment in a charity shop. The CMHT social worker helped sort out Ms C's financial problems and ensured that she got her benefits.*

## Prognosis

Accurate estimates for the long-term outcome of schizophrenia are surprisingly hard to obtain,

because the diagnostic criteria have changed over time and because they depend on how recovery is defined. For example, some patients have persistent symptoms but live a reasonably normal life; others are functionally impaired despite minimal symptoms. Taking both symptoms and functioning into account, only about a third of cases have the stereotyped chronic, deteriorating course; a quarter have a very good outcome; and the remainder have a relapsing, remitting illness (Figure 12.1).

• At least 1 in 20 commit suicide. Previous estimates were higher. The risk is higher after an acute episode, when the patient may have realized the nature of his disorder and its implications, and may have developed a depressive disorder.

• There is an increased mortality from natural causes too, especially cardiovascular disease, though rates of some cancers are lower than expected.

Poor outcome factors are shown in Table 12.7. However, they are only weak predictors and it is impossible to foresee which category in Figure 12.1 someone presenting with schizophrenia will end up in.

• First-rank symptoms have no prognostic significance.

• The outcome of schizophrenia is better in developing than developed countries. The explanation

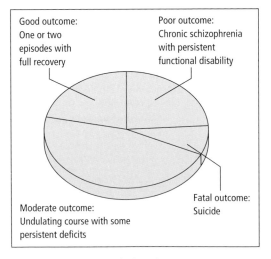

Good outcome:
One or two
episodes with
full recovery

Poor outcome:
Chronic schizophrenia
with persistent
functional disability

Fatal outcome:
Suicide

Moderate outcome:
Undulating course with some
persistent deficits

**Figure 12.1** Outcomes of schizophrenia.

**Table 12.7** Factors associated with poor outcome in schizophrenia.

*Demographic characteristics*
  Young age at onset (e.g. under 25)
  Male
  Isolated, unmarried
  Poor work record
  Premorbid personality disorder
  Substance misuse

*Illness characteristics*
  Insidious onset
  Prolonged untreated psychosis
  Disorganized subtype
  No mood disturbance
  Early negative symptoms
  Non-compliance with medication

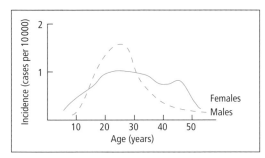

**Figure 12.2** Schizophrenia: age at onset.

is unknown, but probably reflects the importance of the social environment.

## Epidemiology

The lifetime risk for schizophrenia is about 0.8%, with an annual incidence of 0.3 per 1000 and a point prevalence of about 5 per 1000. The onset peaks in early adulthood, though the prodromal symptoms are often in adolescence.

• Men have a slightly higher incidence, and women also have a later and different age of onset profile, with a second peak around the menopause (Figure 12.2). Men tend to have a more severe illness and worse prognosis. Oestrogen's regulation of dopamine receptor sensitivity may explain these gender differences.

• Suggestions of a fall in incidence of schizophrenia over the past 30 years are probably the result of changing diagnostic practice and service provision, not a true decline.

• Some cases of schizophrenia begin later in life. *Late-onset schizophrenia* refers to subjects with onset over age 60. Very little is known about this subtype.

• Other epidemiological associations are considered below.

## Aetiology

There have been many and diverse views of schizophrenia: as a brain disease, as a psychological disorder with no organic basis, and as a myth. Over the past 20 years, its original conception as a genetically influenced neurodevelopmental disorder again prevails.

## Genetic factors

There is an increased risk of schizophrenia in people with a family history of the condition (Figure 12.3). Twin studies show that this is due almost entirely to genetic factors and that the heritability is about 80% (Chapter 6). Adoption studies support this conclusion, in that children of a schizophrenic parent who are adopted by parents without schizophrenia retain their increased (10–12%) risk of illness.

• These studies also show that the genetic predisposition to schizophrenia overlaps with schizotypal disorder and perhaps delusional disorder. These conditions are therefore sometimes grouped together as *schizophrenia spectrum disorders*. There are also genetic overlaps with bipolar disorder, and with autism.

• Several schizophrenia susceptibility genes have now been identified. One common mode of action may be an influence on neurodevelopment and synaptic functioning (Table 12.8). The mode of inheritance is not clear, but probably involves these and many other susceptibility genes, each of small effect. The genes probably interact with each other ('*epistasis*') and affect a person's vulnerability to the environmental risk factors mentioned

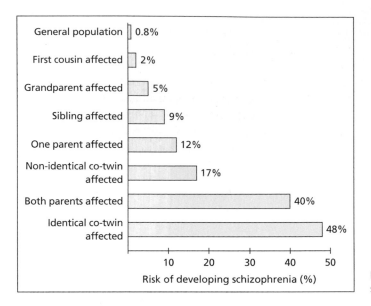

General population ▯ 0.8%

First cousin affected ▯ 2%

Grandparent affected ▭ 5%

Sibling affected ▭ 9%

One parent affected ▭ 12%

Non-identical co-twin affected ▭ 17%

Both parents affected ▭ 40%

Identical co-twin affected ▭ 48%

Risk of developing schizophrenia (%)

**Figure 12.3** Familial risk of schizophrenia.

**Table 12.8** Schizophrenia susceptibility genes and loci.

| Gene name | Chromosomal locus |
| --- | --- |
| Neuregulin-1 | 8p |
| Dysbindin | 6p |
| DISC 1 | 1q |
| MHC locus | 6p |
| ZNF804A | 2q |
| G72 | 13q |

below. For example, variants in some susceptibility genes are associated with a stronger relationship between obstetric complications and schizophrenia, or between early cannabis use and schizophrenia.

• About a quarter of people with velo-cardio-facial syndrome (VCFS), caused by a deletion of one copy of chromosome 22q11, develop schizophrenia.

## Environmental factors

Although quantitatively the most important factor, genes are not the sole cause of schizophrenia. There are many known and suspected environmental risk factors, both biological and social

(Table 12.9). However, the interpretation of many of the factors is unclear. Taken together this information supports the view that schizophrenia has its roots in early development (see below).

• *Obstetric complications.* The risk of developing schizophrenia in people with a history of obstetric complications is increased about 4-fold. Complications associated with foetal hypoxia are particularly implicated. However, it is not known if the relationship is causal, or a sign of a pre-existing foetal abnormality, or a consequence of the mother's antenatal behaviour or physiology.

• *Excess of winter births* (February and March). This is a true seasonal effect, being reversed in Australia (and absent near the Equator). It may be a correlate of viral infections during pregnancy being more common in early winter (especially influenza, which is itself weakly associated with risk), or of reproductive behaviour (i.e. conceiving in the summer) or (in one theory) a reflection of perinatal weather and vitamin D deficiency.

• *Urban birth and upbringing.* This is a dose-dependent relationship (risk increased ~3-fold for a large town compared with a rural area). Its cause is unknown—for example, pollution, noise, overcrowding, infectious agents, etc.

**Table 12.9** Risk factors for schizophrenia.

| |
|---|
| *Family history* (genes) |
| *Social* |
| Urban birth |
| Migration |
| Low social class |
| *Pre- and perinatal* |
| Obstetric complications |
| Winter birth |
| Maternal influenza |
| Maternal malnutrition |
| Rhesus incompatibility |
| *Postnatal* |
| Viral meningitis |
| Epilepsy |
| Learning disability |
| Delayed milestones (walking, talking) |
| Poor child peer relationships |
| Ambiguous handedness |
| Early cannabis use |
| Life events (precipitate onset) |

- *Migration.* There is an increased frequency (relative risk ~4) of schizophrenia in the children of Afro-Caribbeans who came to Britain in the 1950s, and in many other migrant groups in other populations. The risk is particularly high in those immigrants living in areas where they are a 'rare' ethnic group. Its explanation is controversial, with biological (genetic, viral) and sociological (racial prejudice, social deprivation) theories.
- *Early cannabis use* (pre-teens) is a risk factor, but studies have not fully controlled for use of other drugs.
- There is an increased seropositivity for several viruses in schizophrenia (e.g. herpes simplex type 2), but it is unclear when exposure to the virus occurred, and what causal role they played.

## The brain in schizophrenia

### The dopamine hypothesis

The dopamine hypothesis has been the leading biochemical explanation for schizophrenia for over 30 years. It proposes that there is an excess of dopamine transmission ('hyperdopaminergia') in schizophrenia (whether due to too much dopamine, too many receptors, etc.). It was based on three main lines of evidence:

- Antipsychotic drugs are, without exception, dopamine $D_2$ receptor antagonists.
- Dopamine agonists (e.g. amphetamines, L-DOPA) can produce a paranoid psychosis.
- Some CSF and brain studies of schizophrenia indictate abnormal levels of dopamine, its metabolites, enzymes or receptors.

Advancing or refuting the dopamine hypothesis has proved difficult. However, the past few years have seen considerable progress, mostly through PET and SPECT brain imaging studies with dopamine radioligands. Dopamine does indeed appear to be closely linked to the symptoms of schizophrenia, but in a much more subtle way than originally proposed:

- There is good evidence that hyperdopaminergia occurs during acute schizophrenia, in the basal ganglia (striatum). The more 'overheated' the dopamine system, the better the subsequent response to antipsychotics (which is logical, since they are dopamine receptor antagonists). Recent evidence shows that the 'overheating' occurs during the prodrome of the illness.
- As well as the hyperdopaminergia during acute schizophrenia in the striatum, there is probably insufficient dopaminergic activity in the prefrontal cortex in patients with chronic schizophrenia, which contributes to the cognitive and negative symptoms.
- The dopamine system is unlikely to be the primary abnormality. Much evidence suggests that the dopamine changes are downstream of alterations in glutamate transmission. Notably, signalling via the NMDA subtype of glutamate receptor is implicated both by the genetic discoveries and the fact that NMDA receptor antagonists (ketamine, phencyclidine) produce a schizophrenia-like syndrome.

### Functional imaging studies

Abnormalities in regional cerebral blood flow and metabolism occur in schizophrenia, related to particular situations and neuropsychological tests. Such differences support the idea that particular neuronal circuits are impaired in schizophrenia, especially those involving the frontal cortex, hippopcampus, thalamus and cerebellum. For example, patients show:

• Failure to activate the prefrontal cortex when performing tasks requiring its use (*hypofrontality*).

• Greater activation in order to complete a task successfully, due to less efficient processing.

• Abnormal blood flow responses to dopaminergic drugs.

• Characteristic metabolic patterns depending on the predominant symptoms.

• Alterations in functional connectivity between brain regions.

## Structural brain changes

The most robust finding is enlargement of the lateral ventricles and a slight decrease in size of the brain. There may be a preferential involvement of the temporal lobe and a loss of normal cerebral asymmetries.

• The structural brain changes are statistically robust, but not diagnostically useful since there is much overlap with controls, and the same findings can also occur in other disorders.

• Some of the abnormalities are present in people before they get ill; the other changes develop when the person develops psychosis. Thereafter, the progression of brain alterations with the course of the illness remains unclear (and is confounded by medication effects).

• The histological basis of schizophrenia is unknown, though the cytoarchitecture of the cerebral cortex—its neuronal and synaptic organization—appears altered. The white matter and its myelination may also be affected. There is no gliosis (proliferation and activation of glial cells), suggesting an absence of neurodegenerative processes.

## Psychological and social theories

The earlier psychological and social theories of the causation of schizophrenia lack convincing supporting evidence. However, psychological and social factors are clearly important in its outcome, exemplified by the effect on the patient of the emotion expressed by family members. These factors may also precipitate schizophrenia, since there is an excess of life events in the months preceding the first episode.

• Psychological interest is now directed mainly at the neuropsychological mechanisms. For example, one theory views schizophrenia as affecting the ability to distinguish actions generated by internal events (thoughts, feelings) and external stimuli (sensations).

• Schizophrenia is also being viewed as a *salience syndrome*—that is, an inability to decide which stimuli are important (salient) and to respond accordingly. This theory fits in well with the hyperdopaminergia mentioned earlier, since dopamine is a key determinant of how we decide what to respond to and what to ignore.

## The neurodevelopmental model

Putting the various findings together, most researchers now view schizophrenia as a neurodevelopmental disorder. That is, it is caused by abnormalities of brain development, largely driven by genetic predisposition and early environmental factors (Figure 12.4).

• Different versions of the model emphasize the prenatal environment ('doomed from the womb'), adolescence or a combination of both.

• Ongoing factors throughout life may well contribute as well, since a pure developmental model does not explain well the age of onset, the fluctuating clinical course or cases beginning later in life. One notion is that the developmental abnormalities render the brain less able to undergo 'plasticity'—its normal adaptive response to changing environmental demands and stressors.

• Though psychosocial and family factors are neglected in the model, their influence should not be ignored, as mentioned above. These are likely to be mediated via stress and its effects upon the brain.

The evidence in favour of the neurodevelopmental model includes:

**Figure 12.4** The neurodevelopmental model of schizophrenia.

- The fact that the neuropathological findings (e.g. ventricular enlargement) are present before the onset of symptoms.
- The histological abnormalities suggest a prenatal origin.
- Most of the robust environmental risk factors (Table 12.9) act *in utero* or early childhood.
- Children destined as adults to get schizophrenia have impaired behavioural, intellectual and motor development, demonstrable from infancy onwards.
- People with schizophrenia have increased rates of minor physical anomalies and abnormal dermatoglyphics, both of which point to prenatal developmental disturbance.

## Disorders related to schizophrenia

Several other disorders are grouped together with schizophrenia, because:
- they are also psychoses which are not secondary to a mood disorder or organic disorder (in the case of schizoaffective disorder and delusional disorders); or
- they are thought to be causally related (in the case of schizotypal disorder); and

- they do not meet the criteria for diagnosis of schizophrenia (Table 12.1).

## Schizoaffective disorder

### Clinical features

The distinction of schizophrenia from bipolar disorder originated in the belief that these were two discrete disorders. It is reflected in the classification of bipolar disorder as a mood disorder separate from schizophrenia. However, this view is almost certainly wrong (based on epidemiological and genetic considerations). Certainly, many patients have features of both conditions, hence *schizoaffective disorder*.

- Use the diagnosis only for patients who satisfy criteria for schizophrenia *and* mood disorder *during the same episode*. Otherwise, diagnose the predominant syndrome (or neither). For example, one first-rank symptom in mania does not warrant a label of schizoaffective disorder (let alone schizophrenia). Similarly, labile mood is common in acute schizophrenia.
- Overuse of the diagnosis is a common mistake—and often seized upon by examiners.

## Management and prognosis

Mood symptoms and schizophrenic symptoms are treated on their merits. Mood stabilizers and antipsychotics are often used in combination.

- The prognosis is intermediate between schizophrenia and mood disorder. It is better in those whose predominant mood disturbance is manic rather than depressive.

## Delusional disorders (paranoid psychoses)

Many patients have a psychosis without an underlying mood disturbance or organic disorder but do not satisfy the criteria for schizophrenia. Persecutory delusions are the main feature. Hallucinations are rare. Personality remains intact. These disorders are divided into acute and chronic types.

- The disorders in this 'residual' category of psychosis have had a variety of names. The preferred collective term is now *delusional disorder*, though *paranoid psychosis* is still commonly used.

## Acute delusional disorder

These conditions are characterized by their acute onset, clinical features and rapid resolution.

- There are multiple, transient persecutory delusions, a sense of perplexity or suspicion, and a labile mood.
- They may be caused by drugs (in which case they are diagnosed as such) or follow extreme stresses, hence the older terms *psychogenic psychosis* and *brief reactive psychosis*. There is also an evocative French term, *bouffée delirante* (a 'puff of madness').
- Some cases will, of course, turn out to be more persistent psychotic disorders.

## Persistent delusional disorder

A persistent delusional disorder is one lasting more than 3 months. *Chronic paranoid psychosis* and *paranoia* describe similar disorders.

- The delusions are usually *systematized* (i.e. stable and combined into a complex system). They often centre upon alleged (and plausible) injustices. The person may embark on litigation, or occasionally retribution, so it is important to ask about thoughts of aggression and hostility.
- The delusions are often *encapsulated*. The rest of the mental state can be unremarkable to the point that, if the delusional system is not detected, no abnormal features are elicited. Because of this, the disorder can go unrecognized for years, becoming hard to distinguish from paranoid personality disorder (Chapter 15)—though in the latter the paranoid ideas are not truly delusional.
- The appropriate diagnosis may change to one of mood disorder or schizophrenia.
- Onset is usually in middle age. Social isolation, deafness and paranoid personality traits are risk factors.

> *A 50-year-old librarian, Mr Y, was arrested for threatening his boss, having been made redundant after 30 years. He had no psychiatric history. Mr Y was convinced that the boss had plotted against him. His diary revealed an increasing preoccupation with these ideas and included allegations and events known to be false. Hallucinations, thought disorder, mood disorder and substance misuse were excluded. Mr Y was single, without close friends, and had a lifelong interest in spying. He reluctantly agreed to take haloperidol, which gradually resolved the delusions and he stopped pestering his ex-boss. However, the beliefs remained in attenuated form, and he continued to suspect various conspiracies were going on.*

## Specific variants of persistent delusional disorders

The following variants of persistent delusional disorder are mentioned either because of their clinical importance or because they have a memorable eponym and are beloved by examiners.

- *Morbid (pathological) jealousy* is not uncommon, and is potentially dangerous. The patient, usually male, has the delusional belief that his partner is unfaithful. He may go to elaborate lengths to prove this and remains unconvinced by evidence to the contrary. He may threaten and finally attack his partner or the alleged third party. Usually morbid jealousy is a symptom of psychotic depression, schizophrenia, alcoholic psychosis or dementia, but it can be seen in isolation. The risks posed by morbid jealousy (and other psychoses with persecutory delusions with potential for violent acts) sometimes over-rule patient confidentiality so the intended victim can be warned. Full risk assessment (Chapter 4) is mandatory.

- *Monosymptomatic hypochondriacal psychosis (somatic delusional disorder)* is the delusional belief that the person has an illness or deformity. It can lead to a prolonged search for inappropriate medical or surgical treatments. It must be distinguished from hypochondriasis and dysmorphophobia.

- In *De Clèrambault's syndrome (erotomania)*, the patient, usually female, has a delusion that a man of high standing (a pop star, even a psychiatrist) is in love with her. Some stalkers have this disorder.

- In *folie à deux*, two people, often isolated sisters, share the same delusions. One is genuinely psychotic, the other is 'induced' to become so and is said to recover spontaneously when they are separated.

- *Capgras' delusion (illusion des soisies)* is the belief that someone close by has been replaced by an impostor or double. *Fregoli's delusion* is the belief that someone close to them is impersonating other people. Both have been called syndromes, but they are really symptoms (delusional misinterpretations). Both are very rare. They occur in schizophrenia, dementia and after right hemisphere damage.

## Management and prognosis of delusional disorders

Delusional disorders, like all psychoses, usually respond to antipsychotic drugs.

- Acute delusional disorders often resolve within days, especially if the triggering stressor is removed. Full recovery is the rule, although relapses may occur. Continue medication for a few months.

- Persistent delusional disorders can be resistant to treatment (or go untreated) and continue for years. Unlike schizophrenia, negative symptoms rarely occur. It has been claimed that pimozide is more effective than other antipsychotics, but without good evidence. SSRIs can also be useful.

## Schizotypal disorder

Schizotypal disorder is like a chronic, attenuated form of schizophrenia, in which the beliefs stop short of being delusional, and the sensory experiences are not quite hallucinatory. The key features are:

- An aloof and suspicious manner.
- Eccentric behaviour.
- Avoidance of social contact.
- Odd beliefs and magical thinking.
- Vague, rambling or metaphorical speech.
- Tendency to odd ideas and sensory experiences.
- At least three of the above present for more than 2 years.

Schizotypal disorder is diagnosed infrequently, partly because people rarely come into psychiatric contact, and partly because it overlaps with paranoid and schizoid personality disorders.

- Schizotypal disorder appears to have a similar genetic background to schizophrenia.

- There are no specific treatments.

---

**Key points**

- Schizophrenia is a psychosis characterized by specific types of delusions, hallucinations and thought disorder, called first-rank symptoms. By definition, schizophrenia is not secondary to a mood or organic disorder, and the symptoms must have lasted more than a month.

- Some patients progress to a chronic state where social isolation, apathy and poverty of speech predominate. These are called negative symptoms, in contrast to the positive symptoms which characterize the acute episodes. Cognitive deficits also occur and contribute to poor functional outcome.

- Antipsychotic drugs are effective for positive symptoms but they do not prevent or treat negative symptoms. Clozapine is an atypical antipsychotic effective in some otherwise treatment-resistant cases.

- Most patients with schizophrenia need long-term, multidisciplinary support. Psychological and social interventions are an integral part of management.

- Schizophrenia is a neurodevelopmental disorder caused primarily by genetic factors. Many susceptibility genes exist and contribute to the risk. Obstetric complications, urban birth and migration are important environmental risk factors.

## Chapter 13

# Organic psychiatric disorders

Organic psychiatric disorders are those with demonstrable pathology or aetiology, or which arise directly from a medical disorder. They are thereby distinguished from all other psychiatric disorders, which are traditionally called *functional*. This distinction is an oversimplification and conceptually flawed as all disorders have biological, psychological and social contributions (Chapter 1). The term causes both practical and semantic problems, but remains in widespread use, and so is used here:

- The major organic disorders are *dementia* and *delirium*. Like other psychiatric syndromes they are defined by their clinical features. However, unlike other syndromes they are known to arise from different diseases with various aetiologies and pathologies. A complete diagnosis requires the disease as well as the syndrome to be identified. In the case of dementia, this is ideally based on a neuropathological examination post-mortem.
- Other organic disorders are simply psychiatric disorders, of any type, that appear, in a particular case, to be caused by an identifiable medical condition. Sometimes it is the psychiatric symptoms that first bring the person to medical attention.
- Substance misuse disorders are organic, in that there is a specific pharmacological cause.

*Lecture Notes: Psychiatry*, 10e. By Paul Harrison, John Geddes and Michael Sharpe. Published 2010 by Blackwell Publishing Ltd.

By convention they are classified separately (Chapter 14).

- Psychiatric disorders which are considered *psychological reactions* to illness—such as becoming depressed after being told you have cancer—are excluded from the organic category.

## Dementia

### Clinical features of dementia

- Review the core and module approach to assessment of dementia (Chapters 2 and 3).

Dementia is also known as *chronic brain syndrome*. Its cardinal feature is memory impairment (short-term worse than long-term) without impaired consciousness (cf. delirium). The overall clinical profile differs depending on the specific type of dementia, as outlined below, but other common features of dementia are:

- Symptoms present for 6 months, of sufficient severity to impair functioning.
- Personality and behavioural change—for example, wandering, aggression, disinhibition.
- Dysphasias, dyspraxias and focal neurological signs may be present.
- Psychotic symptoms in half of cases at some stage.
- Unawareness of deficits (except early on).
- Nearly always progressive (though this is not a diagnostic criterion).

The incidence of dementia rises rapidly with age, affecting approximately 5% of 65 year olds and more than 20% of 80 year olds. (Exact figures depend on the severity threshold.) The risk of dementia is doubled in those with an affected first-degree relative. Other risk factors depend on the type of dementia concerned.

- The rapid rise with age is typified by Alzheimer's disease (Figure 13.1).
- Dementia in the under 65s is termed *presenile dementia*.
- *Mild cognitive impairment* (MCI) describes people who do not meet the criteria for dementia but who have evidence of a decline in cognitive function. It progresses to dementia within a year in about 30% of cases. There is much interest in this group with a view to early intervention.

## Differential diagnosis of dementia

Established dementia is usually unmistakable, but mild dementia can be confused with (or coexist with) other conditions:

- *Depression*. Poor concentration and impaired memory are common in depression in the elderly, hence *pseudodementia*. Two factors which help distinguish depression from dementia are: Did low mood or poor memory come first? Is the failure to answer questions due to lack of ability or lack of motivation?
- *Delirium*. See next section.
- *Deafness*. Check the person can hear.
- *Dysphasia*. Check they can understand and speak.
- *Amnesic syndrome*. A purer short-term memory defect (see below).
- *Late-onset schizophrenia* (paraphrenia). Check for prominent and preceding symptoms of psychosis.

## The causes of dementia

The common dementias are listed in Table 13.1. Alzheimer's disease accounts for over half of all cases, with the majority of the rest explained by vascular dementia and Lewy body dementia.

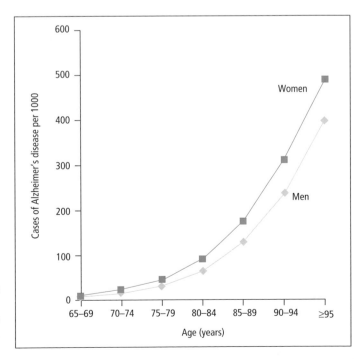

**Figure 13.1** The prevalence of Alzheimer's disease with ageing. Adapted from Nussbaum RL, Ellis CE (2003). *N Engl J Med* **348**, 1356–1364.

**Table 13.1** Causes of dementia.

| |
|---|
| *Alzheimer's disease* (50–60% of cases) |
| *Vascular dementia* (20–25%) |
| *Dementia with Lewy bodies* (10–15%) |
| *Other causes* (<10%) |
| Degenerative disorders |
|    Frontotemporal dementia (including Pick's disease) |
|    Huntington's disease |
|    Prion disease |
|    Progressive supranuclear palsy |
| Metabolic disorders |
|    Alcoholic dementia |
|    Vitamin B12 deficiency |
| Infections |
|    HIV |
|    Syphilis |
| Other causes |
|    Normal pressure hydrocephalus |
|    Intracranial tumours |
|    Subdural haematoma |
|    Head injury |

- The syndromes are not mutually exclusive, and the common ones often coexist.
- In presenile dementia, a much higher percentage of cases are due to rare genetic disorders, or are the consequence of severe head injury.

## Clinical features differentiating the dementias

Careful clinical evaluation identifies the specific dementia (as determined by diagnostic neuropathological examination) in more than 80% of cases (Table 13.2).

- A distinction is sometimes made clinically between *cortical dementia* (e.g. Alzheimer's disease) and *subcortical dementia* (e.g. Huntington's disease) (Table 13.3). However, it is better to try and make a specific diagnosis (and the terms are misleading as most dementias affect both regions of the brain).
- The disorders themselves are discussed in the next section.

## Assessment of dementia

In the history and examination, look for clues pointing towards one of the diagnoses in Table 13.2. For example, a history of a fall (?subdural haematoma) or incontinence (?normal pressure hydrocephalus), rapid fluctuations (?dementia with Lewy bodies); on examination you might find hypertension and a carotid bruit (?vascular dementia). Table 13.4 shows the baseline and specialized tests used in the investigation of dementia. Remember also that a range of memory tests are available as part of the assessment of the presence and severity of dementia, of which the Mini-Mental State Examination is most widely used (Chapter 3).

- Only the baseline blood tests would routinely be ordered, with further investigation depending on the age of the patient and the suggestion of a treatable aetiology (e.g. a brain scan to exclude a subdural haematoma). In the absence of such clues, further tests in an elderly person rarely change the diagnosis, let alone reveal a reversible cause, beyond that provided by a careful history and examination.
- Conversely, in a young person, every effort is made to make a diagnosis—not only in case it is treatable and to inform prognosis, but because the dementia may well be inherited and genetic testing available for the family. Presenile dementia is usually referred to neurologists.
- There is much interest in '*biomarkers*' to diagnose early dementia, or predict its onset, especially Alzheimer's disease. Levels of various proteins in the CSF show promise, as do some MRI measures, and some genetic tests. As yet none has the necessary sensitivity or specificity for routine use.

## Management of dementia

Occasionally, dementia is potentially reversible (e.g. space-occupying lesion, vitamin B12 deficiency) and responds to appropriate treatment. Specific interventions to treat symptoms in Alzheimer's disease are also now available, as discussed below. However, the management of

**Table 13.2**  Clinical features distinguishing between the dementias.

|  | Prominent symptoms and signs | Other clinical features |
|---|---|---|
| Alzheimer's disease | Memory loss, especially short term<br>Dysphasia and dyspraxia<br>Sense of smell impaired early<br>Behavioural changes, e.g. wandering<br>Psychotic symptoms at some stage | Relentlessly progressive<br>Survival 5–8 years |
| Vascular dementia | Personality change<br>Labile mood<br>Preserved insight | Stepwise progression<br>Signs of cerebrovascular disease<br>History of hypertension<br>More common in men, smokers |
| Dementia with Lewy bodies | Fluctuating dementia<br>Delirium-like phases<br>Parkinsonism<br>Visual hallucinations | Antipsychotics worsen condition |
| Frontotemporal dementia | Stereotyped behaviours<br>Personality change<br>Early loss of insight<br>Expressive dysphasia<br>Memory relatively preserved<br>Early primitive reflexes | Slowly progressive<br>Family history common<br>More common in women<br>Onset usually before age 70 |
| Huntington's disease | Schizophrenia-like psychosis<br>Choreiform movements<br>Depression and irritability<br>Dementia occurs later | Presents in the 20s–40s<br>Affected parent and other relatives |
| Normal pressure hydrocephalus | Mental slowing, apathy, inattention<br>Urinary incontinence<br>Problems walking (gait apraxia) | Most common in 50–70 year olds<br>Most common reversible dementia |
| Prion disease | Myoclonic jerks<br>Seizures<br>Cerebellar ataxia | Often presenile<br>Rapid onset and progression<br>Death within a year |

**Table 13.3**  Clinical features of subcortical versus cortical dementias.

|  | Subcortical dementia | Cortical dementia |
|---|---|---|
| Memory loss | Moderate | Severe, early |
| Language | Normal | Affected (dysphasia) |
| Personality | Apathetic, inert | Indifferent |
| Mood | Flat, depressed | Normal |
| Coordination | Impaired | Normal |
| Motor speed | Slowed | Normal |

**Table 13.4** Investigation of dementia.

| Test | What the test may show |
| --- | --- |
| *Blood tests* | |
| Full blood count | Macrocytosis, anaemia |
| Electrolytes | Hypercalcaemia, renal disease |
| Liver function tests | Alcoholic liver disease |
| Thyroid function | Hypothyroidism |
| Vitamin B12 and folate levels | Deficiencies can produce dementia |
| Syphilis serology | Now rare, but overlooked |
| HIV test | Dementia common in AIDS |
| | |
| *Radiography* | |
| Chest X-ray | Bronchial carcinoma with ?cerebral metastases |
| Brain imaging (CT or MRI) | Tumour; infarcts; haematoma; temporal lobe atrophy suggests Alzheimer's; pulvinar hyperintensity suggests prion disease |
| *EEG* | Characteristic 3 Hz 'spike and wave' in prion disease |
| | |
| *Other tests* | |
| Lumbar puncture | Normal pressure hydrocephalus; herpes encephalitis |
| Cerebral blood flow studies | Parietal hypometabolism suggests Alzheimer's |
| Neuropsychological testing | Assess severity; profile of deficits may point to brain region most affected |
| Genetic testing | Available for some familial dementias |
| Brain biopsy | Very rarely done; mainly for suspected prion disease |

dementia generally has more modest goals, the main one being to optimize quality of life for patient and carer. Whatever the cause of the dementia, the following principles and strategies are important:

• Think about the patient, their environment and their carers, as potential targets for intervention.

• Characterize and treat the non-cognitive abnormalities. Simple interventions can improve problems such as wandering (e.g. by regular exercise, or raising the door handle) and incontinence (e.g. by a toileting routine). Non-pharmacological methods should always be employed first.

• Psychotic symptoms respond to low-dose antipsychotics. They should be used sparingly and for brief periods only (reviewed at least every 6 weeks), because psychosis in dementia is usually transient, and because they are associated with more rapid cognitive decline and with sudden death, especially in Lewy body dementia. Antipsychotics may also increase risk of stroke, although absolute risks are low. Because of these concerns, trazodone or carbamazepine are sometimes used instead.

• Antipsychotics should *not* be used long term, nor for sedation, nor for behavioural problems without evidence of a psychotic basis.

• Treat depression. SSRIs are better tolerated than tricyclics.

• A range of other interventions are also sometimes used, including reality orientation, lavender oil aromatherapy, carbamazepine, reminiscence therapy, music therapy, art therapy and memory training. There is some evidence that the first three may be beneficial for behavioural problems.

• Social interventions such as meals-on-wheels, day care and respite admissions help carers cope.

• Patients with dementia should be cautioned about the risks of driving. The DVLA or other relevant authority should be informed when the diagnosis is made.

• Investigate any sudden deterioration. It may be due to a treatable cause [e.g. superimposed delirium due to a urinary tract infection (UTI)].

• In advanced dementia, palliative rather than active treatment is often indicated. Next of kin should be fully involved in these decisions (see vignette in Chapter 8).

• Patients with dementia usually lack capacity, and the requirements of the 2005 Mental Capacity Act should always be taken into account—for example, regarding advance directives and deprivation of liberty safeguards (Chapter 7).

## Prognosis of dementia

Most dementias progress inexorably. Death is usually within 5–8 years of onset, with some dementias, notably prion disease, progressing much more rapidly. Younger cases and those with focal neurological signs or psychotic symptoms have a worse prognosis. Severe dementia has a mean survival of 18 months, with death often associated with pneumonia and other febrile episodes.

• People with dementia should not be blood or tissue donors in view of the risk of transmission of prion disease.

## Specific dementias

This section summarizes the aetiological, pathological and therapeutic factors for the important dementias.

• Their main distinguishing clinical features are summarized in Table 13.2.

## Alzheimer's disease

As the most common dementia, it is fortunate that substantial progress has been made recently in understanding Alzheimer's disease, and the first treatments are now available.

It is a neuropathological diagnosis. The cardinal features are neurofibrillary tangles and senile (amyloid) plaques in the hippocampus and cerebral cortex. Loss of synapses is also important. Neurochemically, the main abnormality is a loss of acetylcholine due to degeneration of the cholinergic neurons of the basal forebrain. The cholinergic deficits and synaptic loss are proportional to the severity of the dementia.

A considerable amount is now known about the causes of the disease (Table 13.5).

• The major risk factor, apart from age, is the E4 (epsilon4) variant of the apolipoprotein E (apoE) gene. Three polymorphisms exist, apoE2, apoE3 and apoE4: 20% of the population carry one copy of apoE4 and have twice the risk of Alzheimer's disease; the 3% who are apoE4 homozygotes (i.e. two copies of apoE4) are at several-fold increased risk. Conversely, the risk is about 40% lower in people without an apoE4 allele, and those with apoE2 alleles may be at lower risk still. The effect of apoE4 is probably that it brings forward the age of onset of dementia, by about a decade. (Note that apoE4 is neither necessary nor sufficient for Alzheimer's disease—it is a risk factor.) Many other genes of small effect probably also contribute.

• Presenile Alzheimer's disease is often familial and (unlike most cases) caused by an autosomal dominant mutation. Three genes have been found so far, with several different mutations in each: amyloid precursor protein (APP), and presenilins PSEN 1 and PSEN 2. Though extremely rare, these cases helped identify the pathways involved in Alzheimer's disease generally (see below).

• A history of treatment with NSAIDs, hormone replacement therapy (HRT) or statins has been associated with a lower risk of developing dementia and Alzheimer's disease. Plausible mechanisms exist to explain these effects. However, it is unclear if the association is genuine, or reflects other factors (e.g. women given HRT tend to be healthier and better educated).

• High educational attainment and mental or physical exercise are both protective factors, perhaps by increasing 'cognitive reserve' and supporting a 'use it or lose it' theory of brain function.

• Plasma homocysteine is an independent, graded risk factor for developing Alzheimer's disease several years later. This may be due to its role in atherosclerotic processes, or in neurotoxicity.

The key process leading to Alzheimer's disease is abnormal metabolism of β-amyloid, the main constituent of senile plaques, and a fragment of the amyloid precursor protein. The abnormality results in formation of insoluble forms and complexes of β-amyloid which accumulate and trigger a range of other harmful biochemical events. This 'amyloid

**Table 13.5** Risk factors for Alzheimer's disease.

| Factor | Comments |
|---|---|
| *Genetic* | |
| Apolipoprotein E (chromosome 19) | ApoE4 allele markedly increases risk |
| APP (chromosome 21); PSEN 1 and 2 (chromosomes 14 and 1) | Autosomal dominant mutations which cause early-onset familial Alzheimer's disease |
| Other genes (chromosomes 6, 10, 11, etc.) | Identity and contribution uncertain |
| Down's syndrome (trisomy 21) | Alzheimer's disease occurs in middle age |
| *Other risk factors* | |
| Increasing age | Predominant risk factor (Fig. 13.1) |
| Females | Slightly higher risk than men (Fig. 13.1) |
| Homocysteinaemia | High plasma homocysteine doubles risk |
| Obesity or diabetes in middle age | Mechanism unclear |
| Head injury | Doubles risk of Alzheimer's disease |
| Latent herpes simplex infection | In people with an apoE4 allele |
| History of depression | Risk of dementia may be increased |
| Aluminium exposure | Controversial, probably false |
| *Environmental—protective factors* | |
| High educational level | 'Cerebral reserve' |
| Physically and mentally active lifestyle | 'Use it or lose it' |
| Non-steroidal anti-inflammatories | ?Retard a chronic inflammatory process |
| Statins | ?Decrease atherosclerotic risk factors |
| Hormone replacement therapy | ?Oestrogens are neuroprotective |

cascade' is promoted in various ways by the causal factors mentioned (Figure 13.2). For example, NSAIDs and apoE4 both affect β-amyloid trafficking or processing.

- The central role of β-amyloid is supported by findings in transgenic mice with Alzheimer's disease-causing mutations in the APP gene. They become demented and get senile plaques, a fate which does not afflict normal rodents.
- Abnormalities in microtubule-associated tau protein (which forms neurofibrillary tangles), oxidative stress and inflammatory processes may also be important. Their connection to β-amyloid is unclear.

## Treatment of Alzheimer's disease

- At present, the 'non-specific' components of dementia management (see above) remain of greater importance than any specific drug or other treatment.

- Cholinesterase inhibitors (e.g. donepezil) are licensed for mild and moderate Alzheimer's disease. They have modest effects against cognitive symptoms, global outcome and activities of daily living. The effect is roughly equivalent to a 6-month delay in cognitive decline. They may also have benefit for behavioural symptoms. In the UK, they must be prescribed by a specialist according to specified diagnostic and severity criteria.
- The rationale for cholinesterase inhibitors is that they ameliorate the cholinergic deficits which occur early in the disease process; the fact they have such a modest effect probably reflects the more widespread, and progressive, disease process.
- Memantine is an NMDA glutamate receptor antagonist licensed for use in moderate to severe Alzheimer's disease. Its therapeutic value in practice is not yet established.
- Several other treatment approaches are in development, most targeted at β-amyloid and its

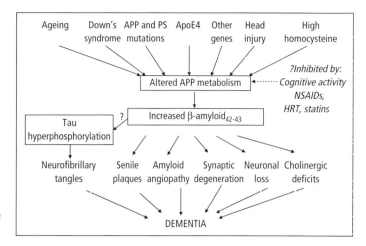

**Figure 13.2** The pathogenesis of Alzheimer's disease.

metabolism. One method is immunization—based on the surprising finding that active and passive immunization against β-amyloid is effective in mouse models of the disease, and with encouraging preliminary data in patients.

• Treatment trials with NSAIDs and folic acid (to lower homocysteine) are also underway.

• Trials of HRT have been negative.

• Any potential preventative or disease-retarding intervention must take into account the fact that the pathology begins in earnest at least a decade before the first symptoms.

## Vascular dementia

An umbrella term for dementia thought to be vascular in origin. One type is caused by multiple small infarcts (hence the earlier name of *multi-infarct dementia*). Others include 'small vessel disease' and Binswanger's disease. It is associated with risk factors for atherosclerosis and cerebrovascular disease.

• An overt stroke leads to dementia in 10% of cases, and in 30% after a second stroke.

• There is no specific treatment for vascular dementia, other than to attend to the cerebrovascular risk factors (e.g. aspirin, smoking).

• Vascular impairment acts synergistically with Alzheimer's disease to produce dementia.

## Dementia with Lewy bodies

Also called *Lewy body disease*, it is the third most common form of dementia. It has a distinctive clinical appearance (Table 13.2). The overlap with Parkinson's disease reflects their common pathology—that is, Lewy bodies (intracellular inclusions made of α-synuclein), but in dementia with Lewy bodies these occur in the cerebral cortex. Its aetiology is unknown, and no genes have been identified.

• Cholinesterase inhibitors are valuable (and appear more effective than in Alzheimer's disease).

• Antipsychotics should be avoided because of the risk of sensitivity reactions and increased mortality.

## Parkinson's disease dementia

Dementia with Lewy bodies merges into *Parkinson's disease dementia*. The convention is that the latter category is used for dementia occurring more than 12 months after onset of parkinsonism. By this definition, dementia occurs in about a third of cases of Parkinson's disease. Other cases of Parkinson's disease have a more circumscribed 'executive dysfunction' syndrome, with failures of attention and short-term memory.

• L-DOPA does not improve the dementia: cholinesterase inhibitors may.

• Clozapine and quetiapine are useful for psychotic symptoms.

• Other psychiatric and behavioural symptoms of Parkinson's disease (with or without dementia) include sleep disturbances, pain, apathy and depression. Pathological gambling can occur in those treated with dopamine agonists.

## Frontotemporal dementia

A spectrum of conditions affecting the frontal and temporal lobes, including *Pick's disease* (characterized by Pick bodies and Pick cells), and dementias associated with motor neuron disease. Causes about 5% of dementia, more so in younger subjects. The clinical picture is characteristic (Table 13.2).

• Some cases, maybe up to a half, are caused by mutations in the tau (MAPT) or progranulin (PGRN) genes, both on chromosome 17. Others are associated with a protein called TDP-43

• There is no specific treatment. Patients are very sensitive to many psychotropic drugs, which should be used with caution to treat depressive or psychotic symptoms.

## Huntington's disease

Also called *Huntington's chorea*. Unlike most psychiatric disorders, it is entirely genetic. It is autosomal dominant, caused by a trinucleotide repeat expansion ('molecular stutter') in the *huntingtin* gene on chromosome 4. Pathologically, there is marked atrophy of the caudate nucleus, and later in the frontal lobe. The abnormal huntingtin protein is thought to be neurotoxic, though the mechanism is not clear.

• Predictive genetic testing is available.

• The psychosis and depression can be treated symptomatically, but the dementia, and the disease itself, remain untreatable.

## Normal pressure hydrocephalus

Accounts for up to 5% of dementia, and is the most common potentially reversible type. The term is a misnomer as CSF pressure is often increased. The clinical triad (Table 13.2) is characteristic, and MRI or CT scanning, showing disproportionate ventricular enlargement, may help diagnostically.

• The dementia is usually mild, and the other symptoms more prominent.

• Treatment is by ventricular shunting; 50% respond well.

## Prion disease

Includes *Creutzfeldt–Jakob disease (CJD)*. Prion disease is caused by an abnormal form of a protein called prion protein. The abnormality can be inherited or acquired, because abnormal prion protein is transmissible, via blood, diet and contaminated surgical instruments.

• Prion disease is exceedingly rare but notable, especially in the UK, because of '*variant CJD (vCJD)*', acquired from cows with bovine spongiform encephalopathy (BSE)—prion disease in cattle—during the 1980s.

• 166 cases of vCJD have been reported in the UK (November 2009). The current best predictions are for hundreds more—earlier estimates were much higher. Unlike typical CJD, these have occurred in young adults and present with prominent psychiatric symptoms, especially depression and personality change. There may be a genetic predisposition to vCJD.

• Any suspected case of prion disease should be referred to the National Surveillance Unit in Edinburgh.

• The prion protein is thought to be a receptor for APP, the protein central to Alzheimer's disease.

• There is no treatment for prion disease.

## Alcoholic dementia

True alcoholic dementia is rare. Visuospatial deficits are often prominent. It is associated with atrophy of the white matter and frontal lobes.

• Dementia in those with alcohol dependence is more often due to Alzheimer's disease or vascular dementia rather than to the alcohol itself.

• Alcoholic dementia does not usually improve with abstinence.

- Alcohol dependence also causes amnesic syndrome (see below).

## Delirium

Also known as *acute confusional state* or *acute brain syndrome*. It is common on medical and surgical wards—a third of elderly patients in hospital have an episode of delirium—so all doctors should be able to recognize and manage it.

- Review the unresponsive patient and cognition modules (Chapter 3).

## Clinical features of delirium

*Clouding of consciousness* is the most important diagnostic sign. It refers to drowsiness, decreased awareness of surroundings, disorientation in time and place, and distractibility. At its most severe the patient may be unresponsive, but more commonly the impaired consciousness is quite subtle.

- Minor degrees of impaired consciousness can be detected by problems estimating the passage of time (e.g. how long the interview has been going on), and with concentration tasks (e.g. counting from 20 down to 1).

Because clouding of consciousness may not be apparent, the first clue to the presence of delirium is often one of its other features:

- Fluctuating course, worse at night.
- Visual hallucinations.
- Transient persecutory delusions.
- Irritability and agitation, or somnolence and decreased activity.
- Impaired concentration and memory.

The differential diagnosis includes dementia (Table 13.6), acute psychosis and depression. Usually the clinical picture (especially the acute onset and rapid fluctuations), and its context, is sufficiently characteristic to make delirium a relatively simple diagnosis. However, differentiating delirium from Lewy body dementia can be difficult in the short term, or without a good history.

## Aetiology of delirium

Recognition of delirium is followed by an urgent search for its cause (Table 13.7).

**Table 13.6** Delirium versus dementia.

|  | Delirium | Dementia |
| --- | --- | --- |
| Onset | Acute | Insidious |
| Short-term course | Fluctuating | Constant |
| Attention | Poor | Good |
| Delusions and hallucinations | Common, simple, fleeting | Less common, more stable |

**Table 13.7** Common causes of delirium.

*Prescribed drugs*
Tricyclic antidepressants
Benzodiazepines and other sedatives
Digoxin
Diuretics
Lithium
Steroids
Opiates

*Other drugs*
Alcohol intoxication
Alcohol withdrawal and delirium tremens

*Medical conditions*
Post-operative hypoxia
Febrile illness
Septicaemia
Organ failure (cardiac, renal, hepatic)
Hypoglycaemia
Dehydration
Constipation
Burns
Major trauma

*Neurological conditions*
Epilepsy (post-ictal)
Head injury
Space-occupying lesion
Encephalitis

- Medication is implicated in a third of cases, mostly drugs with anticholinergic effects (e.g. TCAs) or sedatives.

Several demographic factors predict those who are at high risk of developing delirium (Table 13.8). In these individuals, delirium can follow relatively trivial precipitants (e.g. constipation).

**Table 13.8** Predisposing factors for delirium.

Elderly
Male
Pre-existing dementia
Pre-existing frailty or immobility
Previous episode of delirium
Sensory impairment

**Table 13.9** Management of delirium.

*Environmental components*
Quiet surroundings (side room), constant lighting,
  clock, calendar
Regular routine
Clear simple communications
Limit numbers of staff (e.g. key nurse)
Involve family

*Medical components*
Monitor vital signs
Investigate and treat underlying cause (e.g. antibiotics,
  oxygen, stop drug)
Control agitation or psychotic symptoms with
  antipsychotics

## Management of delirium

Delirium is managed where it occurs—usually in general hospitals. Psychiatrists may be asked to assess the patient, make the diagnosis and give advice. Treatment is directed both at the symptoms and at the cause, and includes both medical and environmental interventions (Table 13.9).

- In practice (and in an exam), emphasize the need both to search for a cause, and for supportive, environmental interventions (as in Table 13.9) whilst this is ongoing. The latter may avoid the need for medication, which can complicate the problem, and which should only be used when necessary.
- Antipsychotics are the first-line pharmacological treatment. Haloperidol is often used, by intramuscular injection if it cannot be taken orally. It can be given intravenously but this is rarely required.
- The exception is for alcohol- or seizure-related delirium, when a benzodiazepine (e.g. lorazepam) is indicated (because of the epileptogenic potential of antipsychotics).

- A delirious person may occasionally be a risk to self, other patients or staff. Call for help, ensure safety and use physical restraint if essential (e.g. to allow drug to be administered).
- Patients with delirium are often incapable of giving informed consent. Treatment is therefore given under the Mental Capacity Act or common law. If continuing interventions without consent are anticipated, the Mental Health Act may be required.

## Prognosis of delirium

Prognosis depends on the cause. Within a week the patient is usually better or has died. A quarter have died by 3 months. There is no good evidence that delirium progresses to dementia (although pre-existing dementia is a risk factor for delirium).

*A 75-year-old lady was found lying on the floor and taken to hospital. She is drowsy, disorientated in time and place, distractable and unable to give any history. She thinks you are trying to kill her. She is febrile and hypotensive, but has no neurological signs or injuries. Blood tests and X-rays are performed. She is given oxygen, and antibiotics for the clinical suspicion of septicaemia. Her agitation worsens but settles with haloperidol. The GP tells you that there is no past history of note. Blood cultures grow an organism sensitive to the antibiotic. Her condition improves over 72 hours. The haloperidol is tailed off and her cognitive function returns to normal.*

## Other organic disorders

Dementia and delirium have been described in detail because they are common. As mentioned at the start of the chapter, there are many other 'organic' conditions which can together present with the whole range of psychiatric disorders. The important principles, and some specific examples, are summarized here.

## Organic psychiatric disorders

The diagnostic rule is to preface the psychiatric label with 'organic' and state the aetiology

(Table 13.10). For example, 'Organic anxiety disorder due to thyrotoxicosis'.

Each organic syndrome is very rare compared with its 'functional' counterpart. In areas with good primary care, psychiatrists rarely see undiagnosed organic psychiatric disorders. However, when an organic syndrome does occur it is essential to recognize it. Detecting an organic disorder requires that you:

- Consider the possibility, with every patient. If this is done, it is easier not to forget to take a brief medical history, conduct a relevant physical examination and order investigations.
- Always include an organic disorder on your list of differential diagnoses in an exam situation.
- Be suspicious if aspects of the psychiatric presentation are unusual. For example, organic syndromes often produce abnormalities in unexpected functions, such as anosmia in depression due to a frontal meningioma.

There may or may not be an effective treatment for the organic disorder. Regardless, the psychiatric symptoms are still treated with the appropriate pharmacological, psychological and social interventions.

**Table 13.10** Organic psychiatric disorders.

| Syndrome | Example of cause |
|---|---|
| Organic brain syndromes | Dementia, delirium, amnesic syndrome |
| Organic delusional (psychotic) disorders | Systemic lupus erythematosus |
| Organic mood disorders | Multiple sclerosis |
| Organic anxiety disorders | Thyrotoxicosis |
| Organic personality disorders | Head injury |

- As a rule, treatment response in an organic disorder is similar to that of its functional equivalent, subject to the progression of the underlying condition—for example, depression responds to antidepressants whether it is organic or not. The presence of the organic disorder may, however, affect the choice of drug (e.g. avoid TCAs in depression following myocardial infarction).

## Amnesic syndrome

Amnesic (or *amnestic*) syndrome completes the triad of conditions (with dementia and delirium) which affect memory and which always have an organic cause. Its features are

- Selective loss of recent memory.
- Confabulation: the unconscious fabrication of recent events to cover gaps in memory.
- Time disorientation.
- Attention and immediate recall intact.
- Long-term memory and other intellectual faculties intact.

Amnesic syndrome is rare and, in practice difficult to distinguish from some dementias. It is due to damage to the mammillary bodies, hippocampus and thalamus. The usual cause is alcohol-induced thiamine deficiency (*Korsakov's syndrome*), which is treated with thiamine and abstinence, and which may follow Wernicke's encephalopathy (Chapter 14). Other causes include herpes simplex encephalitis, severe hypoxia and head injury.

The memory deficits are often irreversible.

## Epilepsy

There are several types of epilepsy (Table 13.11). Epilepsy is usually managed by neurologists, but

**Table 13.11** The main forms of epilepsy.

| Type | Comments | Conscious level during seizure |
|---|---|---|
| *Generalized seizures* | No focal onset | |
| Tonic–clonic (Grand mal) | The 'classic' type of seizure | Unconscious |
| Absence (Petit mal) | Subtle and brief | Impaired |
| *Partial seizures* | Focal onset | |
| Complex partial (psychomotor) | Of most psychiatric significance | Impaired |
| Simple partial | | Unaffected |

**Table 13.12** Psychiatric aspects of epilepsy.

| Category | Example |
|---|---|
| *Psychiatric symptoms related to seizures* | |
| Due to shared aetiology | Temporal lobe tumour |
| At start of seizure | Hallucinations during aura |
| During seizure | Non-convulsive status presenting as a fugue state |
| After seizure | Post-ictal delirium |
| Between seizures | Psychosis of complex partial epilepsy |
| | Pseudoseizures |
| *Psychiatric disorder masquerading as epilepsy* | |
| *Psychiatric disorder associated with epilepsy* | |
| Depression | Common in people with epilepsy |
| Suicide | Several times more common |
| *Psychiatric problems of treatment* | |
| Side-effects of anticonvulsants | Depression with barbiturates |
| Seizures as medication side-effect | Antipsychotics and tricyclic antidepressants |

has many psychiatric aspects. Only the latter are covered here (Table 13.12).

• Consult a neurology text for general coverage of epilepsy.

## Relationship of psychiatric symptoms to seizures

*Complex partial epilepsy* was called *psychomotor epilepsy* because of the frequency of psychiatric symptoms during seizures (Table 13.13). It has also been referred to as *temporal lobe epilepsy*, though this is not always the site of the seizure focus.

• The risk of schizophrenia is several-fold higher in people with complex partial epilepsy, more so if the focus is in the left temporal lobe, and due to an early developmental abnormality.

• The association with sexual dysfunction may be due to the epilepsy, or the medication. Psychiatric presentations can occur with other epilepsies, but are much rarer.

• *Absence seizures* in children produce transient lapses in concentration or simple automatisms, and can be mistaken for a behavioural disorder.

• A *generalized seizure disorder* can present to a psychiatrist if, for example, the person was found wandering in a postictal delirium.

**Table 13.13** Psychiatric symptoms of complex partial seizures.

| |
|---|
| *During the seizure (ictal)* |
| Impaired consciousness |
| Hallucinations and other distorted perceptions |
|     olfactory |
|     somatic—especially epigastric |
| Sense of *déjà vu* |
| Depersonalization and derealization |
| Impaired speech and memory |
| Automatisms and stereotyped behaviour |
| *After the seizure (post-ictal, hours to days)* |
| Transient, florid psychosis |
| *Between seizures (interictal)* |
| Schizophrenia-like psychosis |
| Depression |
| Sexual dysfunction and lack of libido |

## Psychiatric disorders masquerading as epilepsy

*Pseudoseizures (hysterical seizures* or *non-epileptic attack disorder)* is a form of dissociative disorder (Chapter 10). It can be hard to distinguish clinically from a true seizure. EEG monitoring during attacks may be required to make the diagnosis. Pseudoseizures are more common in people who also have epilepsy.

- Other conditions which can be misdiagnosed as epilepsy include panic attacks, hypoglycaemia and schizophrenia. In children, consider temper tantrums and nightmares.

## Psychological problems associated with having epilepsy

Historically, epilepsy has been attributed to demonic possession and its sufferers seen as irritable, self-centred people with criminal tendencies. Although entirely false, persisting negative attitudes, acting in concert with the real disabilities, probably contribute to the higher incidence of psychiatric disorders and suicide in epilepsy.

- The most common psychiatric disorders are anxiety and depressive disorders.
- The suicide risk is increased 5-fold, and more so in those with complex partial seizures.
- Anticonvulsant treatments can compound the psychiatric problems—phenobarbitone causes hyperactivity and irritability in children; phenytoin can produce ataxia and delirium.

## Head injury

Head injury is a major cause of organic psychiatric syndromes in young adults. They can be difficult to treat and services are greatly under-resourced.

- The psychiatric consequences of a head injury depend partly on the nature and location of the injury, and partly on the person's premorbid characteristics. In blunt trauma, the brain suffers contusions at the point of impact, focal damage elsewhere as the brain reverberates in the skull and diffuse axonal damage due to the shearing forces.
- People with an apoE4 allele are at greater risk of persistent deficits following head injury.

A wide range of psychiatric problems can follow a head injury:

- A head injury with loss of consciousness may produce amnesia, either *anterograde* (post-traumatic), for events after the injury, or *retrograde*. Anterograde amnesia lasting more than 24 hours predicts a poor long-term outcome, including persistent cognitive deficits. The impairment ranges from a subtle slowing of thought and distractibility

**Table 13.14** Other medical disorders with psychiatric manifestations.

| Medical disorder | Psychiatric manifestations |
| --- | --- |
| Cerebral tumour | Psychiatric symptoms in 50%, more so if tumour is in frontal or temporal lobes |
| Cerebral abscess | May present with psychiatric symptoms |
| Multiple sclerosis | Mood disturbance in 25%: bland euphoria or depression |
| | Cognitive deficits in 25%: can become severe |
| | Personality change: apathy, irritability |
| Parkinson's disease | Depression in 50%, L-DOPA therapy may cause psychosis |
| SLE and related vasculitides | 5% at presentation, 50% at some stage: mood disorder, psychosis, delirium and seizures |
| HIV | Dementia in 30% with AIDS; psychosis—prevalence uncertain |
| Cushing's disease | Severe depression common; occasionally psychosis and cognitive impairment |
| Addison's disease | Apathy and fatigue in 80%; depression in 50%; cognitive impairment in 50%; psychosis in 5% |
| Hyperthyroidism | Anxiety (common), depression, mania, delirium |
| Hypothyroidism | Mental slowing and depressive symptoms very common; rarely 'myxoedema madness'—delirium, depression, dementia; symptoms may persist despite thyroxine replacement |
| Hypercalcaemia | Psychosis, delirium and mood disorders in 50%; cognitive impairment in 25% |

through to dementia. It tends to improve in the first year, but thereafter deficits are likely to be permanent. There is no specific treatment.

- *Personality changes* are frequent. Typically the changes are indicative of frontal lobe damage: impaired ability to plan or persevere; emotional shallowness and lability; impulsivity; and irritability. Altered sexual behaviour (in any direction) and long-winded speech also occur. Improvement is partial and slow.
- *Mood disorder, anxiety disorders* and *schizophrenia* are more common than expected after head injury. Left- and right-sided frontal lobe damage are associated with depression and mania, respectively.
- *Post-concussional syndrome* describes emotional, cognitive and bodily symptoms occurring after relatively minor head injury. The symptoms are sometimes thought to be 'psychological' or even feigned, related to hopes of compensation, but may reflect subtle brain injury.

## Other medical disorders associated with psychiatric disorders

Table 13.14 lists some medical disorders that often have psychiatric manifestations.

### Key points

- Organic psychiatric disorders are those due to a recognized medical cause or pathology. Dementia and delirium are by definition organic disorders; all other psychiatric disorders can be. Hence consider an organic cause for every psychiatric presentation—epilepsy and endocrine disorders are classic culprits.
- Dementia is characterized by memory loss. It is usually insidious and progressive, sometimes reversible. The most common causes are Alzheimer's disease, vascular dementia and dementia with Lewy bodies.
- Delirium is an acute, fluctuating confusional state, with clouding of consciousness. It has many causes (e.g. drugs, septicaemia). It is usually treatable.
- Treatment of organic disorders is aimed at the underlying cause *and* at the psychiatric symptoms.

# Chapter 14

# Substance misuse

## General issues

Many substances are taken for pleasure. A substance is regarded as being *misused* (or *abused*) if it produces physical, psychological or social harm. Commonly misused substances are shown in Table 14.1. This chapter describes:

- The features of substance misuse.
- Its psychiatric consequences.
- The management of substance misuse and its associated psychiatric disorders.

Substance misuse presents in diverse ways—for example, as depression or morbid jealousy (both associated with alcohol), as an acute psychosis (amphetamines) or as haematemesis (alcoholic cirrhosis). Its various presentations, and frequency, mean that detection of substance misuse, notably of alcohol, is part of every psychiatric assessment.

- Review the substance misuse module (Chapter 3).

Prevalence figures for misuse of substances other than alcohol are likely to be unreliable as use is frequently illegal. Clinic data or statistics about registered addicts give a misleading impression of what is being misused and the common health consequences. Bear this in mind when reading this chapter.

*Lecture Notes: Psychiatry*, 10e. By Paul Harrison, John Geddes and Michael Sharpe. Published 2010 by Blackwell Publishing Ltd.

- In the USA, 1.5% of adults admit to having tried heroin, 7% amphetamines, 8% LSD, 12% cocaine and 30% cannabis. A quarter of each group were regular users.
- A common approach to reducing the recreational use of drugs is to make them illegal. Most countries have legal classifications based on the harmful potential of the drugs to the user and society. The classifications are not described here as they vary between countries and over time. For example, cannabis use is legal in the Netherlands and elsewhere: its legal classification is controversial in other countries. The use of alcohol, which is probably the most important cause of harm in many societies, is not legally restricted for adults in most Western societies.

## Types of substance misuse

There are several categories of substance misuse:

- *At-risk consumption*—(alcohol) intake at a level associated with increased risk of harm.
- *Harmful use*—misuse associated with health and social consequences, but without dependence.
- *Dependence*—prolonged, regular use of some substances (especially alcohol, opioids, amphetamines) can lead to *dependence (addiction)* and *withdrawal* syndromes.
- *Intoxication* is the acute effect of the substance—being drunk (alcohol), tripping (LSD) or stoned

**Box 14.1 Annual costs of alcohol to UK society (2004 figures)**

- Direct NHS costs: £1.7 billion.
- Crime and antisocial behaviour: £7.3 billion.
- Lost productivity: £6.4 billion.
- Specialist alcohol treatment services: £95 million.
- 22 000 premature deaths—deaths from cirrhosis increasing in the UK.
- 30 000 hospital admissions.
- Up to 70% of all presentations to A&E departments.
- 3000 deaths or serious injuries as a result of drink-drive accidents.
- 1.2 million violent incidents.

**Table 14.5** Features of delirium tremens.

| |
|---|
| Onset 24–48 hours after stopping heavy, prolonged drinking |
| Delirium |
| Visual hallucinations |
| Delusions, usually persecutory and transient |
| Fear and agitation, sometimes aggression |
| Coarse tremor |
| Seizures |
| Autonomic disturbance (sweating, fever, tachycardia, hypertension) |
| Insomnia |
| Dehydration and electrolyte disturbance |
| Lasts 3–4 days, followed by exhaustion and patchy amnesia for the episode |

## Clinical features of alcohol misuse

### Dependence

The concept of dependence was introduced in Chapter 3. The diagnosis of alcohol dependence (alcoholism) is made if three or more of the following are present:

- Feeling compelled to drink.
- Primacy of drinking over other activities—for example, eating, family life, work, health.
- Increased tolerance to alcohol—being able to drink quantities that would incapacitate others.
- Relief drinking—drinking to stop or prevent withdrawal symptoms.
- Stereotyped pattern of drinking.
- Reinstatement after abstinence—unable to give up alcohol for long.
- Drinking despite awareness of harmful consequences.
- Withdrawal symptoms.

### Withdrawal and delirium tremens

The main features of alcohol withdrawal are:

- Tremulousness ('the shakes').
- Agitation.
- Nausea and retching.
- Sweating.
- Overwhelming desire to drink (craving).
- Withdrawal symptoms are relieved by alcohol. If untreated, the symptoms may last for several days.

Transient misperceptions and hallucinations may occur.

- Withdrawal symptoms often occur on waking as the blood alcohol concentration falls during sleep.
- The most severe form of withdrawal (5% of cases) is *delirium tremens* (the 'DTs'), a potentially fatal condition (Table 14.5).

### Wernicke's syndrome

An acute encephalopathy presenting with delirium, ataxia, nystagmus and ophthalmoplegia, occurring in the severely alcohol dependent, usually in the context of withdrawal. It is due to thiamine deficiency and requires urgent treatment. It may progress to Korsakov's syndrome (p. 153).

### Harmful alcohol use

About 20% of patients attending GPs drink hazardously (i.e. above the recommended limits)—most of these are 'asymptomatic' and most go undetected. Detection can be improved by:

- Asking about alcohol intake during all medical and psychiatric assessments, including use of FAST, CAGE or AUDIT questionnaires (Chapters 2 and 3).
- Following up on comments suggesting that a patient thinks he drinks too much.

- Unexplained macrocytosis or abnormal liver function tests.
- Noting the presence of one or more of the psychiatric or social consequences of harmful alcohol use (Table 14.4).

## Associated medical disorders

If alcohol misuse has led to a medical disorder, then psychiatric or social impairments (Table 14.4) are likely. Assess and take appropriate action. If an alcohol-related psychiatric disorder is present, check for physical symptoms and signs of alcohol dependency.

## Associated psychiatric disorders

Alcohol misuse is associated with an increased risk of, and worse prognosis for, most psychiatric disorders. These are covered in the respective chapters.

- In *alcoholic hallucinosis*, a heavy drinker experiences recurrent auditory hallucinations, usually of a threatening or derogatory nature. The hallucinations occur in clear consciousness (cf. withdrawal hallucinations). The syndrome is an example of a drug-induced psychosis.
- About 10% of people who are alcohol dependent commit suicide.

## Management of alcohol problems

The focus in this section is on clinical rather than on population-based interventions.

- Figure 14.1 gives an algorithm for management of hazardous, harmful, and dependent drinking.

## Management of hazardous and harmful alcohol use

A brief intervention in primary care is usually sufficient if someone is drinking more than the safe limits but is not dependent and has no specific medical or psychiatric disorder. The components are:

- Assess accurately the amount consumed (use diaries, informants).
- Assess the nature and extent of harm (e.g. liver function tests, work record).
- Provide brief advice of the hazards of excess alcohol intake. Tailor advice to the individual, and reinforce with written information. Advice should be given in a non-judgemental manner.
- Review progress. If problem drinking persists, or is in the harmful range, consider extended brief intervention and/or motivational interviewing.

The FRAMES acronym covers the main approach to giving advice about drinking:

- Structured **F**eedback on risk and harm.
- Emphasis on the patient's **R**esponsibility for change.
- Clear **A**dvice to make a change in drinking.
- Discuss a **M**enu of options for making change.
- Express **E**mpathy and be non-judgmental.
- Reinforce the patient's **S**elf-efficacy.

## Treatment of alcohol dependence

The first requirement is detoxification ('detox', 'drying out'), which is controlled withdrawal, using a reducing course of a benzodiazepine in place of alcohol. This should always be done as part of a care plan which includes after-care and relapse prevention.

- *Mild dependence*—withdraw at home without drugs or with small doses of benzodiazepines.
- *Moderate dependence*—can usually withdraw at home:
  - Day 1 chlordiazepoxide 20 mg four times a day
  - Day 2 chlordiazepoxide 15 mg four times a day
  - Day 3 chlordiazepoxide 10 mg four times a day
  - Day 4 chlordiazepoxide 5 mg four times a day
  - Day 5 chlordiazepoxide 5 mg twice a day
  - Advise the patient to drink plenty of non-alcoholic liquids. Prescribe vitamins (thiamine 300 mg per day—deficiencies are common and withdrawal may precipitate Wernicke's syndrome. Consider parenteral thiamine if risk of Wernicke's syndrome is judged to be high.
- *Severe dependence, or history of complications such as DTs, cognitive impairment, etc.*—may need higher

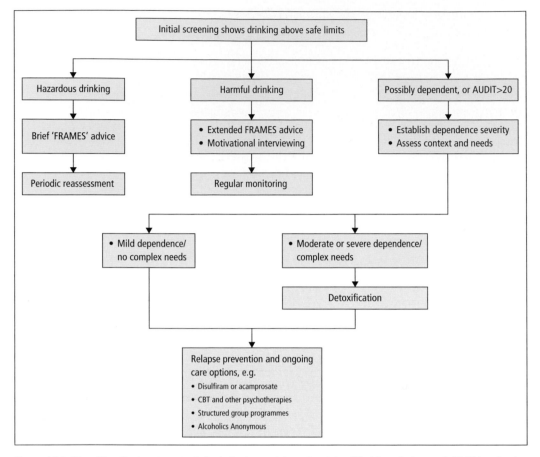

**Figure 14.1 Algorithm for treatment of alcohol misuse**. Adapted and simplified from Parker *et al.*, 2008 (see Further reading for details).

doses of chlordiazepoxide, and/or in-patient treatment. Give parenteral thiamine routinely.

## Maintaining abstinence

Various strategies are used to prevent relapse following withdrawal from alcohol. None has been shown to be very effective.

- Aim for abstinence where possible—it has a better long-term outcome than controlled drinking.
- Regular liver function tests and breath alcohol measurements help monitor progress.
- Encourage attendance at groups run by local community alcohol services or Alcoholics Anonymous.

- Consider disulfiram (Antabuse), acamprosate or opioid antagonists (p. 72).
- Psychological interventions include CBT, social skills training, problem solving and motivational interviewing (helping them make the decision to change their behaviour).
- About 50% of patients will return to drinking again within 6 months of abstinence.

## Treatment of associated medical disorders

Many of the medical syndromes arising from alcohol misuse can present as emergencies (e.g. Wernicke's encephalopathy, bleeding varices), and the admission provides an opportunity for psychiatric intervention. Look out for withdrawal symptoms occurring during hospitalization.

## Treatment of associated psychiatric disorders

The principles are:
- Reduce intake to safe limits, since continuing alcohol misuse acts as a perpetuating factor.
- Treat the psychiatric disorder in the standard manner. Check for interaction of alcohol with prescribed medication (e.g. antidepressants).

## Cannabis

### Epidemiology and pharmacology

- Derived from the hemp plant *Cannabis sativa*. The main psychoactive ingredient is Δ-9-tetrahydrocannabinol (THC), which acts on endogenous cannabinoid receptors in the brain. Cannabis also contains cannabidiol, which to some extent antagonizes the effects of THC.
- The THC content of cannabis varies, and is rising over time in the UK.
- Usually smoked.
- *Marijuana* is the dried flowers and leaves of cannabis plant; *hashish* is the dried resin.
- It is the most widely used illicit recreational drug. Used for millennia for medical and religious purposes, use as a recreational drug has increased dramatically over the past 40 years particularly in adolescents and young adults.
- Used by an estimated 150–200 million adults worldwide.
- 10% of those using the drug become daily users.

The effects of cannabis are shown in Table 14.6.

### Adverse health effects

- Difficult to untangle causality because users of cannabis are more likely to smoke and drink alcohol.
- Anxiety and panic—especially in first-time users.
- Paranoid ideation—especially in first-time users—and occasionally delirium.

**Table 14.6** Effects of cannabis.

| |
|---|
| Dose-related impairment in reaction time, information processing, coordination, motor performance, attention |
| Exaggeration of pre-existing mood |
| Mellowness and increased enjoyment of aesthetic experience |
| Distortion of sense of space and time |
| Reddening of eyes |

- Increased risk of road traffic accidents.
- Increased risk of using other, more harmful, drugs.
- Possible increased risk of respiratory illness.
- Possible mild long-term cognitive impairment in heavy and regular users.
- May provoke angina in people with heart disease.
- Cannabis does not cause dependence or withdrawal, though some tolerance occurs (and use may become so ingrained as to warrant the term 'psychological dependence').
- Early and heavy use of cannabis increases risk for schizophrenia.
- Continued use in schizophrenia is associated with a worse treatment response.

### Treatment

CBT may reduce cannabis use, but there are high rates of re-use within 6–12 months.

## Opioids

### Epidemiology and pharmacology

- Opioids mimic endogenous endorphins and enkephalins and activate opioid receptors.
- They include naturally occurring substances (morphine and codeine) and synthetic opioids (heroin and methadone).
- Highly addictive.
- Heroin is most commonly misused because it causes euphoria—estimated 100 000 regular users in the UK.

**Table 14.7** Effects of opioids.

| |
|---|
| Euphoria |
| Analgesia |
| Drowsiness |
| Respiratory depression |
| Cough reflex suppression |
| Nausea and vomiting |
| Bradycardia and hypotension |
| Lowering of body temperature |
| Pupillary constriction |
| Constipation |

**Table 14.8** Features of opioid withdrawal.

| |
|---|
| Craving |
| Restlessness and insomnia |
| Myalgia |
| Sweating |
| Abdominal pain, vomiting and diarrhoea |
| Dilated pupils, running nose and eyes |
| Tachycardia |
| Yawning |
| 'Goose bumps' |

- There are several modes of use:
  - Intravenous injection ('mainlining'). It is associated with a high risk of infections, thrombosis and phlebitis. Hepatitis B and C, and HIV, should be suspected and testing performed (with informed consent and appropriate counselling) in anyone who has injected drugs.
  - Inhalation—'chasing the dragon': the opiate is melted on metal foil and then inhaled as it vaporizes.
  - 'Snorting'—the opioid is cut into a fine powder and then sniffed.

The effects of opioids are shown in Table 14.7.

## Adverse health and social effects

Opioids have many serious adverse effects.

- They cause high levels of morbidity and mortality—the mortality rate is 12 times that of the general population; most deaths occur in males.
- Different routes have a major influence on bioavailability, speed of onset, severity of dependence and rates of physical complications. Intravenous injecting has the highest risk of overdose and complications.
- Risk of transmission of blood-borne viruses—HIV, hepatitis B and C.
- Psychiatric comorbidity, including misuse of other substances. The suicide rate is increased 14-fold.
- Major negative social effects.

## Clinical features

### Dependence

Tolerance to all opioids rapidly develops. Because of this (and because of batch-to-batch variation in purity), overdose is common and frequently fatal due to respiratory depression.

- Tolerance makes pain management in an opioid user difficult as higher doses may be required.
- High risk of overdose after detoxification—for example, released prisoners.

### Withdrawal

Stopping opioids leads to an extremely unpleasant withdrawal syndrome called 'cold turkey' (Table 14.8). The onset is usually within 8–12 hours of the last dose (longer after methadone), peaking 24–48 hours later and subsiding over 10 days. Though severe, opioid withdrawal is rarely life threatening.

## Management

### Rapid detoxification and abstinence

- In-patient detoxification is more effective than out-patient detoxification—probably because many opioid-dependent people live in chaotic environments (often with other users). Information is given about the nature and course of withdrawal symptoms.
- Prescribe reducing doses of a substitute drug, methadone linctus, which reduces the severity of

the withdrawal symptoms. Clonidine and naltrexone (an opioid antagonist) are also used.

• Post-withdrawal abstinence programmes vary from specific relapse-prevention therapies to residential houses where a network of ex-users helps the recovering addict overcome the craving.

• Even when withdrawal is achieved, the relapse rate is high (40% at 6 months; the majority at a year).

## Harm reduction and maintenance therapy (substitution treatment)

In maintenance therapy for opioid dependence, the priority changes from abstinence to reducing the harm from ongoing opioid use. The first aim is to make services acceptable to users in order to engage them in treatment. Then, the aims are to:

• Reduce injecting.

• Stabilize drug use and lifestyle.

• Reduce criminal behaviour by avoiding need to obtain expensive drugs.

• Reduce the death rate.

Motivational interviewing and contingency management may be helpful when combined with pharmacological management.

The harm reduction approach is pragmatic and includes a range of initiatives such as free needles and syringes and public education. A central feature is *substitute prescribing*. Oral methadone is prescribed to prevent the need for intravenous injections.

Long-term use of the oral drug is usual.

• Substitute prescribing does not suit all opioid users. It is best targeted at those whose social functioning and health have already been seriously affected by drug use, and where abstinence is an unrealistic goal.

## Management of overdose

Early recognition and treatment is vital.

• Patient is unconscious, with pinpoint pupils, bradycardia, hypotension and shallow breathing or snoring. Check for respiratory arrest.

• Place in recovery position. Naloxone (opioid antagonist) 0.4 mg intramuscularly—may need to be repeated

## Stimulants

### Amphetamines

Amphetamines ('speed', 'whizz') may be taken orally, snorted or injected. They produce symptoms similar to those of hypomania: elevated mood, over-talkativeness, increased energy and insomnia. Pulse and blood pressure increase, pupils dilate and mucous membranes become dry.

• *Dependence* occurs. Regular users develop depression and mood swings. The withdrawal syndrome can be severe (a 'crash'), with agitated depression, lethargy, suicidal thoughts and craving.

• Treat intoxication or psychosis with benzodiazepines and antipsychotics; treat depression with TCAs.

• Prolonged use can lead to *paranoid psychosis*, which can last for months after use has ceased.

• Amphetamines are used clinically for attention deficit hyperactivity disorder and narcolepsy.

• Amphetamines are potent dopamine enhancers—they inhibit its reuptake and stimulate its release. NA and 5-HT are also enhanced.

• *'Crystal meth'* (d-methamphetamine hydrochloride) is a particularly addictive form of amphetamine that reaches high brain concentrations when smoked. It is associated with frequent and severe psychiatric symptoms, and withdrawal reactions.

### Cocaine

*Cocaine* produces similar effects to amphetamines, but the features tend to be more dramatic.

• Cocaine is either snorted, or smoked in the form of 'crack' or 'freebase' (cocaine processed to remove the hydrochloride), which increases the intensity of the effect.

• Cocaine misusers often also misuse opioids and alcohol.

• Immunization against the effects of cocaine is currently being tested.

• *'Formication'* or 'cocaine bugs' refers to delusions of infestation, which can lead to numerous scabs from picking at the skin. Also seen with crystal meth.

## 3,4-Methylenedioxymethamphetamine (MDMA, ecstasy)

Ecstasy is a synthetic amphetamine analogue with mild stimulatory and hallucinogenic effects. It is widely used in Britain—30% of teenagers say they've tried it. Tolerance occurs and the best experience is said to be the first. Though safer than amphetamines or cocaine—probably much safer—there is concern about its harmful effects:

• Adverse reactions—hyperpyrexia and acute renal failure due to dehydration, as well as water intoxication in users who overcompensate. There are very rare, but well-publicized, fatalities.

• Acute psychosis—prevalence unknown.

• The drug is neurotoxic to 5-HT fibres (at least in monkeys), and chronic users have lowered central 5-HT levels and some cognitive deficits. There is, therefore, concern that depression and impulsivity may be a long-term consequence, although no good evidence of this has emerged.

Management of stimulant misuse has a very limited evidence base. Use the same approaches as for opioids. Antipsychotics and benzodiazepines are used to treat acute agitation and psychosis.

## Hallucinogens

Hallucinogens alter perception, producing *psychedelic* experiences. They are taken orally. LSD is the main synthetic hallucinogen; similar effects can be achieved using magic mushrooms. Agonism at 5-HT$_2$ receptors is a likely common mechanism.

### Lysergic acid diethylamide (LSD)

The 'trip' starts about 2 hours after consumption, lasts 8–12 hours and consists of distorted sensory perception, alteration of the sense of time and scale, and changes in body image (e.g. out of body experiences). The effects can be very intense—and occasionally terrifying (a 'bad trip').

• Hallucinogens rarely cause dependence or withdrawal. They are associated with *flashbacks* when the sensations of a trip are re-experienced long afterwards.

• Emergency psychiatric referral may occur because of the panic or agitation associated with a bad trip. Reassurance, reorientation and 'talking down' are necessary. Sedation as required with benzodiazepines. The person may also come to harm from responding to the hallucinations.

## Other substances

### Phencyclidine

Phencyclidine (PCP, 'angel dust') and ketamine ('special K') are volatile anaesthetics which in smaller doses produce a sense of drunkenness, hallucinations, disorientation and agitation. The picture resembles schizophrenia. Complications include nystagmus, tachycardia, hypertension and seizures.

• Usage is common in the USA but still rare in the UK.

• The drugs are antagonists at NMDA glutamate receptors.

• When managing PCP intoxication or psychosis, avoid chlorpromazine. The medical complications may need treatment.

### Solvents

Solvent misuse (of glue, aerosols, petrol, etc.) is mainly an adolescent male group activity. The effects are rapid in onset and short-lived—euphoria, disinhibition, blurred vision, ataxia.

• Solvent use comes to medical attention when complications arise—cardiac arrhythmias, inhalation of vomit, coma. Chronic damage to the liver and brain can occur.

### Anabolic steroids

Anabolic steroids are misused mainly by male athletes and bodybuilders. They produce a range of psychiatric effects that can be severe and persistent—euphoria, depression, aggression ('roid rage') and hyperactivity. A form of dependency may result in some users. Clinical suspicion may be raised by the physical appearance.

## Benzodiazepines

Benzodiazepines are taken illicitly, often as part of multiple drug misuse and as an opioid substitute. It can be difficult to decide whether symptoms and side-effects are attributable to the benzodiazepine or to the other drugs being used.

• Iatrogenic benzodiazepine dependence and its management is mentioned in Chapter 7.

## Nicotine and caffeine

Both nicotine and caffeine are addictive—ask any smoker or serious coffee drinker. Each has its own acute actions and side-effects, but psychiatric problems are rare.

• Psychiatric patients smoke more than the population average—90% of people with schizophrenia do so. For unknown reasons they have a lower incidence of lung cancer than other smokers.

• Abstinence rates after nicotine dependence (30% at 6 months) are worse than for opioids, cocaine and alcohol.

### Key points

• For each substance, consider: What are its acute effects? Does it cause dependence and withdrawal? What are the associated psychiatric, medical and social complications?

• Dependence is a combination of physical and psychological effects. It is common in people who regularly use alcohol, opioids or stimulants. Withdrawal occurs if the substance is withheld.

• Substance misuse is widespread. Those in treatment are a small and unrepresentative fraction.

• Substance misuse is often comorbid with psychiatric disorders. Both need to be treated. The combination worsens prognosis.

• Alcohol produces a wide range of psychiatric, medical and social problems. Enquire about alcohol intake and consider a role for alcohol misuse in all patients.

• Management of substance misuse includes psychological, pharmacological and social components. The prognosis for persistent abstinence after being dependent on any substance is poor.

## Chapter 15

# Personality disorders

## Personality and personality disorder

*Personality* describes the characteristic behavioural, emotional and cognitive attributes of an individual. Thus we talk about an aggressive man, a nervous lady, and so on. Such traits are usually apparent by mid-adolescence. Psychiatrists are interested in personality because it forms a major part of the contextual understanding of every case (Chapter 5) and interacts with psychiatric disorders in many ways, as discussed below.

- Although established personality traits are fairly stable (almost by definition) they are exacerbated in the short term by stress (*'decompensation'*), and it is usually at such times that they are medically encountered.

Personality is also of interest to psychiatrists because in some individuals certain personality traits are extreme—being either excessive or deficient—and lead to problems for the person or others. This constitutes *personality disorder*. A formal definition of personality disorder is given in Box 15.1. People with personality disorder come into contact with medical and psychiatric services either because they are concerned about themselves or, more commonly, because others

are concerned or affected by their actions. For example:

- A spinster who has been too timid to ever have a close relationship takes an overdose because she is so lonely.
- A tax inspector whose obsessive need for tidiness at work leads to an industrial dispute and a psychiatric report is requested.
- A young woman who takes impulsive overdoses each time a boyfriend leaves her.

A personality disorder may also be detected during the assessment or treatment of a psychiatric disorder—though it is very important to bear in mind that the person's behaviour and self-description may be modified by the illness and consequently give a misleading impression about their 'normal' personality.

## Core features of personality disorder

This section covers the features common to all personality disorders. The following section deals with the factors specific to particular personality disorders.

### Diagnosis

Diagnosis of personality disorder is based on a marked deviation of one or more aspects of personality. The main effect may be on:

*Lecture Notes: Psychiatry*, 10e. By Paul Harrison, John Geddes and Michael Sharpe. Published 2010 by Blackwell Publishing Ltd.

**Box 15.1 Definitions of personality disorder**

ICD-10: '... a severe disturbance in the characterological constitution and behavioural tendencies of the individual, usually involving several areas of the personality, and nearly always associated with considerable personal and social disruption.'

DSM-IV: 'an enduring pattern of inner experience and behavior that deviates markedly from the expectations of the individual's culture, is pervasive and inflexible, has an onset in adolescence or early adulthood, and leads to distress or impairment.'

**Table 15.1** Areas to cover in assessment of personality disorder

| |
|---|
| *Personality disorder itself* |
| Presence |
| Characteristics and features |
| Severity |
| Treatability |
| |
| *Other issues* |
| Presence of comorbid psychiatric disorders |
| Risk to self |
| Risk to others |
| Drug and alcohol use |
| History of self-harm and violence |
| Current social situation |
| Psychosocial stressors |

- Cognitions (attitudes; ways in which others' actions are interpreted).
- Mood (range, intensity and appropriateness of emotions).
- Impulse control and gratification of needs.
- Relationships and the way interpersonal situations are handled.

In addition, other criteria must be met, which help establish that the disturbance is sufficient to merit a diagnostic label:

- The personality attributes cause distress or dysfunction for the individual or those he interacts with.
- The dysfunction occurs across a range of situations.
- The characteristics are pervasive, stable and recognizable since late adolescence.

The specific personality disorders are diagnosed according to the domain(s) of personality which are most affected, and the most prominent behaviours.

## Assessment

The above features mean that a diagnosis of personality disorder requires that you gather considerable information about the patient's previous behaviour, personal history and mental state (see Chapters 2, 3 and 5). The areas to be covered in the assessment are summarized in Table 15.1.

- Use of an informant is very important to corroborate the history.

- Always describe clearly the characteristics upon which the diagnosis is being based.
- Always seek and record positive as well as negative personality attributes; the former will prove useful in management.
- Carefully examine for the presence of a psychiatric disorder—it may be a differential diagnosis or a comorbid condition.
- Do the same for substance misuse, which exacerbates many personality traits.
- Standardized assessments of personality disorder, such as the Personality Assessment Schedule, are useful, but not widely used in clinical practice.

## Classification

Personality disorder in ICD-10 is divided into 10 types. However, the validity and reliability of these categories is limited. Most patients seem to fit several descriptions or none of them. A simpler option, from DSM-IV, is to use three clusters, which encompass the individual categories (Table 15.2). In practice, both categories and clusters are used by clinicians.

- Personality traits and personality disorders are, in reality, *dimensional*—that is, they merge into each other (and into psychiatric disorders). Consequently, any categorical classification is bound to be problematic. One illustration is that

**Table 15.2** Classification and features of personality disorders.

| Cluster and subtype | Main features |
|---|---|
| **Cluster A (eccentric)** | **Aloof or suspicious, solitary** |
| *Paranoid* | Suspicion and distrust of others |
| | Sensitivity to criticism |
| | Bears grudges |
| | Self-importance |
| *Schizoid* | Emotionally cold and detached |
| | Introspective |
| | Social isolation |
| | Lack of *joie de vivre* |
| **Cluster B (dramatic)** | **Emotionally labile and intense** |
| *Dissocial (= psychopathic, antisocial)* | Callous |
| | Unstable, transient relationships |
| | Low frustration threshold |
| | Irritable and impulsive |
| | Failure to learn from experience |
| | Failure to accept responsibility |
| | Lack of guilt |
| | Tend to be young men |
| *Borderline (= emotionally unstable)* | Multiple, turbulent relationships |
| | Impulsivity |
| | Recurrent emotional crises |
| | Variable, intense mood |
| | Stress-related psychotic-like symptoms |
| | Tend to be young women |
| *Histrionic* | Exaggerated, theatrical displays of emotion |
| | Attention seeking |
| | Vain |
| | Suggestible |
| | Shallow, labile mood |
| | Crushes and fads |
| *Narcissistic* | Grandiose self-importance |
| | Exaggerates achievements and abilities |
| | Exploits others |
| | Arrogant |
| | Expects special praise and respect |
| **Cluster C (anxious)** | **Timid, dependent, low self-esteem** |
| *Anankastic (= obsessional)* | Excessive orderliness |
| | Preoccupation with detail |
| | Inflexible and dogmatic |
| | Humourless |
| *Anxious (= avoidant)* | Persistent tense and apprehensive feelings |
| | Avoid personal contact |
| | Fear of criticism or rejection |
| *Dependent* | Encourage others to make decisions |
| | Excessive need to be taken care of |

several categories formerly included as personality disorders are now considered to be psychiatric disorders—for example, schizotypal disorder (Chapter 12).

• Other difficulties with the concept of personality disorder are covered later in this chapter.

• The vignettes below illustrate the category and cluster approaches to personality disorder.

> *Miss D is 22 and has taken an impulsive overdose. She felt bored and angry with her boyfriend and various others. She has repeatedly self-harmed since early adolescence in response to minor life events—particularly when she feels abandoned. She reports having been sexually abused by her stepfather. Her lifestyle is chaotic and she misuses alcohol. Previous attempts to offer help have been thwarted by her failure to keep appointments. Her one enduring pleasure in life is looking after horses. Two days later she discharges herself; her boyfriend sent her some flowers and she is planning to marry him.*
>
> *Key features*: impulsivity, sensitive to rejection, emotional instability.
>
> *Positive attributes*: the care of animals. Has done unpaid work for an animal charity.
>
> *Cluster*: B (dramatic)
>
> *Subtype*: emotionally unstable (borderline) personality disorder.

> *Dr E is a 60-year-old scientist who has accepted psychiatric referral under protest. He is unmarried and has had several brief, unsatisfactory relationships. He feels strongly that he has been denied the acclaim he deserves and is currently complaining bitterly to his head of department after unsuccessfully applying for promotion. He alleges that other workers steal his ideas. He does not mix with his colleagues and is uneasy in social gatherings.*
>
> *Key features*: socially isolated, suspicious, tendency to exaggerate self-importance.
>
> *Positive attributes*: his research eminence shows a high level of functioning.
>
> *Cluster*: A (eccentric)
>
> *Subtype*: paranoid personality disorder.

## Management

Personality cannot usually be modified to any significant degree in adults. However, there are evidence-based treatments for some personality disorders, as outlined below, and very occasionally, in-patient psychotherapy (a *therapeutic community*) is used as a treatment. The main aspects of standard management are:

• Help the person to avoid situations that cause problems such as intoxication or confrontations

• Help them to find a lifestyle which suits their strengths and minimizes the effects of their personality difficulties

• Be consistent in managing crisis presentations. Admissions are rarely helpful and may reinforce the behaviour. A consistent, limited and community-based approach is usually better.

• Treat any coexisting substance misuse.

• Treat any coexisting psychiatric disorder.

## Prognosis

The fact that personality disorders are considered to be lifelong and stable implies that prognosis is uniformly bad. In fact, considerable fluctuations do occur, and improvement is often observed by middle age. Some clinicians distinguish:

• Mature personality disorders (equating to cluster A—see below), which are first recognizable in late adolescence and which remain stable or worsen with age.

• Immature personality disorders (clusters B and C) which have an onset in childhood and which mellow with age.

Personality disorder is associated with an increased mortality rate. It also worsens outcome of comorbid psychiatric disorder, and increases the risk of violence when comorbid with psychosis.

## Epidemiology

Estimates of the prevalence of personality disorders vary widely—for example, from 2% to 15% in the general population. A recent large survey of British households found:

• 4.4% of people had a personality disorder. Of these, half met the criteria for two or more disorders.

• The most common were obsessive–compulsive, avoidant, schizoid and borderline. No cases of histrionic or narcissistic personality disorder were seen.

• Personality disorders frequently coexist with psychiatric disorders.

The prevalence of personality disorder is much higher in specific populations. For example:

• Prisoners: over 50% of men and 30% of women, with most being antisocial personality disorder.

• Psychiatric patients: about 50%.

• Patients with substance misuse and eating disorder: 70%.

## Aetiology

Very little is known about the aetiology of personality disorders, partly because so little is understood about the determinants of normal personality. Most current research focuses on borderline and dissocial personality disorder, largely because they cause the greatest clinical and forensic difficulties (see below).

• Patterns of childhood behaviour, even as young as infancy, predict personality and personality disorders, albeit only weakly, emphasizing the early origins and stability of personality characteristics.

• Upbringing and childhood experiences have major influences on our personality for better and worse. Adverse childhood events, including sexual and physical abuse, are important risk factors for personality disorder.

• There is a moderate genetic contribution to personality traits (e.g. 35–50% heritability for neuroticism and extraversion) and to some personality disorders, especially anankastic and dissocial types.

• Aggressive behaviour may be slightly more common in men with sex chromosome abnormalities (especially XYY), but much less so than sometimes portrayed.

## Specific personality disorders

• Refer back to Table 15.2 for key features of each personality disorder, and a comparison of clusters and subtypes.

## Cluster A personality disorders ('eccentric')

People with cluster A personality disorder (especially schizoid type) by their nature tend to avoid services, and usually present (as with Dr E in the vignette) when their suspiciousness or persecutory beliefs lead them to behave in a way which concerns others (e.g. making accusations or threatening retribution for a perceived wrongdoing). The key issues are:

• To distinguish the personality disorder from a psychosis, especially chronic delusional disorder (Chapter 12). Paranoid personality disorder is a risk factor for development of a psychosis.

• To decide if there is a significant risk of harm to the person or others (Chapter 4).

• To decide what, if any, treatment should be given for the personality disorder. Low-dose antipsychotics may be tried, with appropriate consent, but compliance is likely to be poor. Similarly, social interventions may be offered, but isolation is rarely perceived as a problem. Psychotherapy is said to be ineffective, even harmful, and is contraindicated.

## Cluster B personality disorders ('dramatic')

There is considerable overlap between the individual disorders in this cluster. In practice, the only widely used categories are borderline (for women) and dissocial (for men).

### Borderline personality disorder

Miss D (see vignette above) fits the typical profile of borderline personality disorder. There may be frequent presentations for a variety of reasons:

• Following an overdose or self-cutting.

• With depressive or 'quasi-psychotic' symptoms or suicidal ideation. The psychiatric presentation and subjective description is often dramatic, yet somewhat out of keeping with the objective impression.

• With a dramatic plea or demand for help of some kind (e.g. admission, medication).

Management can be difficult; clinicians may oscillate between over-reacting and failing to intervene. The principles of management are:

- Careful differentiation, as far as is possible, from mood disorders and psychosis. Bear in mind the symptom profile and the onset and course.
- A written care plan. Ensure good communication between the agencies involved to avoid 'splitting' (disagreements between staff induced by the patient—people with these personality traits induce a range of strong feelings).
- Respond to threats consistently and do not reinforce manipulative behaviour.
- Clear boundaries should be agreed about unacceptable behaviour and about the nature of care that will be provided. For example, recurrent psychiatric admission is probably not helpful.
- A psychotherapeutic assessment should be considered. A very intensive and specific form of psychotherapy, *dialectical behaviour therapy*, is effective in decreasing self-harm. *Cognitive analytical therapy* is also advocated. Group therapy in *therapeutic communities* may occasionally be helpful. None of these therapies is widely available in the NHS.
- Trials of an antidepressant or a mood stabilizer may be indicated even in the absence of a clear depressive episode. TCAs probably do more harm than good, but there is some evidence that SSRIs, low-dose antipsychotics and mood stabilizers may be effective at reducing impulsive behaviour and mood variability. However, although good responses are seen in a few patients, long-term medication is not appropriate for many patients.
- The diagnosis of 'borderline personality disorder' is sometimes applied loosely and pejoratively, especially to young women who self-harm, abuse alcohol, have eating difficulties and have chaotic lifestyles. Use the label carefully, sticking to the principles outlined here.

Borderline personality disorder is under active research investigation at present.

- The key neuropsychological deficits are thought to be *affective instability* and *impulsivity*.
- Brain imaging suggests dopamine and the frontal lobes are important.
- The disorder may be related to, or be a form of, bipolar mood disorder.

- There is an association of borderline personality disorder with childhood sexual abuse, post-traumatic stress disorder and bulimia nervosa. However, these associations are neither as strong nor as specific as sometimes claimed.

## Dissocial (psychopathic, antisocial) disorder

Historically, *psychopathic disorder* (as it is still called in legal circles) has had its own status within the Mental Health Act (Chapter 7). In practice, most general psychiatrists rarely treat people with dissocial personality disorder (with or without consent) as no interventions have been shown to be effective. Admission is usually avoided, as it is often disruptive for other patients. The main goal is to exclude other diagnoses that may be more treatable. Forensic psychiatrists, on the other hand, spend much of their time assessing and managing the disorder.

- The Mental Health Act is used to send some people with dissocial personality disorder who have committed serious crimes to secure psychiatric hospitals rather than to prison. This is controversial, affected by societal and financial influences rather than by evidence of effectiveness. In hospital, prolonged psychotherapy or antipsychotic drugs may be tried.
- The problems of dissocial personality disorder are often worsened by drugs and alcohol.
- The whole range of genetic, developmental, psychological and social factors are thought to be involved in the origins of dissocial personality disorder. A few people have temporal lobe EEG abnormalities. *Minimal brain dysfunction* refers to the view that the disorder results from minor brain injury or delayed maturation.
- As with borderline personality disorder, the core neuropsychological deficits are thought to involve impulsivity and decision making, and relate to abnormalities in the regulation of frontal lobe activity by dopamine and 5-HT.

## Cluster C personality disorder ('anxious')

This cluster rarely presents clinically, and there is little information about how to manage it. If it does, set realistic goals for treatment, try and enhance self-esteem and avoid escalating contact which simply fosters dependency.

- The diagnosis is usually made in someone who presents with a depressive disorder or anxiety disorder. Cluster C personality disorder is a risk factor for both.

## Personality disorder and psychiatric disorder

The interaction between personality (disorder) and psychiatric disorder is important and manifold (Figure 15.1):

- Personality disorder can *predispose to* psychiatric disorder.
- Personality disorder can *coexist with* psychiatric disorder (a type of comorbidity). This worsens prognosis. For example, comorbidity of schizophrenia and personality disorder increases the risk of violence; the comorbidity of depression and personality disorder increases suicide risk. Additional comorbidity with substance misuse further elevates such risks.
- Personality disorder, in reality, *merges into* psychiatric disorder, as illustrated by the reclassification of cyclothymia from a personality disorder to a form of bipolar disorder.

- Personality disorder can be *mistaken for* psychiatric disorder, and vice versa. For example, someone with a depressive disorder may give the impression that they have a personality disorder; a person with borderline personality disorder may be misdiagnosed as having a psychotic disorder.
- Personality can be *affected by* psychiatric disorder. For example, the deterioration in personality in chronic schizophrenia.
- Personality can have a *pathoplastic* effect on psychiatric disorder—that is, it can modify the clinical features even if it has no direct causal role.

## Multiaxial classification

These interactions have led to a *multiaxial* classification system in which psychiatric disorder and personality disorder are coded separately. Other axes record additional information (Table 15.3).

**Table 15.3** Multiaxial classification.

| | |
|---|---|
| Axis I | Psychiatric disorder |
| Axis II | Personality disorder and mental retardation |
| Axis III | General medical conditions |
| Axis IV | Psychosocial and environmental problems |
| Axis V | Global assessment of functioning (rated on a 1–100 scale) |

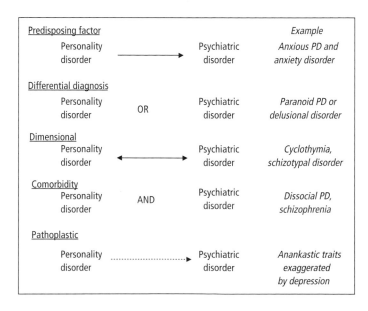

**Figure 15.1** Relationships between personality and psychiatric disorders.

- Multiaxial classification is part of DSM-IV. In the UK it is used mainly in child psychiatry (Chapter 16).

> *A 55-year-old man has lived alone all his life, usually in hostels. He has developed delusions of persecution. He has few interests, is barely literate and has never held down a job. His mobility is limited. He improves moderately with treatment.*
>
> *Axis I: delusional disorder.*
> *Axis II: schizoid personality disorder; mild mental retardation.*
> *Axis III: osteoarthritis.*
> *Axis IV: homelessness, illiteracy.*
> *Axis V: global assessment 25 (on admission), 45 (on discharge).*

## Problems with the concept of personality disorder

The concept of personality disorder has been controversial. Arguments include:

- It isn't a 'disease'. It medicalizes individual differences and implies they can and should be treated by doctors.
- Its diagnosis is unreliable.
- One man's personality disorder is another man's virtue. Many famous people meet the criteria for personality disorder, yet the traits are either tolerated because of, or are actually the basis of, their success.
- The term is pejorative: the label is applied to patients that doctors don't like or find hard to manage, or is used as a justification to avoid trying to help.
- There is no clear distinction to be made between personality disorders and psychiatric disorders.

Some of these arguments raise issues that go well beyond the boundaries of psychiatry. Given the current state of knowledge, psychiatrists must at least ensure that they use the term 'personality disorder' as reliably and usefully as possible.

## Dangerous and severe personality disorder (DPSD)

A particular current controversy in the UK is *dangerous and severe personality disorder (DPSD)*, a concept introduced by the UK government in 1999, largely in response to a high-profile homicide.

- DPSD is not a clinical category. The working definition is: an individual who presents a significant risk of harm to others, with the risk linked to a significant disorder of personality. In reality, it mostly comprises a subgroup of people with dissocial (psychopathic) disorder who are at high risk of violent offending.
- The purpose was to allow such people to be detained—possibly indefinitely. Specific DPSD units have now been set up within prisons. Admission is based on high scores on rating scales for psychopathy, and on a diagnosis of two personality disorders. A range of treatments are offered, and are being evaluated, within the units.

---

### Key points

- Personality is the combination of persistent and relatively stable emotional, cognitive and behavioural traits which characterize each of us. A personality is deemed disordered if these traits are excessive or deficient, and cause problems for the individual or for those around him.
- Personality disorders are classified pragmatically into three clusters: eccentric, dramatic and anxious. Important specific types are paranoid, dissocial (psychopathic) and borderline.
- Always be wary of diagnosing personality disorder solely on the basis of behaviour during an episode of psychiatric illness. Illness can affect how personality is expressed.
- Personality disorder interacts with psychiatric disorder in several ways: as a predisposing factor, a pathoplastic factor, a prognostic factor, a comorbid disorder and as a differential diagnosis.
- Focus treatment on helping the person modify their circumstances, removing exacerbating factors and reinforcing positive behaviours. Medication has a very limited role. Specific psychotherapies may help borderline personality disorder.

# Chapter 16

# Childhood disorders

## Principles of child psychiatry

### Interviewing children

When interviewing a child, the objectives are the same as with adults: to establish rapport, make a diagnosis, understand its context and plan treatment. However, for several reasons, the nature of the interview differs, especially with young children:

- The child may not understand the question or be unable to express himself.
- The range of disorders being sought, and hence the diagnostic focus, is different.
- Parents determine when and how the child presents.
- Family factors contribute to many disorders—so more attention is paid to the family environment.

Child psychiatry interviews have several features:

- Parents are present and are often interviewed alone first.
- The interviewer must be able to jump from one topic to another as led by the child.
- Assessment may start with play and gentle conversation to gain trust.

*Lecture Notes: Psychiatry*, 10e. By Paul Harrison, John Geddes and Michael Sharpe. Published 2010 by Blackwell Publishing Ltd.

- Much information comes from the child's appearance and behaviour.
- Significant others (e.g. teachers, siblings) provide key parts of the history.
- More than one session may be needed to complete the interview.

By adopting these strategies, the interviewer aims to collect information about the topics in Table 16.1.

In addition a paediatric history and neurological examination may be indicated. To complete the assessment, background information is sought from relevant sources, such as teachers or social services.

- Get parental consent at each stage, unless abuse is suspected, in which case the duty of care to the child may over-ride this principle.

### Classification

The major childhood psychiatric disorders are shown in Table 16.2. A *multiaxial* scheme is often used to record the diagnostic information because of the importance of developmental stage, overall abilities and social circumstances:

- Axis I: psychiatric disorder(s) present.
- Axis II: developmental stage and delays.
- Axis III: intellectual level.
- Axis IV: medical problems.
- Axis V: abnormal social situations.

Learning disability in children is covered in Chapter 17.

**Table 16.1** Topics for the child psychiatric interview.

| |
|---|
| *Presenting problem*<br>　Onset, duration, factors affecting it<br>　Associated problems and symptoms<br>　Recent life events<br>　Parents' and child's explanation for it<br><br>*Developmental milestones*<br>　Motor, e.g. sitting, walking<br>　Social, e.g. smiling<br>　Emotional, e.g. attachment behaviour<br>　Cognitive, e.g. talking, reading<br>　Other, e.g. toilet training<br><br>*Emotional profile*<br>　Temperament<br>　Problem behaviours<br>　Likes and dislikes<br><br>*Family*<br>　Relationship with parents and siblings<br>　Problems at home<br>　Separations from parents<br>　Parental and sibling health and personalities<br><br>*Schooling*<br>　Educational record<br>　Attendance<br>　Relationship with peers<br><br>*General health*<br>　Hospital admissions<br>　Previous psychiatric history<br>　Sleep pattern and problems<br><br>*Observation of child*<br>　General appearance<br>　Interactions with interviewer and family members<br>　Attention and concentration<br>　Prevailing mood and range of emotions expressed<br>　Language and motor skills |

**Table 16.2** Classification of childhood psychiatric disorders.

| |
|---|
| *Emotional disorders (neuroses)*<br>　Anxiety disorders<br>　Somatoform disorder<br><br>*Behavioural disorders*<br>　Conduct disorder<br>　Attention deficit hyperactivity disorder (ADHD)<br><br>*Depressive disorder*<br><br>*Developmental disorders*<br>　Autism and other pervasive developmental disorders<br>　Specific (e.g. specific reading disorder)<br><br>*Miscellaneous conditions*<br>　Enuresis<br>　Encopresis<br>　Selective mutism<br>　Tics |

## Epidemiology

Transient symptoms and behavioural disturbances are common in children of all ages. As in adults, making a psychiatric diagnosis requires a persistence and pervasiveness of symptoms, and evidence of dysfunction. The major epidemiological features of childhood psychiatric disorder are:

- Prevalence at age 10 is 7% in rural areas and 13% in urban areas. At age 14 the prevalence is higher.

(These numbers come from a classic, though dated, UK study.)
- Boys are affected twice as often as girls for most diagnoses.
- The most common diagnoses are emotional disorders and conduct disorders.
- Disorders are more common in children with learning disability, epilepsy and chronic physical illnesses.

## Aetiology

The same broad range of aetiological factors operate in childhood as in adulthood (Table 16.3).
- There is a genetic component to most disorders, mediated partly through its influence on temperament and intelligence.
- The major environmental factors are the family and social circumstances.
- Genes and environment are not independent factors, but interact to determine risk.

## Management

Management of children with psychiatric disorders is based upon several principles:

**Table 16.3** Causative factors in child psychiatry.

| Factor | Examples |
|---|---|
| *Genetic* | Autism |
| *Environmental* | |
| Family factors | |
|     Parenting styles | Harsh, critical style associated with conduct disorder |
|     Parental conflict | Increased risk of emotional or conduct disorder |
|     Parental psychiatric disorder | Increased risk of eating disorder |
| Social factors | |
|     Deprivation | Increased risk of conduct disorder |
|     Bullying | School refusal |
| Other factors | |
|     Prematurity | Increased risk of developmental delay and behavioural disorders |
|     Medical disorder | Epilepsy increases risk of most disorders |
|     Physical abuse | Increased risk of emotional and behavioural disorders |

**Table 16.4** Prognosis of psychiatric disorders in childhood.

| Category | Long-term outcome |
|---|---|
| Emotional disorders | Good, two-thirds resolve in a 4-year period |
| Mood disorder | Poor, half have depressive disorder in adulthood |
| Behavioural disorders | |
|     Conduct disorder | Poor, often leads on to personality disorder or substance misuse |
|     ADHD | Variable |
| Developmental disorders | |
|     Autism | Poor, lifelong |
| Other conditions | |
|     Enuresis | Good |
|     Tics | Usually transient (unless Tourette syndrome) |
|     Selective mutism | Uncertain, may have persistent communication problems |

- Take the child's developmental stage and overall level of functioning into account.
- Most problems are treated initially with advice, support and behavioural interventions.
- Involve the family.
- Avoid removal from school or home wherever possible.
- Medication has little or no role in most disorders.
- Further details are discussed in the sections describing the specific disorders.
- Psychodynamic approaches continue to play a greater role in child psychiatry than in adult psychiatry.

- The organization of child psychiatric services, through which treatments are delivered, was mentioned in Chapter 8.

## Prognosis

Childhood psychiatric disorders have a variable outcome, in part because of the influence of the child's ongoing development and experiences. The basic pattern is summarized in Table 16.4.

### Emotional disorders (neuroses)

Neuroses (emotional disorders) were described in Chapter 10. In children, the disorders are in many ways similar but there are important differences too:

- 'Emotional disorder', not neurosis, is the usual term.
- Some subtypes are different (e.g. separation anxiety).
- Medication is rarely if ever used.
- Equal male to female ratio (cf. 1 : 2 in adults).
- Most affected children do not become affected adults.

## Anxiety disorders

Crying when mummy goes out, or becoming fearful of spiders, are anxieties which children normally experience at particular developmental stages, especially at times of stress and transition. They must be distinguished from persistent, significant symptoms warranting a diagnosis of anxiety disorder. The latter affect 5% of children at some time. As in adults, anxiety manifests with behavioural, psychological and physical symptoms (Table 16.5).

### Separation anxiety

Among 5–11 year olds, 3–4% have excessive anxiety when faced with separation from parents or others they are attached to. The child clings— literally or metaphorically—to the person and tries to avoid being separated from them. Sleep disturbance and nightmares occur. Older children may

describe being fearful that the person will be harmed and will not return. Separation anxiety often begins at times of stress, such as after the death of the family dog. Some parents are noted to be overprotective. Management includes:

- Working with the family to explain and reassure.
- Identification and resolution of stressors.
- Ensuring the parents are not reinforcing the problem (e.g. by appearing anxious when about to leave the child).
- Use of specific interventions for secondary problems that develop, such as school refusal.

## Somatoform disorder

Children readily develop somatic symptoms, especially when stressed. Non-specific abdominal pain and headaches are the most common and may lead to a paediatric referral. As in adults, *somatoform disorder* describes bodily symptoms that are unexplained by a medical condition. The assessment of these requires:

- Exclusion of a medical disorder that fully explains the symptoms.
- Exclusion of emotional or depressive disorder.
- Identification of likely precipitating and perpetuating factors. For example, the child may be unhappy at home, is worried about a sick sibling or is using the symptoms to gain attention.

Management is aimed at avoiding reinforcing the symptoms (e.g. by teaching the parents how not to do this inadvertently) and at tackling the underlying stresses. The prognosis is variable. Some children proceed to somatoform disorder as adults.

## Other emotional disorders

*Obsessive–compulsive disorder* in children is rare clinically, but has a prevalence of 1 in 400 in British 5–15 year olds. It is sometimes associated with *Tourette syndrome* (see below). It may sometimes occur as an autoimmune reaction to a streptococcal infection, though this remains uncertain.

- OCD is the only childhood emotional disorder with good evidence that antidepressants (clomi-

**Table 16.5** Symptoms of anxiety in children.

*Behavioural*
  Clinging to parent (or other carer)
  Unwilling to leave house
  Unwilling to go to bed
  Actions designed to avoid feared event (e.g. hiding)

*Psychological*
  Feeling worried
  Nightmares

*Physical*
  Abdominal pain
  Headaches

**Table 16.6** Assessment of suspected school refusal.

*Why is the child absent from school?*
School refusal
Truancy
Parents keeping child at home
Physical illness

*What does the school refusal reflect?*
Reluctance to leave home (i.e. secondary to separation anxiety)
A specific 'school phobia' (e.g. of getting there, or being bullied)
A more generalized disorder (e.g. social phobia, depressive disorder)

*What other factors are relevant?*
Recent life events (e.g. bereavement)
Recent events at school (e.g. change of class)
Parental characteristics (e.g. overprotective)

**Table 16.7** Distinguishing school refusal from truancy.

| School refusal | Truancy |
|---|---|
| Younger (<11 years old) | Older (>11 years old) |
| Underlying emotional disorder | Underlying conduct disorder |
| Good school record | Poor school record |
| Good prognosis | Poor prognosis |
| Parents overprotective | Broken home |

pramine, fluoxetine) and psychological (cognitive behavioural) therapy are effective, and for which antidepressants are still widely used. Nevertheless, the prognosis in severe cases is quite poor.

Children also suffer from the other emotional disorders seen in adults (Chapter 10). For example, they can get *specific phobias* or develop emotional disorders following particular stresses (*adjustment reactions*).

• *Chronic fatigue syndrome* is also now well recognized in children. As in adults, its aetiology and management remain controversial. Pending better evidence, treatment is based on the same principles of graded return to activities and cognitive behavioural methods, with the close involvement of the family.

## School refusal

School refusal is not a psychiatric disorder, but it is a common cause of referral to a child psychiatrist and is frequently attributable to an emotional disorder. Its assessment is summarized in Table 16.6.

• Exclude truancy and parental behaviour as causes for the absence from school. The characteristics of school refusal and truancy are different (Table 16.7).

School refusal is usually due to separation anxiety, often provoked by recent events at home or at school. In older children, school refusal may reflect bullying; it can also herald a more pervasive problem such as social phobia or depressive disorder.

Management of school refusal is aimed at a rapid return to school before avoidance is too ingrained. Sometimes a graded re-exposure is needed. Address any specific fears or stresses, and treat any associated psychiatric disorder.

The prognosis in younger children is good. In older children, the problem may become prolonged and other psychiatric problems emerge. It may recur at times of transition (e.g. moving schools). There is a slightly increased risk of anxiety disorder in adulthood.

## Mood disorders

The existence of mood disorders in pre-pubertal children used to be disputed. It is now clear that they occur, even in young children.

• Prevalence estimates are variable. They increase dramatically after puberty, when the higher rate in females first appears.

• The occurrence of bipolar mood disorder pre-pubertally is more controversial, but gaining acceptance (especially in the USA, where some argue it may be related to the widespread use of stimulants for ADHD).

When evaluating mood and mood disorder in a child, apply the same principles as in adults:

• Symptoms should be present for at least 2 weeks and associated with distress and dysfunction.

- If there are also symptoms of an emotional disorder, attempt to distinguish the primary diagnosis.
- Children, especially adolescents, may present in crisis or after self-harm, with isolated or transient depressive symptoms, which (as in adults) are better viewed as an adjustment reaction than as a depressive episode.
- Childhood depressive disorders are classified using the adult system (Chapter 9).
- As in adults, depression in post-pubertal children carries an increased suicide risk. In severe cases, psychotic symptoms may occur.
- The main difference from adults concerns young children, who may not experience depression in the same way or be unable to articulate their feelings. Much diagnostic attention must therefore be placed on their appearance and behaviour both in the interview and elsewhere (e.g. school work, activities, sleep pattern).

The aetiology of childhood depressive disorder involves the same mixture of genes, life events and unknown influences as prevail in adult cases.

Management includes support, monitoring and reducing stressors. Neither antidepressants nor psychological treatments have been shown unequivocally to be effective.

- Despite the lack of evidence, SSRIs have been widely prescribed to children and adolescents, but their use is now very restricted because of concern that they may increase suicide risk. Only fluoxetine is currently allowed (in the UK) for use in under 18s.
- Admission may be needed for severe or psychotic depression. ECT is very occasionally used.

The prognosis of childhood depressive disorder is often poor. The condition may become chronic, and half go on to suffer from depressive disorder in adulthood.

## Behavioural disorders

Behavioural disorders are diagnosed in children who have persistent problematic and antisocial behaviour. The main distinction is between behavioural problems that result mainly from overactivity (ADHD) and those that do not (conduct disorder)—though in practice the boundary is blurred.

- Neither label should be applied unless the diagnostic criteria are met—all children are naughty and 'hyper' from time to time.

## Conduct disorder

Conduct disorder is the most common psychiatric disorder of childhood and adolescence. Prevalence estimates range from 1% to 15%. It occurs mainly in boys (sex ratio 5:1). Conduct is disturbed and antisocial well beyond the range of misbehaviour normally observed for that age group (Table 16.8). Diagnosis is usually made after age 7, though problems have often been apparent much earlier. The term *oppositional defiant disorder* may be used for these younger children.

- A distinction is sometimes made between *socialized conduct disorder*, where the activities occur within a peer group, and *unsocialized conduct disorder*, where the child acts in isolation.

In adolescence, conduct disorder has a strong relationship with juvenile delinquency and substance misuse. There is often repeated police contact and convictions for theft, criminal damage or assault. Conduct disorder is associated with a variety of indices of social deprivation and poor

**Table 16.8** Clinical features of conduct disorder.

| |
|---|
| *In pre-school children* |
|     Aggressive behaviour |
|     Poor concentration |
| *In mid-childhood* |
|     Lying |
|     Stealing |
|     Disruptive and oppositional behaviour |
|     Bullying |
| *In adolescence* |
|     Stealing |
|     Truancy |
|     Promiscuity |
|     Substance misuse |
|     Vandalism |
|     Reckless behaviour |

parenting (Table 16.9). Any genetic contribution is small.

The long-term prognosis is poor; 50% of cases progress to dissocial personality disorder, and persistent substance misuse and criminality are common. Those who form stable relationships have a better outcome. There is no standard therapeutic approach, and a mixture of attempts to shape and reward behaviour are used, with varying degrees of evidence:

- Family-focused treatments seek to identify and remedy causes for the behaviour, improve the home environment, and includes teaching parents how to cope with the behaviour and reduce conflict ('parental training'). There is evidence that this is effective for younger children with comorbid ADHD.
- Praise and rewards for positive behaviour.
- Setting out clear rules and commands, with consistent and calm responses to unwanted behaviour.
- Anger management.
- 'Problem-solving skills training' is a recent approach that focuses on the child rather than the parents. It is based on evidence that children with ADHD are poor at problem solving and interpersonal skills.
- Alternative outlets for energies and behaviours (e.g. youth clubs, car workshops).
- Tackle associated problems such as truancy and substance misuse.

**Table 16.9** Factors associated with conduct disorder.

| |
|---|
| *Family factors* |
| Parental personality disorder |
| Paternal alcoholism |
| Parental disputes and violence |
| Harsh, inconsistent parenting |
| Being in care early in life |
| Large family size |
| |
| *Social factors* |
| Inner cities |
| Deprivation and overcrowding |
| |
| *Individual factors* |
| Brain damage |
| Epilepsy |
| Specific reading disorder |

- Stimulant medication is increasingly being used, especially if there are coexistent ADHD features.
- Residential care is occasionally unavoidable.

## Attention deficit hyperactivity disorder (ADHD)

The clinical features are shown in Table 16.10. As with conduct disorder, the diagnosis requires that the problem is both persistent and extreme. In Britain, the prevalence is 2%; three-quarters are boys. In the USA, where less stringent criteria are used, prevalence and treatment rates are correspondingly higher.

- *Hyperkinetic disorder* is sometimes used interchangeably with ADHD. Strictly, it refers to a severe subgroup of ADHD in which all three core signs (inattention, hyperactivity and impulsiveness) are present, pervasive and with onset before age 7.
- ADHD is often comorbid with conduct disorder, anxiety, depression and tic disorders. ADHD symptoms may also be seen in pervasive developmental disorders.

**Table 16.10** Features of attention deficit hyperactivity disorder (ADHD).

| |
|---|
| *Core features* |
| Hyperactivity |
| Poor attention and concentration |
| Impulsivity |
| Present for at least 6 months |
| Evidence for impaired functioning in two or more settings |
| Onset by age 9, usually by 5 |
| |
| *Other features* |
| Distractibility |
| Poor at planning and organizing tasks |
| Learning difficulties |
| Clumsiness |
| Low self-esteem |
| Socially disinhibited |
| Unpopular with other children |
| Non-localizing neurological signs |
| Conduct disorder coexists in 50% |

The aetiology of ADHD is multifactorial:

- There is a significant genetic contribution (heritability ~70%), including genes affecting dopamine and serotonin functioning in the brain. Families also show increased rates of depressive disorder, learning difficulties, alcoholism and dissocial personality disorder.
- A neurodevelopmental abnormality is suspected, on the basis of the soft neurological signs and learning difficulties, and from brain imaging and EEG findings.
- There is an association with social deprivation, though less striking than for conduct disorder.
- Other risk factors include maternal smoking and alcohol intake.
- Many parents blame food allergy, but this is rarely substantiated when investigated properly.

The management of ADHD involves:

- Support and psychoeducation for the child and family.
- Specific educational approaches, including attention to associated learning difficulties.
- Firm adherence to behavioural principles (to reward good behaviour and discourage hyperactive behaviour).
- Psychostimulants (e.g. methylphenidate, atomoxetine) have an important role and are recommended in UK guidelines as part of a comprehensive treatment programme. This seemingly paradoxical treatment originated from the (incorrect) belief that there is a failure of cortical arousal in ADHD. Their main neurochemical effect is to increase dopamine in the synapse. Side-effects are insomnia, poor appetite and headaches. Concerns about addiction and growth retardation have not been noted in practice.
- Modafinil is an attention-enhancing drug also used in ADHD. Its mechanism is unknown.
- Dietary restriction (e.g. of food additives or colourings) is not generally recommended.

ADHD has a variable prognosis. Gradual improvement occurs in adolescence, and a third of cases resolve. The rest have residual hyperkinetic features, especially in those with learning difficulties or conduct disorder. Dissocial personality disorder and substance misuse commonly develop. It is unclear how long treatment should continue into adulthood,

- There is increasing interest in adult-onset ADHD, but no consensus on its diagnostic status or management.

## Developmental disorders

Developmental disorders can be *pervasive* or *specific*. The former, typified by *autism*, affect many aspects of psychological and neurobiological development; in the latter, there is impairment in only one domain (e.g. reading) relative to overall development. These seemingly diverse conditions are grouped together for three reasons:

- The child is seemingly normal until late infancy or early childhood, at which point progress stops or reverses.
- The abnormality is thought to be directly related to aberrant brain development.
- Their course lacks the fluctuations of most psychiatric disorders.

### Pervasive developmental disorders

Current classification divides this category into several distinct disorders, as outlined here. However, the concept of *autistic spectrum disorders* is increasingly being used, recognizing that all share core impairments in social interactions, language and communication, and the child's range of interests and activities.

### Autism

Autism is a syndrome characterized by a failure to develop normal communication, especially social and emotional communication. Autistic children have a delayed, restricted and deviant use of language. They seem oblivious to non-verbal cues and emotional expressions, with little desire to interact with others or form relationships. Instead, they demonstrate a limited range of solitary, repetitive behaviours and resist attempts to change their routine. Most also have a degree of learning disability. The features are summarized in Table 16.11.

**Table 16.11** Features of autism.

| |
|---|
| 1 in 1000 children—though estimates vary several-fold |
| 80% are boys |
| Age of onset <3 years |
| |
| *Core features (the 'autistic triad')* |
|   No emotional warmth (autistic aloneness) |
|   Impaired language and communication |
|   Solitary, repetitive behaviours |
| |
| *Associated and comorbid features* |
|   Learning disability in 75% |
|   Epilepsy in ~25% |
|   Mannerisms and rituals |
|   Hyperactivity |
|   Anxiety and OCD-like symptoms |
|   Sleep disturbance |
|   Hypotonia |

• A very few autistic children (and adults), called *idiot savants*, have remarkable abilities in discrete areas, such as complex mental arithmetic (as in the film *Rain Man*).

The diagnosis is made based on a careful history and observations. Various checklists and structured interviews are also used.

• The differential diagnosis of 'true' autism comprises other disorders with autistic features such as Asperger's and Rett's syndromes (see below), and fragile X syndrome and tuberous sclerosis complex (Chapter 17). These other disorders account for only about 10% of autism.

• Remember other causes of a failure to develop communication which may be mistaken for autism, such as specific language disorder and deafness.

The aetiology of autism is strongly genetic.

• Many known or suspected autism susceptibility genes exist, including neuroligins 3 and 4, and other genes that probably converge upon synaptic development. There may also be microscopic structural abnormalities of the chromosomes, called *copy number variation* (CNV). The genetic basis of autism overlaps with that of schizophrenia.

• No confirmed environmental risk factors are known. Despite public concern, there is now good

evidence that vaccines do not cause autism. Neither do mercury amalgam fillings.

• Similarly, there has not been a genuine rise in prevalence of autism, merely greater awareness and/or a loosening of the diagnostic category.

• MRI scans show increased brain size early in life, suggestive of an aberrant growth trajectory. Neuropathological studies suggest cellular alterations in several brain areas, notably Purkinje cells in the cerebellum, also the brainstem and hippocampus. Neurochemically, excess 5-HT (serotonin) function affecting neurodevelopment has been postulated.

• Psychologically, the main hypothesis is a failure to develop a '*theory of mind*'—that is, the ability to attribute mental states and beliefs to others. This is thought to underlie their behaviour and lack of social engagement.

The prognosis is poor. Speech eventually develops in some, but communication remains limited and the core abnormalities rarely improve. Seizures can occur later in childhood. Most autistic children need special schooling and residential care, and only a minority are ever able to live independently.

There is no specific, evidence-based treatment for autism. The main components of management are:

• Make the diagnosis, and support the family in understanding autism and its implications.

• Consider interventions that are aimed to improve socialization, communication and behaviour. Families also often seek out a variety of complementary therapies.

• Provide appropriate education and, if required, accommodation.

• Deal with associated medical problems (e.g. epilepsy).

• Medication is sometimes used, despite very limited evidence. For example, SSRIs for repetitive behaviours, or atypical antipsychotics for irritability.

## Asperger's syndrome

Asperger's syndrome (also called *autistic psychopathy*) is like a milder version of autism, with similar abnormalities in social communication and repetitive, isolated behaviours. The child, virtually always a boy, is solitary, clumsy and eccentric. Unlike autism, intelligence and language are unremarkable, and seizures are not a feature. The prevalence is uncertain, with estimates from 1 to 50 per 10 000.

- The aetiology is unknown. It may or may not be causally related to autism.
- Asperger's syndrome persists into adulthood, and sometimes first presents at that time, when it may be mistaken for schizotypal or schizoid personality disorder, or schizophrenia.

## Rett's syndrome

Rett's syndrome is a rare, progressive and severe disorder occurring almost exclusively in girls. The main features are autism, learning disability, seizures, loss of speech and movements, and irregular breathing. It is usually caused by sporadic mutations in the MeCP2 gene on the X chromosome, and is fatal by early adulthood.

## Specific developmental disorders

Specific developmental disorders are conditions in which there is marked delay in one area of development relative to the child's overall IQ. The most common problem is with reading (80% of cases), but also disorders selectively affecting arithmetic, language or motor skills. Though the disorders are not really 'psychiatric', they are often referred to (or detected by) child psychiatric services because of associated emotional or behavioural difficulties.

- Specific speech and language disorder is related to the FOXP2 gene.

## Specific reading disorder

In specific reading disorder, reading skills are significantly (>2 standard deviations) below that predicted by the child's overall performance. Visual impairment or lack of education must be excluded as the cause. It affects 2–10% of 10 year olds, and is four times more common in boys than in girls.

- It is associated with conduct disorder in a third of cases, also with ADHD, low social class and a disturbed family background. The direction of causality between these factors is unclear.
- Assessment should be by an educational psychologist using standardized tests.
- Management involves enhancing self-esteem and appropriate expert educational help.
- Nutritional supplements (fish oils) are being advocated by some researchers and families.
- Prognosis is poor, with reading abilities often remaining well below average.

## Other conditions

### Enuresis

Enuresis is urinary incontinence after the age at which bladder control is expected (*primary enuresis*; must be at least 5 years old) or after previous normal continence (*secondary enuresis*). It usually presents as bedwetting in the first half of the night (*nocturnal enuresis*). It affects 15% of 5 year olds, 2% of 10 year olds and 1% of 14 year olds. Boys outnumber girls 3:1.

- Enuresis can cause great distress, affect self-esteem, interfere with normal activities (e.g. sleepovers) and can lead to bullying or intolerant parenting.

In the assessment, exclude UTI, diabetes or neurological disorder. Enuresis may be a sign of sleep apnoea. Search for recent stressors and symptoms of emotional disorder (twice as common as expected in those with enuresis). There is often a history of enuresis in male relatives.

The management of enuresis includes:
- Reassurance, explanation and limiting fluid intake in the evening.
- Treatment of associated psychiatric or medical disorder.
- Behavioural methods are the main treatment. A *star chart* is best for younger children; they are rewarded for achieving a realistic target (which may not be a 'dry bed' initially) with stars or other suitable token. An *enuresis alarm* ('pad and buzzer') is a moisture-sensitive pad worn by the child. When urine is passed, a buzzer goes off which

wakes the child in time to go to the toilet to finish. He also participates in changing the sheets. An alarm is usually effective if persisted with for several weeks, especially in children over 7 years old.

• Pharmacological methods are sometimes used, though behavioural methods are preferred. Intranasal desmopressin is the usual first-line drug, with moderate success and few side-effects. The TCA imipramine is licensed for enuresis from the age of 6, but is of limited efficacy, potentially dangerous and not recommended. Relapse is common with both methods.

The prognosis is good, though a few boys remain enuretic into adulthood.

## Encopresis

Encopresis is the passing of faeces in an inappropriate place after age 4. As with enuresis it can be primary or secondary. Children may soil their pants, pass faeces in hidden places or occasionally smear them. At assessment, exclude physical problems (e.g. constipation, Hirschsprung's disease) and learning disability.

• There is often a history of inadequate or harsh toilet training combined with recent stresses and emotional disorder in the child.

Management is by reassurance, help with associated problems and ensuring that the parents do not become punitive. The standard behavioural manoeuvre is to toilet the child after each meal, and to reward him for staying there, for producing a motion and for not soiling. Most encopresis resolves with treatment within a year. Occasionally it persists into adolescence.

## Tics

Tics are involuntary, rapid, spasmodic movements, usually repeated blinking and grimacing. They are common, especially in young boys, and may begin after an emotional upset. They are generally transient and need no specific treatment. However, some tics become severe, prolonged and incapacitating.

The main tic disorder is (*Gilles de la*) *Tourette syndrome*, in which tics are accompanied by vocal grunts and sometimes by stereotyped phrases, movements or expletives (*coprolalia*). Obsessive–compulsive and ADHD symptoms often occur. Boys are affected more than girls (3 : 1). The incidence is usually considered to be around 1 in 2000, but much higher figures exist.

Mild cases need no treatment. Troublesome tics are controlled by low-dose antipsychotics. Obsessional and hyperactivity symptoms can be treated as appropriate. Though the tics tend to diminish in adulthood, some symptoms persist.

• Tourette syndrome has a genetic basis, which overlaps with that of OCD. Autoimmune processes may also contribute. Abnormalities in basal ganglia pathways and the dopamine system are implicated.

## Selective mutism

In selective (also called *elective*) mutism, children refuse to speak although able to do so. Speech is usually normal in one setting (e.g. at home) but absent elsewhere. Non-verbal communication is preserved. Onset is from 4 to 8 years old. Affected children tend to be shy, anxious and isolated in most settings, but aggressive and disturbed at home. The disorder is rare, and unusual in being more common in girls than boys. It is said to be associated with overprotective parents and depressed mothers.

• Selective mutism is increasingly being viewed as an anxiety disorder.

• There is no specific treatment; a range of behavioural interventions may be tried.

• Selective mutism can persist for several years, and residual social anxiety and communication problems are common.

## Sleep disorders

Children, like adults, can suffer from sleep problems secondary to psychiatric disorders, and from sleep disorders. The sleep disturbance can impair the child's behaviour and development, and affect the whole family. A sleep history is part of the assessment (Table 16.1).

- Childhood sleep problems are particularly common in those with learning disability (Chapter 17).

## Psychoses in childhood and adolescence

*Schizophrenia* may begin in adolescence, and occasionally in younger children. *Bipolar disorder* can also start in adolescence.

- The disorders are treated in a similar fashion to adult-onset cases, and are one of the few clear indications for medication in child psychiatry. The prognosis of childhood-onset psychosis is poor.

## Special groups

### Toddlers

Toddlers are notorious for *temper tantrums*. Reassurance that this normal, and simple advice on setting limits, are usually all that is needed. Consistency in the parents' response to the behaviour is crucial. Self-help books are available.

*Sleep disturbances* are common, either refusal to settle or night-time waking due to *night terrors* and *nightmares*. Use reassurance and a consistent bedtime routine. Psychiatric referral is rare, though occasionally the disturbances herald an emotional or behavioural disorder.

### Teenagers

Contrary to the stereotype, neither emotional turmoil nor delinquency is normal for teenagers. Persistently withdrawn, disruptive or bizarre behaviour should be assessed to exclude psychiatric disorder. Diagnostically, adolescents get the tail end of childhood disorders and the early onset of adult disorders (Table 16.12), so the clinician must know about both, and the continuities between them. This has led to *adolescent psychiatry* as a subspecialty.

**Table 16.12** Important psychiatric disorders of adolescence.

| |
|---|
| Conduct disorder |
| Eating disorder |
| Substance misuse disorders |
| Depressive disorder |
| Anxiety disorder |
| Schizophrenia |
| Bipolar disorder |
| Deliberate self-harm |

## Children in institutions

Children in care, especially in children's homes, have increased rates of psychiatric disorder, notably conduct disorder, substance misuse and self-harm. This may be both a cause and a consequence of being in care.

- Teenagers in detention facilities have extremely high rates of psychiatric disorder, with conduct disorder, substance misuse and self-harm again prominent.

## Children with physical illness

Children with any chronic illness are at increased risk of psychiatric disorder. This is especially true for organic brain syndromes and epilepsy. The associations may partly reflect a common aetiology, but also the effects of physical illness on the child's intellectual, psychological and social development.

- Close cooperation between those involved in the psychiatric and medical disorders is essential.

## Children with psychiatrically ill parents

If a parent has a psychiatric disorder, the child is at risk of psychiatric problems via an increased likelihood of inadequate or abnormal parenting, as well as from inheritance of a genetic predisposition. Hence the mental health (and personality) of parents is part of the child psychiatric assessment (Table 16.1). Specific parental problems associated with particular outcomes in the child include:

- Maternal substance misuse affects foetal development.
- Paternal alcoholism and development of conduct disorder.
- Maternal depression impairs infant bonding.
- Maternal eating disorder and abnormal feeding of the child.
- Factitious illness by proxy (sometimes called *Munchausen syndrome by proxy* or *Meadows' syndrome*)—the parent fabricates symptoms or signs in the child.

## Abused children

Children can be abused sexually, physically or emotionally. The abuse has psychiatric as well as medical and legal repercussions. Key points concerning the psychiatric aspects of child abuse are:
- Take specialist advice whenever abuse is suspected. This may be obtained from paediatricians, child psychiatrists and social services' child protection teams.
- Your responsibility is first and foremost to protect the child. This may over-ride the usual duty of confidentiality.
- Children who are being abused may show physical, psychological or behavioural signs.
- Managing abused children is difficult and needs multidisciplinary input. Child psychiatrists have particular roles in identifying and treating the psychological consequences of the abuse. It is unknown whether intervention alters the long-term prognosis.
- Physical abuse (non-accidental injury) causes significant morbidity and mortality. Either the child or the abuser may need to be removed from the home. Physical abuse leads to higher rates of emotional and behavioural disorder.
- Children who are emotionally abused or neglected have delayed psychological and physical development and increased rates of emotional disturbance. In extreme cases, they may present with failure to thrive (*deprivation dwarfism*).

The effects of child abuse may continue into adulthood:
- Women who were sexually abused have double the risk of psychiatric disorder and five times higher rates of psychiatric admission. Borderline personality disorder and possibly bulimia nervosa appear to be particularly common.
- There are no good data on the outcome of sexually abused boys, apart from their risk of becoming abusers and perpetuating the cycle.
- Emotional abuse may lead to persistent low self-esteem, relationship difficulties and personality disorder.

## Refugee children

Children who find themselves in a foreign country, with strange customs, a language they may not understand and often with major social deprivation and other stressors, are a vulnerable and neglected group. Their psychiatric needs are not well met by most services.

### Key points

- Conduct disorder and emotional disorder are the most common childhood psychiatric diagnoses. The former tends to do badly, the latter well.
- The principles of child psychiatry and psychiatric assessment are the same as in adults. However, more attention must be paid to the child's developmental history, and to the home and school environment.
- The risk of child psychiatric disorder is greater in urban areas, in boys, in those in care and in children with learning disability or chronic illness.
- Most disorders arise from an interaction between genetic and environmental factors.
- Treatment is usually behavioural and, given the degree of influence the parents have on a child's behaviour, must be aimed at the family as well as at the child.
- Medication is limited mainly to ADHD and psychosis. Antidepressants should not be used without a specialist opinion.

# Chapter 17

# Learning disability (mental retardation)

## Principles

### Definition and key features

*Mental retardation, mental handicap, developmental disability, intellectual disability* and *learning disability* are synonyms. *Mental retardation* is the official term in ICD-10 and DSM-IV. *Learning disability* is usually preferred, and is used here.

Learning disability is defined as:

- IQ below 70.
- Impairment across a wide range of functions.
- Onset before 18 years old.

The features of learning disability are shown in Table 17.1. It must be distinguished from:

- Lower than average intelligence but IQ >70.
- Specific developmental disorders (Chapter 16).
- Intellectual impairment secondary to an adult organic syndrome (Chapter 13).

The incidence of learning disability has declined because of medical advances (e.g. immunization) and termination of affected pregnancies. However, the prevalence has not changed because of improved survival.

Mild learning disability represents the tail end of the normal population distribution for intelligence and, as such, results from an interaction between multiple genetic and environmental factors. A specific cause is more often identifiable for severe cases.

### Clinical features

Learning disability can be *mild, moderate, severe* or *profound* depending on IQ (Table 17.2). Its cause, if known, is coded separately.

### Assessment of learning disability

The presence of learning disability may be suspected:

- Before birth—from antenatal tests or pregnancy complications.
- At birth—from the physical appearance.
- In infancy or childhood—as a result of developmental delay.

Assessment of a child with suspected learning disability encompasses:

- Making the diagnosis—establish its presence, severity and likely cause. This may involve paediatricians, paediatric neurologists and clinical geneticists.
- Evaluating the level of adaptive functioning.
- Evaluating comorbid psychiatric problems.

The areas of assessment are listed in Table 17.3. The procedures necessary depend on the child's age and the circumstances of the assessment. Compared with the standard psychiatric assess-

*Lecture Notes: Psychiatry*, 10e. By Paul Harrison, John Geddes and Michael Sharpe. Published 2010 by Blackwell Publishing Ltd.

ment there is a special emphasis on the obstetric and neurodevelopmental history and on the physical examination.

## Psychiatric aspects of learning disability

Children and adults with learning disability have high rates (~40%) of behavioural disturbance and psychiatric disorder. The risk of these problems is higher with coexistent epilepsy, and lower in Down's syndrome.

## Psychiatric disorder in learning-disabled children

All the main psychiatric disorders are more common in learning-disabled children. The assess-

**Table 17.1** Features of learning disability.

| |
|---|
| Mild, moderate, severe and profound forms |
| Prevalence is ~2%, with a male : female ratio of 3 : 2 |
| Usually untreatable |
| Often accompanied by: |
|    Psychiatric disorder |
|    Behavioural disturbance |
|    Medical problems (e.g. epilepsy) |
| Caused by: |
|    Chromosomal abnormalities |
|    Genetic mutations |
|    Environmental factors |
|    Most common specific causes are Down's syndrome and fragile X syndrome |

ment of these follows the principles of the child psychiatric assessment, but modified according to intellectual level (Table 17.4).

## Psychiatric disorder in learning-disabled adults

An adult with learning disability may require psychiatric assessment for a number of reasons:

- To assess the level of functioning and nature of current problems in order to help plan future management (e.g. placement).
- To investigate a suspected psychiatric disorder, such as schizophrenia and depression. These occur more commonly than in the general population. Their recognition may be difficult because of the learning disability. Various scales have been devised to help but sometimes the effect of a trial of medication may be needed.
- To assess and characterize a behavioural problem—called a *challenging behaviour*—such as shouting or inappropriate sexual activities, and to determine if it is secondary to a psychiatric diagnosis (e.g. depression).
- As part of a forensic or risk assessment. People with learning disability sometimes commit arson or other dangerous behaviours.
- To assess a decline in abilities. This may reflect the progressive nature of the condition or a superimposed disorder (e.g. depression). Also, dementia is more common than expected in learning disability (not just in Down's syndrome).

**Table 17.2** Comparison of mild, moderate, severe and profound learning disability.

| | Mild | Moderate | Severe/profound |
|---|---|---|---|
| IQ range | 69–50 | 49–35 | <35 (profound ≤20) |
| Percentage of cases | 85% | 10% | 5% |
| Ability to self-care | Independent | Need some help | Limited |
| Language | Reasonable | Limited | Basic or none |
| Reading and writing | Reasonable | Basic | Minimal or none |
| Ability to work | Semi-skilled | Unskilled, supervised | Supervised basic tasks |
| Social skills | Normal | Moderate | Few |
| Physical problems | Rare | Sometimes | Common |
| Aetiology discovered | Sometimes | Often | Usually |

**Table 17.3** Assessment of a child with learning disability.

| |
|---|
| *History* |
| Details of pregnancy |
|    Foetal growth |
|    Infections, trauma, eclampsia |
|    Alcohol or substance misuse |
|    Exposure to other drugs, toxins |
| Delivery |
|    Gestational age |
|    Complications |
|    Condition of baby |
| Child's development |
|    Milestones |
|    Physical difficulties |
| Family history |
|    Mental retardation |
|    Physical anomalies |
|    Consanguinity of parents |
| |
| *Examination* |
| General |
|    Overall health |
|    Weight, height, head circumference |
|    Physical anomalies |
|    Skin |
| Neurological |
|    Tone, posture, power, reflexes |
|    Cranial nerves |
|    Motor skills |
|    Comprehension and use of language |
| |
| *Neuropsychological testing* |
|    Intelligence quotient |
|    Language development |
| |
| *Laboratory investigations* |
|    Karyotyping and genetic testing |
|    Biochemical studies |
|    Brain imaging |
|    EEG |

**Table 17.4** Psychiatric assessment in learning disability.

| |
|---|
| *Background* |
|    Overall level of functioning |
|    Associated physical handicaps |
|    Cause of learning disability |
| |
| *Psychiatric history* |
|    Normal temperament and behaviours |
|    Recent changes in environment |
|    Recent changes in behaviour |
| |
| *Examination* |
|    Interactions |
|    Attention |
|    Perseverance |
|    Mood |
|    Presence and nature of emotional expression |
|    Features of autism |
| |
| *Investigations* |
|    Behavioural rating scales |
|    Autistic rating scales |

**Table 17.5** Diagnostic system for psychiatric disorders in adults with learning disabilities.

| |
|---|
| Axis I: severity of learning disability |
| Axis II: cause of learning disability |
| Axis III: psychiatric disorders |
|    Level A: developmental disorders |
|    Level B: psychiatric illness |
|    Level C: personality disorders |
|    Level D: problem behaviours |
|    Level E: other disorders |

Psychiatric diagnoses in adults with learning disability follow ICD-10 criteria, in a modified, multiaxial approach (Table 17.5).

## Management

Half of those with learning disability do not require any specific service provision, mostly because they are at the mild end of the spectrum. Their psychiatric problems tend to be managed by general psychiatry services. Amongst the rest, the nature and amount of intervention needed is determined by:

- Overall level of functioning.
- Ability in specific domains (e.g. communication, socialization, daily living tasks).
- Physical handicaps (including epilepsy) and motor skills.
- Coexisting psychiatric disorder.
- Prevailing temperament and behaviour.
- Support available from the family.

The management of learning disability is based on the approaches employed elsewhere in psychiatry:

- The large majority of children with learning disability now live at home. Most adults with severe learning disability live in well-supported group homes. Long-stay institutional care has now virtually disappeared in the UK.
- Care is provided by multidisciplinary community learning disability teams using a framework similar to CMHTs (Chapter 8).
- Most local services have a few in-patient beds for the assessment and treatment of behavioural and psychiatric disorders. Forensic services for people with learning disability are provided regionally.
- Voluntary agencies play an important role.

Four principles guide the current strategy for care of people with learning disability:

- Legal and civil rights—to a decent education, to marry, to have children, to vote, etc.
- The right to independence—independence, not dependence, is the default position.
- The right to choice—in where to live, what work to do, who cares for them.
- The right to inclusion—in mainstream services and local communities.

*'Essential lifestyle planning'* is one approach by which to find out what the person thinks about these decisions, and to provide the right package of care and support to help them achieve their goals.

## Specific conditions associated with learning disability

The main individual causes of learning disability are mentioned here. Chromosomal and genetic factors predominate. By and large, the aetiology does not markedly affect management, but it may have major implications for prognosis, and the likelihood of similar problems arising in other family members.

- A useful concept is *behavioural phenotype*—that is, the association of a certain profile of behaviours with a genetic condition, such that recognition of the profile gives useful clues as to the cause of the learning disability. For example, self-injury suggests Lesch–Nyhan syndrome, and overeating suggests Prader–Willi syndrome.

## Chromosomal abnormalities

A range of chromosomal microdeletions, translocations and aneuploidies can cause mental retardation. In total they explain 5–35% of cases.

- Many of the abnormalities can be detected by routine karyotyping. Others require specialist tests, such as subtelomeric analyses, which assess the ends of chromosomes (telomeres) that are relatively common sites of abnormality (5–10% of severe learning disability).
- Much smaller chromosomal abnormalities, called *copy number variants* (CNVs), as described for autism (Chapter 16) are also common in learning disability and may well account for many hitherto unexplained cases.

## Down's syndrome

Down's syndrome (trisomy 21) produces learning disability and characteristic physical features (Table 17.6). The diagnosis is usually made at, or

**Table 17.6** Features of Down's syndrome.

| |
|---|
| Moderate or severe learning disability |
| Placid temperament |
| Physical features |
|    Slanted eyes and epicanthic folds |
|    Small mouth with furrowed tongue |
|    Flat nose |
|    Flattened occiput |
|    Stubby hands with single transverse palmar crease |
|    Hypotonia |
| Associated medical problems |
|    Cardiac septal defects |
|    Gastrointestinal obstruction |
|    Atlantoaxial instability |
|    Susceptibility to infection |
| Increased risk of |
|    Leukaemia |
|    Hypothyroidism |
|    Autoimmune disorders |
|    Alzheimer's disease |

before, birth. It is the most common cause of learning disability. Its 'true' incidence is 1 in 650 live births (though this has fallen to 1 in 1000 in the UK due to antenatal testing and pregnancy termination). The risk is strongly dependent on maternal age, rising from <1/2000 at age 20 to 1/30 at age 45.

The aetiology in 95% of cases is triplication of chromosome 21, with the syndrome presumed to result from expression of the extra copy of the genes on the chromosome. The remainder are due to a translocation involving chromosome 21 or to mosaicism (a mixture of normal and trisomic cells).

• The prognosis has improved with better medical management. Many now survive to middle age, when intellectual decline due to Alzheimer's disease is common. The association between the two disorders was crucial in the discovery of the latter's genetic basis (Chapter 13).

## Fragile X syndrome

Fragile X syndrome is so called because of a fragile site on the long arm of the X chromosome seen when cells are grown in a folate-deficient medium. It occurs in about 1/1500 births and is the second most common cause of learning disability (~10% of cases). Its exact prevalence is uncertain because its phenotype (Table 17.7) is variable and accurate genetic testing has only recently become possible.

Most fragile X syndrome is due to a trinucleotide (triplet) repeat mutation in the FMR1 gene, impairing the gene's normal role in regulating expression of other genes. Being on the X chromosome, the syndrome is more common in boys than in girls. Along with several other X-linked disorders, it explains much of the higher rate of learning disability in males. However, the unusual nature of the FMR1 mutation means that some males who have the mutation are normal, and more females are affected than would be expected. Female carriers also have an increased risk of psychiatric disorders.

The disorder gets worse in succeeding generations (*anticipation*).

• Genetic detection of affected individuals and carriers is feasible.

**Table 17.7** Features of fragile X syndrome.

| |
|---|
| More common in males (>2 : 1) |
| All features are particularly variable |
| Learning disability |
|    May be mild, moderate, severe or profound |
|    Gets worse late in childhood |
|    Performance IQ affected more than verbal IQ |
|    Litany speech—repetitive, lacking in themes or content |
|    Poor attention and concentration |
|    Autistic features common |
| Physical features |
|    Large, protruding ears |
|    Long face with high-arched palate |
|    Flat feet |
|    Lax joints |
|    Soft skin |
|    Large testes (after puberty) |
|    Mitral valve prolapse |

• There is no specific treatment. *Methylphenidate* and *folic acid* may improve the attentional deficits.

• FMR1 regulates genes involved in the formation of synapses and dendrites, and this function is impaired in fragile X syndrome because of the mutation.

## Other chromosomal abnormalities

Severe learning disability is common with other abnormalities of the autosomes, but less frequent in sex chromosome aneuploidies.

• *Prader–Willi syndrome* is learning disability together with compulsive eating, obesity, disruptive behaviour, hypogonadism and psychosis. It is due to deletion of part of chromosome 15. *Angelman syndrome* (severe learning disability, puppet-like movements, laughter and a big tongue) is caused by the same abnormality when inherited from the mother rather than from the father.

• *Williams syndrome*, also known as infantile hypercalcaemia, affects 1 in 15 000 infants. Most cases are sporadic, and due to deletion of part of chromosome 7, including the elastin gene. Children show an 'elfin-like' appearance, and a moderate to severe learning disability. Verbal abilities are much better preserved—especially expressive language—than are visuospatial skills.

• *Velo-cardio-facial syndrome or di George syndrome*, is due to deletion of part of chromosome 22q. It is usually sporadic, and is relatively common (1 in 2000 infants). The physical appearance is characteristic (prominent nose, small head or jaw, short stature, long hyperextensible fingers, plus cardiac and pulmonary abnormalities. Speech and language problems are common and 90% have learning disability. It is also a risk factor for schizophrenia and other psychiatric disorders (Chapter 13).

## Single gene disorders

There are over 1000 different genes known to cause learning disability, often via effects on metabolism or brain development. Most are very rare.

### Phenylketonuria

Phenylketonuria (PKU) is the classic inborn error of metabolism (Table 17.8). The amino acid phenylalanine cannot be converted into paratyrosine because of a defective converting enzyme. It is autosomal recessive and affects 1 in 10 000 live births.

• PKU is one of the few treatable causes of severe learning disability. A rigorous low phenylalanine diet must be started in the first months of life to prevent deterioration—hence the neonatal screening for phenylalanine levels. Carriers can be detected.

## Other inherited errors of metabolism

Learning disability can result from disorders of other metabolic pathways (Table 17.9). The frequency of each is low and varies between ethnic groups. Most are associated with failure to thrive, and hepatic and/or renal dysfunction.

• In *Lesch–Nyhan syndrome*, self-mutilation by biting is characteristic.

All the cited examples are autosomal recessive and most can be detected prenatally. A few can be ameliorated by diet.

## Other genetic disorders

*Neurofibromatosis* and *tuberous sclerosis complex* are neurocutaneous syndromes. Both are autosomal dominant, but spontaneous mutations are also common.

• *Neurofibromatosis* (von Recklinghausen's disease) affects 1 in 4000 births. Diagnostic features are *cafe au lait* spots on the skin and multiple neurofibromas. Mild learning disability occurs in about 50% of cases of type 1 neurofibromatosis, which is due to mutations in the NF1 (neurofibromin) gene on chromosome 17.

• *Tuberous sclerosis complex* occurs in 1 in 6000 births. There are several characteristic skin lesions and multiple tumours (hamartomas) in the brain and elsewhere. Epilepsy and progressive mental retardation occur in 60%. Autistic features are often seen. It is caused by two genes, TSC1 (hamartin) on chromosome 9 and TSC2 (tuberin) on chromosome 16, which affect cell growth and proliferation.

• *Autism* is covered in Chapter 16.

**Table 17.8** Features of untreated phenylketonuria.

| |
|---|
| Severe learning disability |
| Tantrums and unpredictable aggression |
| Abnormal movements and mannerisms |
| Fair skinned |
| Short stature |
| Associated medical problems |
|   Eczema |
|   Vomiting |
|   Seizures |

**Table 17.9** Examples of metabolic disorders associated with learning disability.

| Metabolic category | Example |
|---|---|
| Amino acids | Homocysteinuria |
| Lipids | Tay–Sachs disease |
| Mucopolysaccharides | Hurler's syndrome |
| Carbohydrates | Galactosaemia |
| Purines | Lesch–Nyhan syndrome |

**Table 17.10** Pre- and perinatal environmental causes of learning disability.

| Category | Comment |
|---|---|
| *Obstetric complications* | |
| *In utero* infections | |
|     Rubella | Greatest risk (50%) if infection is in first trimester |
|     HIV | Learning disability in 50% of infected children |
|     Syphilis | |
|     Cytomegalovirus | |
|     Toxoplasmosis | |
| Foetal alcohol syndrome | In some offspring of mothers who drink heavily |
| Other drugs and toxins | For example, methylmercury |
| Placental insufficiency | |
| Placental abruption | |
| Eclampsia/toxaemia | |
| Birth complications | May be a consequence of earlier foetal abnormality |
| Ventricular haemorrhage | |
| *Perinatal factors* | |
| Hypothyroidism (cretinism) | An important cause in areas with low iodine diets |
| Hyperbilirubinaemia | |
| *Other factors* | |
| Cerebral palsy | |
| Hydrocephalus | |
| Spina bifida | |

**Table 17.11** Postnatal causes of learning disability.

| Infections |
|---|
|     Meningitis |
|     Encephalitis |
| Brain tumours |
| Head injury |
|     Accidental |
|     Non-accidental |
| Hypoxia (e.g. anaesthetic accident) |
| Lead poisoning |
| Rare idiopathic syndromes |
|     Disintegrative psychoses |

## Environmental factors

Learning disability can be caused by a variety of environmental insults. Most act pre- or perinatally (Table 17.10) but postnatal factors are also recognized (Table 17.11).

**Key points**

- Learning disability (mental retardation) is defined as an IQ below 70, with functional impairments in several areas and a childhood onset. It affects about 2% of the population, boys more commonly than girls.
- Psychiatric and behavioural problems are common, especially in those who also have epilepsy.
- Severe learning disability is usually caused by genetic or chromosomal abnormalities (e.g. Down's syndrome, fragile X). Mild retardation is often idiopathic and multifactorial.
- Learning disability is rarely treatable. Management is aimed at maximizing potential and quality of life, and at treating concurrent psychiatric and behavioural problems.
- Most people with learning disability live in the community.

## Chapter 18

# Psychiatry in other settings

The most important message of this book is that psychiatry is an integral part of medicine—there is nothing unique about psychiatric patients or psychiatric disorders. Rather it is the traditional separation of psychiatric services from the rest of medicine that has made this appear to be the case (Chapters 1 and 8). We have also emphasized that the conventional view of psychiatry, often gained from attachments to hospital-based psychiatric teams, is potentially misleading as most people with psychiatric disorder present to, and are managed by, other doctors in other settings. All doctors must therefore have basic skills in psychiatric assessment and management. This chapter discusses the implications of the following facts:

- Psychiatric disorders are very common in the population, and thus in all areas of medical practice.
- Outside specialist psychiatric services, somatic symptoms are often the presenting feature of psychiatric disorder.
- Psychiatric disorders frequently coexist with medical illnesses.

## Epidemiology of psychiatric disorder in different settings

### In the population

Epidemiological surveys show that at least 20% of the adult population has a psychiatric disorder at any one time. Neuroses and substance misuse account for most of this morbidity, and psychosis is relatively rare (Table 18.1).

- Overall psychiatric morbidity is strongly associated with social deprivation. Rates are twice as high in areas of deprivation.
- The neuroses are twice as common in women as men; the reverse is true for substance dependence.
- The prevalence of personality disorder, childhood psychiatric disorder and learning disability is covered in Chapters 15, 16 and 17, respectively.

Population prevalence is not the same as demand on services. Many of the individuals in Table 18.1 will never present to any service with their disorder. The difference between the population prevalence and the number who seek medical help is the first step on the pyramid, the peak of which is the tiny and unrepresentative percentage of cases that become psychiatric in-patients. Various 'filters' explain why so few make it to the top (Figure 18.1).

### General practice

Most psychiatric disorder is seen and managed in general practice.

*Lecture Notes: Psychiatry*, 10e. By Paul Harrison, John Geddes and Michael Sharpe. Published 2010 by Blackwell Publishing Ltd.

**Table 18.1** Approximate population prevalence of psychiatric disorders.

| Disorder | Prevalence (%) |
|----------|----------------|
| Mixed anxiety–depression | 8 |
| Alcohol dependence | 5 |
| Generalized anxiety disorder | 3 |
| Specific anxiety disorders | 3 |
| Depressive disorder | 2 |
| Drug dependence | 2 |
| Dementia | 1 |
| Eating disorders | <1 |
| Psychosis | 0.4 |

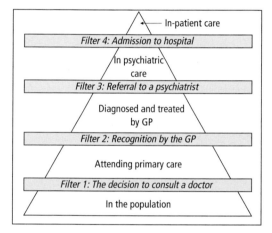

**Figure 18.1** Psychiatric disorders in different settings and the filters to psychiatric care. Not everyone with a psychiatric disorder presents to a doctor. The decision to do so—the first filter to psychiatric care—depends on several factors—for example, awareness that the symptoms may signify psychiatric disorder, their severity, choosing to see a practitioner of alternative medicine, stigma, etc. Of those who do see a doctor (in the UK, usually a GP), the psychiatric disorder is recognized and treated in about half. This filter is determined by the doctor's diagnostic and treatment decisions. About 10% of patients are referred to psychiatric services; this filter depends on the nature of the disorder, the doctor's characteristics and the availability of resources. A tiny minority at some stage have a psychiatric admission. This last filter is based mainly upon the diagnosis, the risk of harm (Chapter 4), and availability of psychiatric beds and alternative treatment options. This figure emphasizes that one's perspective on psychiatry depends largely on whereabouts on the pyramid you are standing.

- The most common psychiatric disorders in general practice are the neuroses and somatoform disorders, depression and substance misuse. Patients with psychosis are rare—most GPs have only a few on their books, and these are usually also under specialist care.

## Psychiatry as seen from general practice

Since psychiatrists and GPs see a different profile of psychiatric disorder it is not surprising that they may have differing views about priorities. For example, a GP may wish to allocate resources to manage neurotic disorders—which fill her surgeries—whereas her local psychiatrist will probably argue that rarer, but more severe, disorders—which dominate his caseload—take priority. This difference may cause tensions when psychiatrists and GPs are jointly involved in planning services in a cash-limited health service.

Integration and coordination between primary and secondary psychiatric care can be improved by:
- Regular meetings (e.g. a psychiatrist regularly visiting general practices in his sector).
- Trainee GPs spending time in psychiatry (and vice versa).
- Good communication, to ensure consistent management of cases by GPs and psychiatrists.
- Local guidelines for the management of common psychiatric disorders.

## A&E departments

Deliberate self-harm is the major psychiatric problem in A&E departments (Chapter 4). Although only a minority of these patients has persistent psychiatric disorder, many have stress-related disorders and some have depressive disorders. Intoxication and delirium related to alcohol and drugs are common, particularly in inner city hospitals and in people involved in accidents.

- Some patients with somatoform disorders and a few with factitious disorders (Chapter 10) are frequent users of A&E departments.

## Medical and surgical out-patient clinics

A third of medical and surgical out-patient clinic attendees have a psychiatric disorder. Half of these have depressive and anxiety disorders, and the remainder have somatoform disorders.

• Adequate recognition and treatment of their psychiatric disorder should be an integral part of management, since this has been shown to improve outcome.

• Depression is a common cause of apparent worsening of a medical condition.

• Panic disorder (Chapter 10) is an important cause of medically unexplained symptoms such as chest pain, dizziness and tingling.

## Medical and surgical wards

About 20% of medical and surgical in-patients have a depressive or anxiety disorder coexisting with their medical disease, 10% have a significant alcohol misuse problem and a third of elderly in-patients have an episode of delirium.

• Some patients with severe somatoform disorders get admitted and undergo multiple investigations and even surgery before the diagnosis is made.

• Remember alcohol withdrawal as a possible cause of delirium in in-patients.

## Psychiatric and medical comorbidity

Many patients with medical disease *also* have psychiatric disorder—the two occur together much more often than would be expected by chance. Chapter 13 covered the situations where a medical condition such as hyperthyroidism or Cushing's disease can produce psychiatric symptoms as part of its pathophysiology. However, there are several other reasons why medical and psychiatric disorders frequently coexist:

• Psychiatric symptoms may be a response to the physical disease. For example, depression associated with cancer; sexual dysfunction after myocardial infarction; a body image disturbance after limb amputation.

• Psychiatric disorder may cause medical illness. For example, anorexia nervosa may cause osteoporosis.

• There may be a shared cause, such as a major life event precipitating both a stroke and depression.

The coexistence of a psychiatric disorder and a medical disorder is clinically important because it:

• Magnifies suffering and disability.

• Prolongs medical care and increases overall health costs.

• Worsens outcome. For example, the mortality of heart disease, cancer or stroke is higher in those with a comorbid depressive disorder.

## Presentations of psychiatric disorder in a medical setting

Some cases of psychiatric disorders that present in medical settings do so with psychological symptoms or behavioural disturbance. However, many others present in ways that are less obviously 'psychiatric', with:

• Somatic symptoms.

• A medical management problem.

• An apparent exacerbation of an established medical condition.

### Presentation with somatic symptoms

#### Psychiatric disorder and somatic symptoms

A significant minority of patients seen in general practice and in hospital out-patient clinics have somatic symptoms which cannot be explained by medical disease; many of these have a psychiatric disorder. The important diagnoses are depressive, anxiety and somatoform disorders.

• Figure 18.2 shows a simple diagnostic approach to medically unexplained somatic symptoms.

#### Depression and anxiety and somatic symptoms

Depression is associated with somatic symptoms such as fatigue, weight loss and pain. Similarly, anxiety produces the bodily symptoms of autonomic arousal, which include palpitations, breathlessness and sensory symptoms.

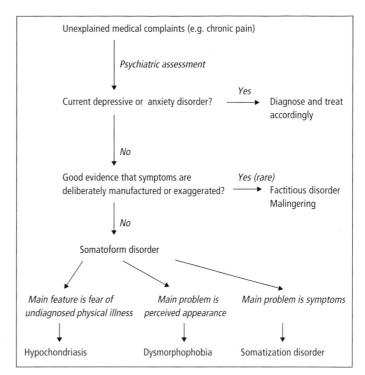

**Figure 18.2** Psychiatric assessment and diagnostic pathway in people with unexplained medical complaints.

For any patient who presents with bodily symptoms that are not adequately explicable by a medical diagnosis, consider the possibility that the patient may have a depressive or anxiety disorder. This psychiatric diagnosis may be the only diagnosis or it may be complicating a medical condition, in which case two diagnoses must be made. When assessing a patient with somatic symptoms it is important both to carry out the appropriate investigations to exclude physical disease and also to seek evidence of depression or anxiety.

• The converse situation—a misdiagnosis of depression or anxiety in a patient whose symptoms are caused by a medical disease—though much rarer, must not be overlooked (Chapter 13).

*Ms M went to her doctor because of abdominal pain. She was upset, but both she and the doctor saw her distress as being a result of the pain. An urgent laparotomy was performed and a normal appendix removed. Only after she took an overdose the following month was a further history taken which revealed that she had been having problems with her relationship with her mother and had developed symptoms of depressive disorder (low mood, anhedonia and poor sleep) prior to the pain starting. She was given an antidepressant drug, helped to address the family conflict and made a full recovery.*

## Somatoform disorders and somatic symptoms

Patients with medically unexplained somatic symptoms who do *not* have a depressive or anxiety disorder may be regarded as having a somatoform disorder (Chapter 10).

*Mr H has attended a gastroenterology clinic intermittently for years with abdominal discomfort and flatulence. No significant abnormalities have been found despite numerous investigations throughout the length of his gastrointestinal tract. Trials of antispasmodics, laxatives and antiulcer drugs have not produced sustained effects. A new junior doctor reviews his case and sees a connection between stresses at home or work and the exacerbation of abdominal as well as anxiety symptoms. Mr H is unwilling to countenance a psychological basis for his problems but agrees to see a liaison psychiatrist who works closely with the clinic. Mr H embarks on a course of problem-solving therapy and attends a stress management class. His irritable bowel syndrome improves markedly and he agrees (for the first time) that further medical interventions are not necessary.*

## Presentation with a medical management problem

Psychiatric disorders may also present as a problem in medical management. For example:
• An old lady repeatedly pulls out her drip in the orthopaedic ward.
• A young woman is repeatedly admitted with an infected operative wound.
• A woman with diabetes refuses to take adequate insulin.
• A young man has thumped a doctor in surgical out-patients.

The diagnosis in all these cases proved to be psychiatric. It was, respectively: delirium, factitious disorder, depression and personality disorder. The cases illustrate that any psychiatric disorder can present with a medical management problem, and that a psychiatric assessment, even if brief (Chapter 2), is essential.

## Psychiatric disorder presenting as an apparent worsening of a medical disease

An exacerbation of symptoms or disability in a patient with a chronic medical condition may erroneously be attributed to a worsening of the disease process, when it is in fact due to the development of a comorbid psychiatric disorder. For example:
• A man with previously stable angina repeatedly presents with severe chest pain.
• A woman with previous hypothyroidism suffers a recurrence of severe lethargy.
• A woman with arthritis becomes housebound.

The diagnosis in these cases proved to be, respectively: panic disorder, depression and agoraphobia. The danger is that such patients are given unnecessary and potentially hazardous medical treatment instead of appropriate psychiatric management.

## Management of psychiatric disorder in medicine

There are three main requirements for the effective management of psychiatric disorder in medical settings. These requirements serve to emphasize the knowledge, skills and attitudes which all doctors should have (Chapter 1):
• To be able to recognize it.
• To be able to treat it appropriately.
• To know how and when to refer to specialist psychiatric services.

## Recognition

The diagnosis of psychiatric disorder in non-psychiatric settings is often missed. This error may be attributable to the doctor, the patient or the circumstances (Table 18.2).

Doctors will be better at the detection and assessment of psychiatric disorder if they:
• Realize that somatic symptoms are not always due to medical conditions.
• Always do a brief psychiatric assessment—even if just a few questions (Table 2.2).

**Table 18.2** Reasons psychiatric diagnoses are missed in medical settings.

*Doctor*
Failure to consider the possibility
Failure to ask about psychiatric symptoms—through lack of effort or skill

*Patient*
Reports only their somatic symptoms
Hides emotional distress and psychosocial stresses from the doctor

*Circumstances*
Lack of time
Lack of privacy
Clinics geared solely toward the detection of physical disease

- Ask the patient about their worries and concerns.
- Enable the patient to express emotions.

## Treatment

The treatment of psychiatric disorder in medical settings follows the same principles as treatment in psychiatric settings. It also requires that:

- The psychiatric diagnosis is explained to the patient in a way that they can accept. This is achieved by emphasizing that it is a real illness, that it is an understandable reaction and not a sign of weakness, and that it can be treated effectively.
- Effective evidence-based treatment is available. Some doctors will regularly use simple psychological therapies themselves. Others will have ensured that they have members of the clinical team, such as specialist nurses or counsellors, who they can ask for assistance.
- The doctor has confidence in prescribing the main psychotropic drugs.

## Referral to specialist psychiatric services

A small but important minority of patients will require a referral to specialist psychiatric services. The main indications for referral are:

- Request for second opinion.
- Failure of first-line management.
- Need for specialist treatment, such as ECT.
- Serious suicide risk.
- Presence of a condition, such as psychosis, requiring specialist services.
- Severe substance misuse.
- Need for compulsory treatment.

From primary care, referrals will usually be made to the local general psychiatric services, unless the problem falls into the remit of one of the subspecialties (Chapter 8). For patients in general hospitals there may be a hospital liaison psychiatry service that will assist both in management and in making appropriate referrals.

- Referrals, other than of exceptional emergencies, should only be made after the doctor has: (a) completed a basic assessment themselves; (b) explained and agreed the referral with the patient.
- Following the referral, good communication between all the agencies involved is essential if problems are to be avoided.

---

### Key points

- Patients with psychiatric disorders are encountered in all medical settings. Neurotic, somatoform, adjustment, depression and anxiety disorders are all common in general practice and general hospitals. In these settings they often present with somatic symptoms.
- Medical disease is frequently accompanied by psychiatric disorder. The combination worsens disability and prognosis if not effectively managed.
- Management of psychiatric disorder is based on the general principles described in this book, plus: (a) attention to the patient's medical condition and treatment; and (b) necessary adaptation to the medical setting.
- Because psychiatric disorders are so common in the general population, all doctors must be:
  - alert to the possibility of psychiatric disorder in all patients;
  - aware that psychiatric disorder often presents with somatic symptoms;
  - aware of the prevalence of psychiatric disorder in the physically ill;
  - able to screen for psychiatric disorder;
  - able to use simple psychological treatments;
  - able to use antidepressants;
  - aware when and how to refer to psychiatric services.

# Multiple choice questions

1. **Hallucinations:**
   a. Can occur in severe depression.
   b. Are misperceptions of external stimuli.
   c. Which are visual suggest an organic disorder.
   d. Voices talking to the person are characteristic of schizophrenia.
   e. Which occur while waking from sleep are called 'hypnopompic'.

2. **Alzheimer's disease:**
   a. Usually presents in the seventh decade.
   b. Is usually inherited as an autosomal recessive disorder.
   c. Death occurs on average 2–3 years after diagnosis.
   d. Is associated with the apolipoprotein E4 genetic variant.
   e. Drug therapy is aimed at reducing excessive cholinergic neurotransmission.

3. **In dementia:**
   a. Incontinence and ataxic gait suggests normal pressure hydrocephalus.
   b. A fluctuating course and visual hallucinations suggests Pick's disease.
   c. Antipsychotics are first-line treatment for behavioural symptoms (e.g. shouting, agitation).
   d. Myoclonic jerks are characteristic of Creutzfeldt–Jakob disease.
   e. About 90% of cases are caused by Alzheimer's disease.

4. **Compared with conventional antipsychotics, atypical antipsychotics:**
   a. Produce fewer extrapyramidal side-effects.
   b. Cause less weight gain.
   c. Tend to be more selective for the dopamine $D_2$ receptor.
   d. Are less sedative.
   e. Decrease suicide rates.

5. **When choosing an antidepressant:**
   a. Nausea is more common with SSRIs than tricyclics.
   b. SSRI-induced sexual dysfunction is usually transient.
   c. Avoid clomipramine in combination with other drugs.
   d. After recovery, halve the dose for maintenance therapy.
   e. Continuing antidepressants after recovery halves the risk of relapse.

6. **First-rank symptoms:**
   a. Were described by Bleuler.
   b. If prominent are diagnostic of schizophrenia.
   c. Are a poor prognostic sign in schizophrenia.
   d. Can occur in mania.
   e. Are rare in developing countries.

7. **Cognitive behavioural therapy:**
   a. Is usually carried out by psychiatrists.
   b. Sometimes includes analysis of dreams.
   c. Usually involves homework and diary keeping.
   d. Is not effective in schizophrenia.
   e. In clinical trials is effective in 80–85% of cases of depression.

8. **In patients taking lithium:**
   a. Liver function tests are needed regularly.
   b. A fine tremor is a sign of lithium toxicity.
   c. She may experience a metallic taste.
   d. Hypothyroidism is a recognized side-effect.
   e. Plasma levels should be kept below 0.5 mmol/l.

9. **Electroconvulsive therapy:**
   a. Has fewer side-effects when given to the non-dominant hemisphere.
   b. Can only be given to patients under the Mental Health Act.

c. Should not be given to those over 70 years old.

d. Is only effective if a seizure is induced.

e. Can be given to patients currently taking antidepressants.

10. **Sleep problems:**

a. Initial insomnia is characteristic of depression.

b. Are a recognized side-effect of SSRIs.

c. Hypersomnia is characteristic of atypical depression.

d. Sleep hygiene is an effective intervention.

e. Narcolepsy usually presents before age 10.

11. **Eating disorders:**

a. Anorexia nervosa is the most common subtype.

b. Many patients have features of both anorexia and bulimia nervosa.

c. Cognitive behavioural therapy is the most effective treatment for bulimia.

d. Are three times as common in women as in men.

e. Anorexia nervosa has approximately a 10-fold increased mortality rate.

12. **Causes of mood disorders:**

a. Bipolar and unipolar mood disorders have similar heritabilities.

b. Early life adversity and recent life events are interacting risk factors for depression.

c. Depression is a common feature of Cushing's disease.

d. Prolonged depression is associated with atrophy of the thalamus.

e. Raised cortisol levels are present in 90% of subjects with moderate to severe depression.

13. **In post-traumatic stress disorder:**

a. Debriefing is an effective preventative treatment.

b. Hyperarousal is a principal feature.

c. Alcohol misuse frequently occurs.

d. Antidepressants are usually effective.

e. Most cases resolve within a few months.

14. **In the treatment of mania:**

a. Lithium carbonate is the standard monotherapy.

b. Antipsychotics should be limited to those with delusions or hallucinations.

c. Depressive symptoms often coexist.

d. Delusions which occur are usually nihilistic.

e. Afterwards, mood stabilizer medication is normally prescribed.

15. **Autism:**

a. Has a similar incidence in boys and girls.

b. About 25% suffer from epilepsy.

c. Is associated with large ears and blonde hair in boys.

d. Is an X-linked recessive disorder.

e. About a third are mentally retarded.

16. **Which of the following are first-rank symptoms of schizophrenia?**

a. Thought disorder.

b. Thought insertion.

c. Thought block.

d. Thought withdrawal.

e. Thought broadcasting.

17. **Which of these drugs is a recognized cause of depressive symptoms?**

a. Amphetamines.

b. Digoxin.

c. L-DOPA.

d. Anticholinergics.

e. Diuretics.

18. **Which of these medical disorders is a recognized cause of depressive symptoms?**

a. Systemic lupus erythematosus.

b. Addison's disease.

c. Hypothyroidism.

d. Cushing's disease.

e. Multiple sclerosis.

19. **Epidemiology of depression:**

a. The lifetime risk of a depressive episode in men is 2–3%.

b. Bipolar disorder has an equal sex incidence.

c. 20% of medical in-patients meet criteria for a mood disorder.

d. Suicide occurs in 1 in 20 patients with mood disorder.

e. At least 50% of people with unexplained physical symptoms meet criteria for depression.

20. **Conduct disorder:**
    a. Is usually part of attention deficit hyperactivity disorder.
    b. Is the most common psychiatric disorder of childhood.
    c. The diagnosis is usually made around puberty.
    d. About half progress to dissocial personality disorder.
    e. Behavioural therapy is an effective intervention.

21. **Delirium:**
    a. Is usually associated with a disturbed sleep–wake cycle.
    b. Place disorientation usually occurs before time disorientation.
    c. Occurs in at least 10% of medical in-patients.
    d. Can be caused by urinary retention.
    e. Low-dose antipsychotics are the first-line drug treatment.

22. **Which of the following are psychotic disorders?**
    a. Hypochondriasis.
    b. Paranoid personality disorder.
    c. Somatoform disorder.
    d. Korsakoff's syndrome.
    e. De Clèrambault's syndrome (erotomania).

23. **Suicide:**
    a. Is more common in married men than in unmarried men.
    b. 70% of those who deliberately self-harm are suffering from major depression.
    c. Is more common in retired than in younger people.
    d. Occurs eventually in 20% of those who have previously self-harmed.
    e. About 50% of suicide victims have a history of alcohol abuse or dependence.

24. **Learning disability:**
    a. Is defined by an IQ of less than 60.
    b. Self-biting is characteristic of fragile X syndrome.
    c. Is caused by a chromosomal abnormality in the majority of cases.
    d. Is associated with an increased risk of developing dementia.

    e. Phenylketonuria can be treated by removing phenylalanine from the diet.

25. **In prophylaxis of bipolar disorder:**
    a. Lithium should not normally be prescribed for more than 2 years.
    b. Carbamazepine is about as effective as sodium valproate.
    c. Elderly patients should not be prescribed lithium.
    d. Cognitive therapy reduces relapse rates.
    e. Thyroid function should be tested regularly in patients taking lithium.

26. **Heritability of psychiatric disorders:**
    a. Refers to the penetrance of a gene.
    b. Is measured using adoption studies.
    c. Heritability of schizophrenia is about 40%.
    d. Heritability of depression is about 40%.
    e. Heritability of anxiety disorders is less than 10%.

27. **Complex partial epilepsy:**
    a. Olfactory hallucinations are characteristic.
    b. Used to be called petit mal epilepsy.
    c. Schizophrenia is more common than expected.
    d. Is associated with a several-fold increase in suicide.
    e. The seizure focus is usually in the thalamus.

28. **Personality disorder:**
    a. Cluster A is called 'eccentric'.
    b. Dialectic behaviour therapy is effective in borderline personality disorder.
    c. Psychodynamic psychotherapy is effective in schizoid personality disorder.
    d. Anankastic personality disorder is also called avoidant personality disorder.
    e. Persecutory delusions are a feature of paranoid personality disorder.

29. **Substance misuse:**
    a. Phencyclidine (PCP) mainly blocks 5-HT receptors.
    b. Ecstasy may damage 5-HT fibres in the brain.
    c. LSD is addictive.
    d. Cannabis can be detected in the urine for several weeks.

e. Chronic amphetamine use is associated with mood swings.

30. **A patient with borderline personality disorder:**
    a. Is unlikely to benefit from any treatments.
    b. May experience brief psychotic symptoms.
    c. Is at a lower risk of suicide compared with patients with other personality disorders.
    d. Usually first shows signs of the disorder in their 30s.
    e. Is likely to misuse alcohol and drugs.

31. **In ICD-10:**
    a. Hypochondriasis is classified as an anxiety disorder.
    b. Dysthymia is classified as a personality disorder.
    c. Dementia and delirium are forms of organic disorder.
    d. Depressive disorder is a form of neurosis.
    e. Symptoms must be present for at least 1 month to diagnose schizophrenia.

32. **Which of the following are used to treat attention deficit hyperactivity disorder?**
    a. Methylphenidate.
    b. Methylprednisolone.
    c. Atomoxetine.
    d. Zopiclone.
    e. Modafinil.

33. **Which of the following are features of dementia with Lewy bodies?**
    a. Parkinsonism.
    b. Visual hallucinations.
    c. Rapidly fluctuating mental state.
    d. Autosomal recessive inheritance.
    e. Can be transmitted by blood products.

34. **Medically unexplained somatic symptoms:**
    a. About 25% have a depressive disorder.
    b. Antidepressants are effective in treating chronic pain.
    c. Briquet's syndrome nearly always occurs in women.
    d. Mortality rate is significantly increased.
    e. Are rarely due to somatoform disorder.

35. **Which of the following are antidepressants?**
    a. Lofepramine.
    b. Loperamide.
    c. Sertraline.
    d. Clomipramine.
    e. Venlafaxine.

36. **In patients with personality disorder:**
    a. Prognosis of any comorbid psychiatric disorder is worsened.
    b. More than one personality disorder is often present.
    c. Their mortality rate is unaltered.
    d. Dangerous and severe personality disorder is a new diagnostic category.
    e. Dissocial personality disorder is synonymous with psychopathic disorder.

37. **The Mental Health Act (1983/2007):**
    a. Section 2 is used for admission for assessment of a mental disorder.
    b. Is only used if the patient lacks capacity.
    c. Only applies in psychiatric settings.
    d. Only applies to patients in hospital.
    e. Section 3 lasts for 6 months in the first instance.

38. **The Mental Capacity Act (2005):**
    a. Is 'trumped' by the Mental Health Act.
    b. Is only relevant to psychiatrists and psychiatric patients.
    c. Requires mental capacity to be assessed in all patients.
    d. Does not apply in Scotland.
    e. Capacity is assumed until proven otherwise.

39. **Attention deficit hyperactivity disorder (ADHD):**
    a. Is synonymous with hyperkinetic disorder.
    b. Is associated with maternal smoking during pregnancy.
    c. Stimulants are contraindicated.
    d. Dopamine genes contribute to its aetiology.
    e. The heritability is estimated at 20%.

40. **Which of these dementias are considered reversible?**
    a. Pick's disease.
    b. Normal pressure hydrocephalus.
    c. Vascular dementia.
    d. Dementia with Lewy bodies.
    e. Alcoholic dementia.

41. **Which of the following are treatments for Alzheimer's disease?**
    a. Modafinil.
    b. Memantine.
    c. Methylphenidate.
    d. Donepezil.
    e. Rivastigmine.

42. **Which of these syndromes is due to a chromosomal abnormality?**
    a. Phenylketonuria
    b. Velo-cardio-facial syndrome.
    c. Williams syndrome
    d. Down syndrome.
    e. Tay–Sachs disease.

43. **Which of the following are autosomal dominant disorders?**
    a. Pick's disease.
    b. Huntington's disease.
    c. Hurler's syndrome.
    d. Autism.
    e. Lesch–Nyhan syndrome.

44. **Physical dependence has been demonstrated for:**
    a. Tricyclic antidepressants.
    b. SSRIs.
    c. Benzodiazepines.
    d. Venlafaxine.
    e. Antipsychotics.

45. **On a general medical ward:**
    a. 5% of patients have a depressive or anxiety disorder.
    b. 30% of elderly patients have an episode of delirium.
    c. Mental Health Act Section 5(2) may be used.
    d. Mental Health Act Section 136 may be used.
    e. The Mental Capacity Act applies.

46. **The following drugs are recognized causes of delirium:**
    a. Diazepam.
    b. Digoxin.
    c. Steroids.
    d. Thiazide diuretics.
    e. Tricyclic antidepressants.

47. **Which of the following are recognized consequences of alcohol abuse:**
    a. Wernicke's encephalopathy.
    b. Morbid jealousy.
    c. Supranuclear palsy.
    d. Korsakov's syndrome.
    e. Dementia.

48. **Ecstasy (MDMA):**
    a. Can lead to hypothermia.
    b. Causes selective degeneration of noradrenaline neurons.
    c. Produces its effects mainly by inhibiting dopamine release.
    d. Is an analogue of amphetamine.
    e. Is a 5-HT$_2$ receptor agonist.

49. **Which of these are variants of persistent delusional disorder?**
    a. de Clerambaut's syndrome.
    b. Cotard's syndrome.
    c. Capgras' delusion.
    d. Morbid jealousy.
    e. Briquet's syndrome.

50. **Schizophrenia:**
    a. Is more common in those born in cities.
    b. Is more common in immigrants.
    c. Rarely has its onset after the age of 35.
    d. Is more common in those who learn to walk later than average.
    e. Is associated with birth complications.

51. **Which of the following are symptoms of psychosis?**
    a. Illusory perceptions.
    b. Paraesthesia.
    c. Delusions.
    d. Obsessions.
    e. Hallucinations.

52. **Which of the following are features of obsessions?**
    a. They are resisted.
    b. They are diagnostic of obsessive–compulsive disorder.
    c. They are also known as overvalued ideas.
    d. They are often secondary to compulsive behaviours.
    e. They are perceived as intrusive.

53. **Which of the following personality disorders are in cluster C?**
    a. Anxious (avoidant).
    b. Schizoid.
    c. Paranoid.

d. Borderline.

e. Anankastic (obsessional).

54. **Which of the following are features of Down syndrome?**

a. Hypertonia.

b. Placid temperament.

c. Autoimmune disorders.

d. Cardiac septal detects.

e. Single palmar crease.

55. **Which of the following are features of fragile X syndrome?**

a. Girls can be affected.

b. Large ears.

c. Mitral valve prolapse.

d. Performance IQ affected more than verbal IQ.

e. Lax joints.

56. **Which of the following are antipsychotic drugs?**

a. Quetiapine.

b. Chlormethiazole.

c. Chlordiazepoxide.

d. Chlorpromazine.

e. Sertraline.

57. **Which are recognized psychosocial interventions for schizophrenia?**

a. Cognitive behavioural therapy.

b. Dialectic behaviour therapy.

c. Cognitive remediation therapy.

d. Family therapy.

e. Psychodynamic psychotherapy.

58. **Which of these factors in schizophrenia predicts poor outcome?**

a. Mood disturbance.

b. Disorganized (hebephrenic) subtype.

c. Female.

d. Insidious onset.

e. Positive family history.

59. **Which of the following are more appropriate for bipolar than unipolar depression?**

a. Lamotrigine.

b. Quetiapine.

c. MAOIs.

d. Venlafaxine.

e. SSRIs.

60. **Which of the following are more common with SSRIs than with TCAs?**

a. Lack of libido.

b. Dry mouth.

c. Urinary retention.

d. Nausea.

e. Arrhythmias.

# Answers to multiple choice questions

1. **Hallucinations:**
   a. True
   b. False (True = false perception)
   c. True
   d. False (True = talking about the person)
   e. True

2. **Alzheimer's disease:**
   a. False (True = more common in eighth and ninth decade)
   b. False (True = usually non-Mendelian (complex) inheritance)
   c. False (True = 5–8 years)
   d. True
   e. False (True = enhance cholinergic neurotransmission)

3. **In dementia:**
   a. True
   b. False (True = dementia with Lewy bodies)
   c. False (Avoid whenever possible)
   d. True
   e. False (True = 50–60%)

4. **Compared with conventional antipsychotics, atypical antipsychotics:**
   a. True
   b. False
   c. False
   d. False
   e. False (True = only for clozapine)

5. **When choosing an antidepressant:**
   a. True
   b. False
   c. True
   d. False (True = the dose that got you better keeps you better)
   e. True

6. **First-rank symptoms:**
   a. False (True = Schneider)
   b. False (True = indicative but not pathognomonic)

c. False (True = no prognostic value)
   d. True
   e. False (True = similar occurrence worldwide)

7. **Cognitive behavioural therapy:**
   a. False (True = psychologists or other health professionals)
   b. False
   c. True
   d. False (True = effective against residual delusions and hallucinations)
   e. False (True = 60–70%)

8. **In patients taking lithium:**
   a. False (True = renal function tests)
   b. False (True = coarse tremor)
   c. True
   d. True
   e. False (True = between 0.4 and 1.0 mmol/l)

9. **Electroconvulsive therapy:**
   a. True
   b. False
   c. False
   d. True
   e. True

10. **Sleep problems:**
    a. False (True = early morning waking)
    b. True
    c. True
    d. True
    e. True

11. **Eating disorders:**
    a. False (True = atypical eating disorder)
    b. True
    c. True
    d. False (True = 10-fold)
    e. True

12. **Causes of mood disorders:**
    a. False (True = bipolar disorder is much more heritable)
    b. True

c. True

d. False (True = atrophy of the hippocampus)

e. False (True = less than 50%)

13. **In post-traumatic stress disorder:**

  a. False

  b. True

  c. True

  d. False

  e. True

14. **In the treatment of mania:**

  a. False (True = antipsychotic)

  b. False (True = effective in non-psychotic mania too)

  c. True

  d. False (True = grandiose)

  e. False (True = only after two manic episodes)

15. **Autism:**

  a. False (True = 80% are boys)

  b. True

  c. False (True = fragile X syndrome)

  d. False

  e. False (True = about 75%)

16. **Which of the following are first-rank symptoms of schizophrenia?**

  a. False

  b. True

  c. False

  d. True

  e. True

17. **Which of these drugs is a recognized cause of depressive symptoms?**

  a. True

  b. True

  c. True

  d. False (True = delirium)

  e. True

18. **Which of these medical disorders is a recognized cause of depressive symptoms?**

  a. True

  b. True

  c. True

  d. True

  e. True

19. **Epidemiology of depression:**

  a. False (True = closer to 10%)

  b. True

c. True

d. False (True = 1 in 8)

e. True

20. **Conduct disorder:**

  a. False (True = differential diagnosis)

  b. True

  c. False (True = usually by age 7)

  d. True

  e. False (True = no proven interventions known)

21. **Delirium:**

  a. True

  b. False (Time disorientation is characteristic)

  c. True

  d. True

  e. True (Except in delirium tremens)

22. **Which of the following are psychotic disorders?**

  a. False (True = neurotic disorder)

  b. False

  c. False

  d. True

  e. True

23. **Suicide:**

  a. False

  b. False (True = this figure applies to completed suicide)

  c. True

  d. False (True = about 5%)

  e. True

24. **Learning disability:**

  a. False (True = 70)

  b. False (True = Lesch–Nyhan syndrome)

  c. False (True = 5–35%)

  d. True

  e. True

25. **In prophylaxis of bipolar disorder:**

  a. False (True = aim for minimum of 2 years)

  b. False

  c. False

  d. True

  e. True

26. **Heritability of psychiatric disorders:**

  a. False (True = proportion of a disorder in the population due to genes)

  b. False (True = twin studies)

  c. False (True = 80%)

d. True

e. False (True = 30%)

27. **Complex partial epilepsy:**

a. True

b. False (True = psychomotor epilepsy)

c. True

d. True

e. False (True = temporal lobe)

28. **Personality disorder:**

a. True

b. True

c. False

d. False (True = obsessional)

e. False

29. **Substance misuse:**

a. False (True = NMDA glutamate receptors)

b. True

c. False

d. True

e. True

30. **A patient with borderline personality disorder:**

a. False

b. True

c. False

d. False

e. True

31. **In ICD-10:**

a. True

b. False

c. True

d. False

e. True

32. **Which of the following are used to treat attention deficit hyperactivity disorder?**

a. True

b. False

c. True

d. False

e. True

33. **Which of the following are features of dementia with Lewy bodies?**

a. True

b. True

c. True

d. False

e. False

34. **Medically unexplained somatic symptoms:**

a. True

b. True

c. True

d. False

e. False

35. **Which of the following are antidepressants?**

a. True

b. False

c. True

d. True

e. True

36. **In patients with personality disorder:**

a. True

b. True

c. False (It is increased)

d. False (It is a UK government category)

e. True

37. **The Mental Health Act (1983/2007):**

a. True

b. False (Capacity is not defined in the Act)

c. False (e.g. Section 5(2))

d. False (Community Treatment Orders)

e. True

38. **The Mental Capacity Act (2005):**

a. False (They are separate)

b. False (Applies in all settings)

c. True

d. True (Separate legislation applies)

e. True

39. **Attention deficit hyperactivity disorder:**

a. False (Hyperkinetic disorder is a subgroup)

b. True

c. False (Widely used)

d. True

e. False (High—about 80%)

40. **Which of these dementias are considered reversible?**

a. False

b. True

c. False

d. False

e. False

41. **Which of the following are treatments for Alzheimer's disease?**

a. False

b. True

c. False
d. True
e. True

**42. Which of these syndromes is due to a chromosomal abnormality?**

a. False (Specific gene mutation)
b. True
c. True
d. True
e. False (Specific gene mutation)

**43. Which of the following are autosomal dominant disorders?**

a. False (Autosomal recessive, or unknown)
b. True
c. False (Autosomal recessive)
d. False (Polygenic)
e. False (Autosomal recessive)

**44. Physical dependence has been demonstrated for:**

a. False
b. False
c. True
d. False
e. False

**45. On a general medical ward:**

a. False (About 20%)
b. True
c. True
d. False
e. True

**46. The following are recognized causes of delirium:**

a. True
b. True
c. True
d. True
e. True

**47. Which of the following are recognized consequences of alcohol abuse:**

a. True
b. True
c. False
d. True
e. True (But rare)

**48. Ecstasy (MDMA):**

a. False (Hyperpyrexia)
b. False

c. False
d. True
e. False.

**49. Which of the following are variants of persistent delusional disorder?**

a. True
b. False (Occurs in psychotic depression)
c. True
d. True
e. False (A somatoform disorder)

**50. Schizophrenia:**

a. True
b. True
c. False
d. True
e. True

**51. Which of the following are symptoms of psychosis?**

a. False
b. False
c. True
d. False
e. True

**52. Which of the following are features of obsessions?**

a. True (At least initially)
b. False (Also occur in other disorders)
c. False
d. False (The other way round)
e. True

**53. Which of the following personality disorders are in cluster C?**

a. True
b. False
c. False
d. False
e. True.

**54. Which of the following are features of Down syndrome?**

a. False (Hypotonia)
b. True
c. True
d. True
e. False

**55. Which of the following are features of fragile X syndrome?**

a. True

b. True

c. True

d. True

e. True

56. Which of the following are antipsychotic drugs?

a. True

b. False

c. False

d. True

e. False

57. Which are recognized psychosocial interventions for schizophrenia?

a. True

b. False

c. True

d. True

e. False

58. Which of these factors in schizophrenia predicts poor outcome?

a. False

b. True

c. False

d. True

e. False

59. Which of the following are more appropriate for bipolar than unipolar depression?

a. True

b. True

c. False

d. False

e. False

60. Which of the following are commoner with SSRIs than with TCAs?

a. True

b. False

c. False

d. True

e. False

# Appendix 1

# ICD-10 classification of psychiatric disorders

| Category | Category | Example |
|----------|----------|---------|
| F00–09 | Organic disorders | F02.2 Huntington's disease |
| F10–19 | Substance use disorders | F10.2 Alcohol dependence |
| F29–29 | Schizophrenia and other psychoses | F20.0 Paranoid schizophrenia |
| F30–39 | Mood disorders | F32.1 Moderate depressive episode |
| F40–49 | Neurotic and stress-related disorders | F45.2 Hypochondriasis |
| F50–59 | Eating, sleep and related syndromes | F50.2 Bulimia nervosa |
| F60–69 | Disorders of personality and behaviour | F60.2 Dissocial personality disorder |
| F70–79 | Mental retardation (Learning disability) | F72.0 Severe mental retardation |
| F80–89 | Developmental disorders | F84.0 Autism |
| F90–99 | Childhood disorders | F94.0 Elective mutism |

# Appendix 2

# Keeping up to date and evidence based

Textbooks and articles can be biased and rapidly outdated. The following are sources of up-to-date, good quality evidence in psychiatry.

- To hone your skills in evidence-based medicine (EBM) we recommend an EBM textbook such as *Evidence-based Medicine. How to Practice and Teach EBM*, 3rd edition. Straus SE, Richardson WS, Glasziou P, Haynes RB (2005). Churchill Livingstone.

## Finding the evidence

Access to high quality evidence in psychiatry is improving all the time.

- NHS Evidence (www.evidence.nhs.uk) is a website maintained by the National Institute for Health and Clinical Excellence (NICE) that brings together many good resources including the Cochrane Database of Systematic Reviews, the British National Formulary, Clinical Evidence and Medline. Access to these resources is free to practitioners in the UK.

- Emerging new evidence in psychiatry is summarized in *Evidence-based Mental Health*—a quarterly journal from the BMJ Publishing Group. The content of the journal is also available on line (http://ebmh.bmjjournals.com/).

## Clinical practice guidelines

Clinical practice guidelines (CPGs) are recommendations on the appropriate treatment and care of people with specific disorders. CPGs can be a useful help, but should augment rather than replace clinical expertise and experience. Before using a CPG, make sure that it is properly evidence based, and relevant to your patients.

- In the UK, the NICE prepares national evidence-based guidelines. As of December 2009, mental health guidelines have been published for a wide range of mental disorders including schizophrenia, bipolar disorder, depressive disorder and eating disorders. All NICE clinical practice guidelines are available at www.nice.nhs.uk.

# Further reading

For general reading, we recommend the *Shorter Oxford Textbook of Psychiatry*, Gelder M, Harrison P, Cowen P (2006), 5th edition, Oxford University Press. For a detailed reference textbook, see the two-volume *New Oxford Textbook of Psychiatry*, Gelder MG, Andreasen NC, Lopez-Ibor J, Geddes JR (2009), 2nd edition, Oxford University Press. We recognize our conflict of interest in both recommendations!

## Chapter 1

Royal College of Psychiatrists (1997). Core psychiatry for tomorrow's doctors. *Psychiatr Bull* **21**, 522–524.

Crisp AH, Gelder MG, Rix S, *et al.* (2000). Stigmatisation of people with mental illness. *Br J Psychiatry* **177**, 4–7.

McParland M, Noble LM, Livingston G, *et al.* (2003). The effect of a psychiatric attachment on students' attitudes to and intention to pursue psychiatry as a career. *Med Educ* **37**, 447–454.

Prince M, Patel V, Saxena S, *et al.* (2007). No health without mental health. *Lancet* **370**, 859–877.

## Chapters 2 and 3

Kopelman MD (1994). Structured psychiatric interview. *Br J Hosp Med* **52**, 93–98 and 277–281.

Crimlisk H, Taylor M (1996). How to cope with a neuropsychiatric case. *Br J Hosp Med* **56**, 103–107.

Kipps CM, Hodges JR (2005). Cognitive assessment for clinicians. *J Neurol Neurosurg Psychiatry* **76**, 22–30.

Oyebode F (2008). *Symptoms in the Mind. An Introduction to Descriptive Psychopathology*, 4th edition. London, Saunders.

Phelan M, Blair G (2008) Medical history-taking in psychiatry. *Adv Psychiatr Treat* **14**, 229–234.

## Chapter 4

Maden A (1996). Risk assessment in psychiatry. *Br J Hosp Med* **56**, 78–82.

Atakan Z, Davies T (1997). Mental health emergencies. *BMJ* **314**, 1740–1742.

Hirschfeld RMA, Russell JM (1997). Assessment and treatment of suicidal patients. *N Engl J Med* **337**, 910–915.

Szmukler G (2001). Violence risk prediction in practice. *Br J Psychiatry* **178**, 84–85.

## Chapter 5

Kendell RE (1975). *The Role of Diagnosis in Psychiatry*. Oxford, Blackwell Scientific.

Sharpe M (1990). The use of graphical life charts in psychiatry. *Br J Hosp Med* **44**, 44–47.

Maguire P, Pitceathly C (2002). Key communication skills and how to acquire them. *BMJ* **325**, 697–700.

## Chapter 6

Cawley RH (1993). Psychiatry is more than a science. *Br J Psychiatry* **162**, 154–160.

Zachar P, Kendler KS (2007). Psychiatric disorders: a conceptual taxonomy. *Am J Psychiatry* **164**, 557–565.

Hyman SE (2007). Can neuroscience be integrated into the DSM-V? *Nat Rev Neurosci* **8**, 725–732.

## Chapter 7

Nicholson TRJ, Cutter W, Hotopf M (2008). Assessing mental capacity: the Mental Capacity Act. *BMJ* **336**: 322–325.

Stahl SM (2008). *Essential Psychopharmacology*, 3rd edition. Cambridge, Cambridge University Press.

Tyrer P, Silk K, eds. (2008). *Cambridge Textbook of Effective Treatments in Psychiatry*. Cambridge, Cambridge University Press.

Taylor D, Paton C, Kapur S (2009). *The Maudsley Prescribing Guidelines*, 10th edition. London, Informa Healthcare.

www.medicines.org.uk—Invaluable website including provides Summaries of Product Characteristics and Patient Information Leaflets for UK approved medicines. A definitive reference resource.

## Chapter 8

Burns T (1997). Case management, care management and care programming. *Br J Psychiatry* **170**, 393–395.

White K, Roy D, Hamilton I (1997). Community mental health services. *BMJ* **314**, 1817–1820.

## Chapter 9

Muller-Oerlinghausen B, Berghofer A, Bauer M (2002). Bipolar disorder. *Lancet* **359**, 241–247.

Alexopoulos GS (2005). Depression in the elderly. *Lancet* **365**, 1961–1970.

Mann JJ (2005). The medical management of depression. *N Engl J Med* **353**, 1819–1834.

Timonen M, Liukkonen T (2008). Management of depression in adults. *BMJ* **336**, 435–439.

## Chapter 10

Sharpe M, Mayou R (2004). Somatoform disorders: a help or a hindrance to good patient care? *Br J Psychiatry* **184**, 465–467.

Prins JB, van der Meer JWM, Bleijenberg G (2006). Chronic fatigue syndrome. *Lancet* **367** 346–355.

Bisson JI (2007). Post-traumatic stress disorder. *BMJ* **334**, 789–793.

Gale C, Davidson O (2007). Generalised anxiety disorder. *BMJ* **334**, 579–581.

Abramowitz J, Taylor S, McKay D (2009). Obsessive–compulsive disorder. *Lancet* **374**, 491–499.

## Chapter 11

Margison FR (1997). Abnormalities of sexual function and interest: origins and interventions. *Curr Opin Psychiatry* **10**, 127–131.

Fairburn CG, Harrison PJ (2003). Eating disorders. *Lancet* **361**, 407–416.

Seteia MJ, Nowell PD (2004). Insomnia. *Lancet* **364**, 1959–1973.

## Chapter 12

Van Os J, Kapur S (2009). Schizophrenia. *Lancet* **374**, 635–645.

Weinberger DR, Harrison PJ (2010). *Schizophrenia*, 3rd edition. Oxford, Wiley Blackwell.

## Chapter 13

Burns A, Gallagley A, Byrne J (2004). Delirium. *J Neurol Neurosurg Psychiatry* **75**, 362–367.

Gauthier S, Reisberg B, Zaudig M, *et al.* (2006). Mild cognitive impairment. *Lancet* **367**, 1262–1270.

Hardy JA (2006). A hundred years of Alzheimer's disease research. *Neuron* **52**, 3–13.

Holsinger T, Deveau J, Boustani M, *et al.* (2007). Does this patient have dementia? *JAMA* **297**, 2391–2404.

David A, Fleminger S, Kopelman M, *et al.* (2009). *Lishman's Organic Psychiatry*, 4th edition. Oxford, Wiley Blackwell.

## Chapter 14

Schuckit MA (1997). Substance use disorders. *BMJ* **314**, 1605–1608.

Parker AJR, Marshall EJ, Ball DM (2008). Diagnosis and management of alcohol use disorders. *BMJ* **336**, 496–501.

Hall W, Degenhardt L (2009). Adverse health effects of non-medical cannabis use. *Lancet* **374**, 1383–1391.

## Chapter 15

Tyrer P (2001). Personality disorder. *Br J Psychiatry* **179**, 81–84.

Lieb K, Zanarini MC, Schmahl C, *et al.* (2004). Borderline personality disorder. *Lancet* **364**, 453–461.

Banerjee PJM, Gibbon S, Huband N (2009). Assessment of personality disorder. *Adv Psychiatr Treat* **15**, 389–397.

## Chapter 16

Bassarath L (2001). Conduct disorder: a biopsychosocial review. *Can J Psychiatry* **46**, 609–616.

Biederman J, Faraone SV (2005). Attention-deficit hyperactivity disorder. *Lancet* **366**, 237–248.

Levy SE, Mandell DS, Schultz RT (2009). Autism. *Lancet* **374**, 1627–1638.

## Chapter 17

King BH, DeAntonio C, McCracken JT, *et al.* (1994). Psychiatric consultation in severe and profound mental retardation. *Am J Psychiatry* **151**, 1802–1808.

Battaglia A, Carey JC (2003). Diagnostic evaluation of developmental delay/mental retardation: an overview. *Am J Med Genet* **117C**, 3–14.

Fraser W, Kerr M (2003). *Seminars in the Psychiatry of Learning Disabilities*, 2nd edition. London, Gaskell Press.

Chelly J, Khelfaoui M, Francis F, *et al* (2006). Genetics and pathophysiology of mental retardation. *Eur J Hum Genet* **14**, 701–713.

## Chapter 18

Craig TK, Boardman AP (1997). Common mental health problems in primary care. *BMJ* **314**, 1609–1612.

Ramirez A, House A (1997). Common mental health problems in hospital. *BMJ* **314**, 1679–1681.

Moussavi S, Chatterji S, Verdes E, *et al.* (2007). Depression, chronic diseases, and decrements in health. *Lancet* **370**, 851–858.

Wang PS, Aguilar-Gaxiola S, Alonso J, *et al.* (2007). Use of mental health services for anxiety, mood, and substance disorders in 17 countries in the WHO world mental health surveys. *Lancet* **370**, 841–850.

# Index

Page numbers in *italics* represent figures, those in **bold** represent tables

# Keep up with critical fields

Would you like to receive up-to-date information on our books, journals and databases in the areas that interest you, direct to your mailbox?

Join the **Wiley e-mail service** - a convenient way to receive updates and exclusive discount offers on products from us.

## Simply visit **www.wiley.com/email** and register online

We won't bombard you with emails and we'll only email you with information that's relevant to you. We will ALWAYS respect your e-mail privacy and NEVER sell, rent, or exchange your e-mail address to any outside company. Full details on our privacy policy can be found online.

**WILEY-BLACKWELL**

www.wiley.com/email

17841